Guide to
Diagnostic Testing

Guide to Diagnostic Testing

Fauzia Khan, MD
Assistant Professor of Pathology
Director of Pathology Informatics
Department of Hospital Laboratories
UMass Memorial Medical Center
Worcester, Massachusetts

Howard J. Sachs, MD
Associate Professor of Clinical Medicine
Department of Medicine
UMass Memorial Medical Center
Worcester, Massachusetts

Liberto Pechet, MD
Director
Hematology Laboratory
Professor Emeritus of Medicine and Pathology
UMass Memorial Medical Center
Worcester, Massachusetts

L. Michael Snyder, MD
Chairman
Department of Hospital Laboratory
Professor of Pathology and Medicine
UMass Memorial Medical Center
Worcester, Massachusetts

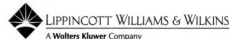
LIPPINCOTT WILLIAMS & WILKINS
A **Wolters Kluwer** Company
Philadelphia · Baltimore · New York · London
Buenos Aires · Hong Kong · Sydney · Tokyo

Editor: Neil Marquardt
Development Editor: Bridget Hilferty
Marketing Manager: Scott Lavine
Project Editor: Paula C. Williams
Designer: Risa Clow
Compositor: Peirce Graphic Services, Inc.
Printer: Vicks Lithograph & Printing

Printed in the United States of America

Library of Congress Cataloging-in-Publication Data
Guide to diagnostic testing / [edited by] Fauzia Khan ... [et al.].
    p. ; cm.
  Includes bibliographical references and index.
  ISBN 0-683-30725-8
    1. Diagnosis—Handbooks, manuals, etc. 2. Diagnosis, Laboratory—Handbooks, manuals, etc. I. Khan, Fauzia.
    [DNLM: 1. Diagnostic Techniques and Procedures. 2. Medical History Taking. 3. Physical Examination—methods. WB 141 G9455 2002]
  RC71 .G86 2002
  616.07'5—dc21

                                                                    2002016203

The publishers have made every effort to trace the copyright holders for borrowed material. If they have inadvertently overlooked any, they will be pleased to make the necessary arrangements at the first opportunity.

To purchase additional copies of this book call our customer service department at **(800) 638-3030** or fax orders to **(301) 824-7390.** International customers should call **(301) 714-2324.**

Visit Lippincott Williams & Wilkins on the Internet: http://www.lww.com. Lippincott Williams & Wilkins customer service representatives are available from 8:30 am to 6:00 pm, EST, Monday through Friday, for telephone access.

02 03 04
1 2 3 4 5 6 7 8 9 10

To Usmann, Mustafa, Mansoor, and Mohsins
Fauzia Khan

To my loving children, Emily, Christie, and Matthew
Howard Sachs

To Inna, for her infinite patience
Liberto Pechet

To Barbara, for her long-time understanding and support
Michael Snyder

Contents

CONTENTS

CONTENTS

Contributors

Ahmad-Samer Al-Homsi, MD
Assistant Professor of Medicine
UMass Memorial Medical Center
Worcester, Massachusetts

Medical Director
Simonds-Sinon Regional Cancer Center
Fitchburg, Massachusetts

Omar Ali, MD
Department of Cardiology
UMass Memorial Medical Center
Worcester, Massachusetts

Eric J. Alper, MD
Assistant Professor of Medicine
Department of Medicine
UMass Memorial Medical Center
Worcester, Massachusetts

Caroline J. Baltimore, MD
Assistant Professor of Medicine
Division of General Medicine, Primary
   Care, and Geriatrics
UMass Memorial Medical Center
Worcester, Massachusetts

Rohit Bhalla, MD, MPH
Medical Director
Quality Management
Montefiore Medical Center
Bronx, New York

Suzanne Blood, MD, MPH
Assistant Professor of Medicine
Department of General Internal Medicine
UMass Medical School
Worcester, Massachusetts

Mark P. Callery, MD, FACS
Chief, Division of General Surgery
Pancreatic, Hepatobiliary, and
   Gastrointestinal Surgery
Beth Israel Deaconess Medical Center
Associate Professor of Surgery
Harvard Medical School
Boston, Massachusetts

Erika Cappelluti, MD, PhD
Fellow
Pulmonary, Allergy, and Critical Care
   Medicine
UMass Memorial Medical Center
Worcester, Massachusetts

Nancy Chun, MD
Department of Medicine
UMass Memorial Medical Center
Worcester, Massachusetts

David M. Clive, MD
Professor of Medicine
Department of Medicine
UMass Medical School
Worcester, Massachusetts

Frederick J. Curley, MD
Associate Professor
Department of Pulmonary and Critical
   Care
UMass Medical School
Worcester, Massachusetts

Medical Director
Pulmonary and Critical Care
Milford Regional Hospital
Milford, Massachusetts

Peter J. Dain, MD
Instructor
Internal Medicine
UMass Medical School
Worcester, Massachusetts

Jennifer S. Daly, MD
Clinical Chief, Infectious Diseases
UMass Memorial Medical Center
Worcester, Massachusetts

Associate Professor of Medicine
UMass Medical School
Worcester, Massachusetts

Raul Davaro, MD
Assistant Professor of Medicine
Department of Infectious Diseases
UMass Memorial Medical Center
Worcester, Massachusetts

Alicia DeTraglia, MD
Fellow
Department of Hematology/Oncology
UMass Memorial Medical Center
Worcester, Massachusetts

Khoa D. Do, MD
Fellow
Department of Gastroenterology
UMass Memorial Medical Center
Worcester, Massachusetts

Stephen B. Erban, MD, MPH
Associate Professor of Medicine
Department of Medicine
UMass Memorial Medical Center
Worcester, Massachusetts

Daniel Ervin, DO
Central Mass Otolaryngology
Private Practice
Fitchburg, Massachusetts
Clinical Associate
UMass Memorial Medical Center
Worcester, Massachusetts

Elaine R. Evans-Metcalf, MD, FACOG, FRCSC
Department of Obstetrics and Gynecology
Newton-Wellesley Hospital
Newton, Massachusetts

W. Christopher Fang, MD, MHSc
Resident
Department of General Surgery
UMass Medical School
Worcester, Massachusetts

Armando E. Fraire, MD
Professor
Department of Pathology
UMass Medical School
Worcester, Massachusetts

Thomas M. Frates, MD
Assistant Professor of Medicine
Internal Medicine
UMass Medical School
Worcester, Massachusetts

Julia M. Gallagher, MD
Instructor of Medicine
Internal Medicine
UMass Memorial Medical Center
Worcester, Massachusetts

David F. Giansiracusa, MD, FACP, FACR
Professor of Medicine, Vice Chair
Department of Medicine
UMass Medical School
Worcester, Massachusetts

Richard H. Glew, MD
Professor of Medicine
Molecular Genetics and Microbiology
Vice Chair for Clinical Affairs
Department of Medicine
UMass Medical School
Worcester, Massachusetts

Kathleen Jennison Goonan, MD
Women's Health Center
Division of Primary Care and Geriatrics
UMass Medical School
Worcester, Massachusetts

Leslie R. Harrold, MD, MPH
Assistant Professor of Medicine
Department of Medicine
UMass Medical School
Worcester, Massachusetts

David Hatem, MD
Associate Professor of Clinical Medicine
Division of General Medicine and Primary Care
UMass Memorial Medical Center
Worcester, Massachusetts

Lauren Hiestand, MD
Assistant Professor
Department of Pathology
Director, Immunology
Department of Hospital Laboratories
UMass Memorial Medical Center
Worcester, Massachusetts

Pauline I. Himlan, RNC, BSN, MEd
Nurse Practitioner
Department of Infectious Diseases
UMass Memorial Medical Center
Worcester, Massachusetts

Allison E. Howard, BS
Research Assistant, Urogynecology
Department of Obstetrics and
    Gynecology
UMass Memorial Medical Center
Worcester, Massachusetts

Eric S. Iida, MD
Associates in Nephrology
Brockton, Massachusetts

Daniel Y. Kim, MD
Chief, Head and Neck Surgery
Department of Otolaryngology
UMass Memorial Medical Center
Worcester, Massachusetts

Robert Lebow, MD, FACP
Chair, Internal Medicine Service
Harrington Memorial Hospital
Southbridge, Massachusetts

Associate in Medicine
UMass Medical School
Worcester, Massachusetts

Richard Lerner, MD
Assistant Professor of Medicine
Department of Medicine
UMass Memorial Medical Center
Worcester, Massachusetts

Gertrude W. Manchester, MD
Associate Professor of Clinical
    Medicine
Department of Medicine
UMass Memorial Medical Center
Worcester, Massachusetts

Michael J. McCormick, MD
Assistant Professor of Medicine
Division of Pulmonary, Allergy, and
    Critical Care Medicine
UMass Medical School
Worcester, Massachusetts

Cliff A. Megerian, MD, FACS
Associate Professor
Director of Otology and Neurotology
Department of Otolaryngology, Head and
    Neck Surgery
UMass Medical School
Worcester, Massachusetts

Michael Mitchell, MD
Director, Microbiology Services
Department of Hospital Laboratories
UMass Memorial Medical Center
Worcester, Massachusetts

Wendy Lawler Mitchell, MD
Chief Medical Resident
Internal Medicine
UMass Memorial Medical Center
Worcester, Massachusetts

Aftab Mohsin, MBBS, FRCP
Associate Professor of Medicine
King Edwards Medical College
Lahore, Pakistan

Majaz Moonis, MD, MRCP, DM
Assistant Professor
Department of Neurology
UMass Medical School
Worcester, Massachusetts

Guy T. Napolitana, MD, FACP
Vice Chairman
General Internal Medicine
Lahey Clinic
Burlington, Massachusetts

Ira S. Ockene, MD
David and Barbara Milliken Professor of
    Preventive Cardiology
Director, Preventive Cardiology Program
Associate Director, Division of
    Cardiovascular Medicine
Department of Medicine
UMass Medical School
Worcester, Massachusetts

Richard Palken, MD
Assistant Professor of Medicine
Department of Internal Medicine and Geriatrics
UMass Medical School
Worcester, Massachusetts

CONTRIBUTORS

John A. Paraskos, MD
Professor of Medicine
Director of Ambulatory Cardiology
Department of Medicine
UMass Medical School
Worcester, Massachusetts

Catherine A. Phillips, MD
Associate Professor
Department of Neurology
UMass Memorial Medical Center
Worcester, Massachusetts

Christian L. Potter, MD
Department of Medicine
UMass Memorial Medical Center
Worcester, Massachusetts

Marjorie Safran, MD
Professor of Clinical Medicine
Division of Endocrinology
Department of Medicine
UMass Medical School
Worcester, Massachusetts

Stacia Remsburg Sailer, MD, DABSM
Co-director, Sleep Disorders Center
Pulmonary, Critical Care Medicine
UMass Memorial Medical Center
Worcester, Massachusetts

Oren P. Schaefer, MD
Associate Professor of Medicine
Division of Pulmonary, Allergy, and
    Critical Care Medicine
UMass Memorial Medical Center
Worcester, Massachusetts

Sandra L. Senno, MSW, MD
Chief Resident
Physical Medicine and Rehabilitation
Tufts University School of Medicine
New England Medical Center
Boston, Massachusetts

Christopher Sorli, MD
Medical Director
Backus Diabetes Management Center
Director of Endocrinology
Williams W. Backus Hospital
Norwich, Connecticut

Rebecca Spanagel, MD
Internal Medicine
UMass Memorial Medical Center
Worcester, Massachusetts

Guenter L. Spanknebel, MD
Director of Continuing Medical Education
Associate Director, Division of Digestive
    Diseases and Nutrition
Internal Medicine
UMass Memorial Medical Center
Worcester, Massachusetts

Mira Sofia Torres, MD
Affiliate Physician
Internal Medicine
Saint Luke's Medical Center
Quezon City, Philippines

Bruce Weinstein, MD
Associate Professor of Medicine
Department of Medicine
UMass Medical School
Worcester, Massachusetts

Michael D. Wertheimer, MD
Professor of Surgery
UMass Memorial Medical Center
Worcester, Massachusetts

Michael Wollin, MD
Assistant Professor in Urology
UMass Memorial Medical Center
Worcester, Massachusetts

Majid Yazdani, MD
Assistant Professor
Department of Medicine
UMass Memorial Medical Center
Worcester, Massachusetts

Stephen B. Young, MD, FACOG
Chief, Division of Urogynecology and
    Reconstructive Pelvic Surgery
Associate Professor, Department of
    Obstetrics and Gynecology
UMass Memorial Medical Center
Worcester, Massachusetts

Michael Zavarin, MD
Head of Inpatient Medical Service
Internal Medicine
Jordan Hospital
Plymouth, Massachusetts

Robert B. Zurier, MD
Professor of Medicine
Director, Rheumatology Division
Department of Medicine
UMass Medical School
Worcester, Massachusetts

Preface

Guide to Diagnostic Testing is a practical guide that will benefit all those involved in clinical care, including medical students, residents, physicians, physicians' assistants, nurse practitioners, and nurses. This book has a unique multidisciplinary approach to making a diagnosis, bridging the gap between clinical medicine and diagnostic testing. The initial emphasis is on performing a detailed medical history and physical examination. Based on the patient's symptoms and signs, diagnostic tests are recommended and their results are interpreted, leading to the generation of a differential diagnosis. Information provided under diseases may then be used to rule in (or out) the final diagnosis.

The format of this book evolved over the course of 3 years as we experimented with a variety of layouts. We are confident that the result is a presentation that is both applicable and highly efficient in meeting your quick-reference needs. More than any previous text, this book follows the techniques used in bedside teaching and medical rounds. The goal is to provide not only relevant, up-to-date information, but also a format that is quick and easy to read. The text has been arranged in the outline format, and numerous tables and algorithms have been used to assist the clinician in initiating an appropriate patient workup.

More than 60 physicians contributed to the 13 different sections of this book. Most chapters are written by primary care physicians in areas in which they are adept, based not only on their experience but also on the principles of evidence-based medicine. The editorial board had the considerable challenge of distilling the information provided by the author team into a pocket-sized reference that includes only the most essential information for laboratory testing and diagnosis. Discussions of pathophysiology and therapy are purposely omitted. We also focused on keeping the organization as consistent as possible from chapter to chapter, with the intent on making the information easy for you to find and use in your daily practice. When appropriate, common pitfalls and limitations of current diagnostic evaluations are addressed.

One part of the job is done, and what you have in your hands is the first edition. However, we think the most important part of the process is your feedback. We welcome you to log on to our Web site, www.DiagnosisOne.com* and join us on this journey.

Fauzia Khan
Howard Sachs
Liberto Pechet
Michael Snyder

*This site is neither affiliated with Lippincott Williams & Wilkins, Inc., nor does Lippincott Williams & Wilkins, Inc., exercise any control over its content or availability.

Acknowledgments

First and foremost, we would like to thank Samia Naseem for her dedication, creativity, and linguistic abilities. She spent many hours formatting the text and algorithms. We would also like to thank Marie Boire for formatting the text and designing the algorithms. Also, special thanks to Cindie Gaston for her invaluable secretarial support. We would also like to thank the staff at Lippincott Williams & Wilkins for their support and input, especially Bridget Hilferty, Elizabeth Nieginski, and Charlie Mitchell.

Introduction

L. Michael Snyder, MD

Guide to Diagnostic Testing is based upon the principles of evidence-based medicine as applied to laboratory medicine. This implies that a request for a diagnostic test is part of a decision-making process. It further means that a test has met quality measurements, is selective, and is clinically relevant.

While each clinical problem is unique, the following four aspects guide the underlying critical thinking: **technical performance, diagnostic performance, clinical utility, and economic impact.**[1]

Technical aspects of precision, accuracy, analytical range, and interference are well recognized. However, an appreciation of pre-analytical factors, which may influence test results independent of the laboratory, is often lacking. For instance, requiring a correct proportion of whole blood to anticoagulant in clotting tests is of the utmost importance. Alteration in this proportion results in misleading results. Another example is of drug levels drawn incorrectly (i.e., shortly after a dose has been administered). This may result in misleading, falsely elevated blood levels, which may lead to dire consequences. Thus, pre-analytic errors can limit the value of test results and lead incorrectly to dissatisfaction with the laboratory.[1]

Diagnostic performance of a test dictates its clinical utility. The parameters used to measure diagnostic performance include:

a. **Sensitivity:** The number of people correctly having the disease: true positive divided by (true positive + false negative).
b. **Specificity:** The number of people who do not have the disease: true negative divided by (true negative + false positive).
c. **Predicted value:** The probability of the disease being present if the test is positive [true positive divided by (true positive + false positive)] or not being present if the test is negative [true negative divided by (true negative + false negative)].
d. **Accuracy:** True positive + true negative divided by total tests.

The contribution of the clinical laboratory to the **clinical and therapeutic strategy** is equally important. For instance, the use of HbA1c for monitoring diabetic control has a major impact on cost and clinical outcomes. Similarly, microalbumin used in detection of early nephropathy in the diabetic patient allows for the timely initiation of angiotensin-converting enzyme (ACE) inhibitors.[1]

The **economic impact** of ordered tests, individually and the cost-benefit analysis on policy issues, is becoming increasingly important in today's environment. For instance, the result of ordering cardiac enzymes on an emergency room patient with chest pain will help decide whether to admit or discharge the patient. Moreover, if the results are positive, among other procedures, a decision may be made to treat with expensive thrombolytic therapy.

In addition to solving clinical problems, another area of testing concentrates on **screening asymptomatic individuals,** the purpose of which is to uncover disease before it becomes symptomatic, so that timely therapy can be instituted, resulting in improved long-term clinical outcomes. It is important to note that screening is clinically and economically useful, mostly when the condition is common in the population. We recommend "smart testing" based on prevalence of disease in specific populations. An example is the screening with serum cholesterol for hyperlipidemia starting at age 20 because the estimate of lipid abnormalities is in the vicinity of 20% in the general population. Recently, it has been shown that intervention in patients with hyperlipidemia does have a positive effect on subsequent development of coronary artery disease.[2]

There are other examples of applying selective testing in populations at risk (i.e., routine fasting blood sugars in obese patients with a family history of diabetes mellitus because it will significantly increase the yield of detection of new diabetic patients than if it would be in screening the general population. Screening for thyroid disease in women older than 65 years of age, where the prevalence of thyroid disease is 5%–10%, is a worthwhile test to perform. However, since Medicare does not reimburse for thyroid-stimulating hormone (TSH) screening tests, a routine history and physical examination is crucial to uncover subtle findings to justify ordering TSH. The prevalence of hemochromatosis is now recognized to be as high as 5% in the general population. Therefore, a periodic serum ferritin is warranted in patients with a family history, but again, there needs to be some reconciliation regarding reimbursement by Medicare for this test.

Tests that are inappropriately ordered, without clear clinical benefits, can be wasteful and run the risk of false-positive results. For example, if 12 tests are ordered in a "normal" individual, the probability is that only 54% of all tests will be normal. When 100 tests are ordered, there is only a 0.6% probability that all tests will be normal. Thus, abnormal test results in "normal" people may lead to added expense and confusion both for the healthcare provider and for the patient. Because of that, the current trend is not to order screening profiles in healthy populations in the absence of symptoms or risk factors for disease.

It is hoped that this handbook will be useful in helping clinicians, as well as anyone involved with a diagnostic process, to reach a diagnosis efficiently.

REFERENCES

[1.]Price CP: Evidence-based laboratory medicine: Supporting decision-making. *Clin Chem* 46:8,1041–1050, 2000.

[2.]Takemura Y, Ishida H, Inoue Y, et al: Opportunistic discovery of occult disease by use of test panels in new, symptomatic primary care outpatients: Yield and cost of case finding. *Clin Chem* 46:8,1091–1098, 2000.

SECTION I

Cardiovascular System

1

Hypertension
Howard Sachs

I. Introduction

A. Definition. A patient is considered to have hypertension when two or more blood pressure readings are elevated (systolic > 140 mm Hg or diastolic > 90 mm Hg).

    1. Readings must be taken in an **unstressed environment,** and must be separated by at least 2 minutes.

    2. Elevated readings must be reproduced at **two or more visits separated over time** (generally a week or more should elapse between readings).

    3. The patient should **refrain from caffeine and nicotine** for at least 30 minutes prior to the blood pressure determination.

B. Treatment considerations. In patients who are newly diagnosed with hypertension, cardiovascular risk factors, secondary causes, target organ damage, and comorbid conditions will influence treatment decisions.

II. Clinical Approach

A. Essential hypertension. The vast majority of patients have essential hypertension, which requires little additional study beyond the initial screen. Commonly cited indications for more **detailed investigation** include:

    1. Age of onset (younger than 20 years of age or older than 55 years of age)

    2. Abrupt onset of **stage III hypertension or hypertensive crisis**

    3. Escape in a **previously stabilized patient**

B. Secondary hypertension. All patients with hypertension should be screened for **secondary causes** (see III).

    1. Although there is an impressive array of evaluation methods for secondary causes, most cases of hypertension will never require detailed study.

    2. In spite of this, the clinician needs to be vigilant for clues that may be suggestive of these less common secondary forms.

C. **Refractory hypertension** warrants a more detailed investigation. Refractory hypertension is defined as failure to respond to a three-drug combination (one of which is a diuretic) given at maximal doses for a sufficient period (approximately 4 weeks in the absence of hypertensive crisis).

1. More than 40% of patients thought to have refractory hypertension are, in fact, being treated with **suboptimal regimens.** A common error is the failure to control plasma volume with appropriate diuretic therapy.

2. Approximately 10% of patients with refractory hypertension will have a **secondary cause.** Medication use and compliance, nonpharmacologic management strategies, and excessive alcohol use are frequently overlooked causes.

D. **Hypertensive crisis** is defined as a severe elevation in blood pressure (diastolic > 120 mm Hg). Hypertensive crisis is estimated to occur in less than 1% of Americans with hypertension.

1. **Classification.** Hypertensive crises are classified as **hypertensive emergencies** in the presence of acute or ongoing end-organ damage or as **hypertensive urgencies** in the absence of end-organ damage.

2. **Organ involvement** may include the central nervous system (CNS) [encephalopathy, infarction, hemorrhage], myocardium (ischemia, infarction, pulmonary edema), vasculature (aortic dissection), hematologic (microangiopathic hemolytic anemia), ophthalmologic (retinopathy, papilledema), or renal deterioration (azotemia, hematuria).

III. Secondary Hypertension

A. Differential diagnosis

1. **Renal parenchymal disease**
2. **Renovascular disease** (1%–5% of hypertension cases)

   a. Renal artery stenosis (RAS)
   b. Vasculitis
   c. Aortic coarctation

3. **Endocrinopathies**

   a. Cushing's syndrome
   b. Hyperthyroidism
   c. Pheochromocytoma (0.1% of hypertension cases)
   d. Primary aldosteronism ($< 2\%$ of hypertension cases)

      (1) Adrenal adenoma
      (2) Bilateral adrenal hyperplasia
      (3) Adrenal carcinoma (rare cause)
      (4) Glucocorticoid-remedial aldosteronism (autosomal dominant trait)

   e. Renin-secreting tumors
   f. Hypercalcemia

4. **Neurologic disorders,** such as a CNS mass or autonomic hyperreflexia
5. **Medications,** such as sympathomimetics, nonsteroidal anti-

inflammatory drugs (NSAIDs), oral contraceptives, corticosteroids, psychotropics, erythropoietin, cyclosporine, alcohol, or illicit drugs

B. Notes on the differential diagnosis

1. **Renal parenchymal disease** is the most common cause of secondary hypertension.

2. **RAS** is the most common renovascular cause of secondary hypertension. Identification of RAS holds particular relevance given that treatment may lead to a reversal of hypertension, or at least improved blood pressure control.

   a. **Causes of RAS:** Atherosclerosis is the most common cause of RAS, followed by fibromuscular dysplasia (in young women).

   b. **Clinical predictors** of atherosclerotic RAS in patients with refractory hypertension include:

      (1) Vascular disease (especially an abdominal bruit)
      (2) Azotemia [baseline or precipitated by an angiotensin-converting enzyme (ACE) inhibitor]
      (3) Renal asymmetry (incidentally discovered on imaging)
      (4) Advancing age

   c. **Complications:** Untreated RAS may lead to a progressive decline in renal function. Progressive hypertension occurs in 40%–50% of patients with RAS.

3. **Endocrinopathies**

   a. **Primary aldosteronism** (see Chapter 16)

   b. **Glucocorticoid-remedial aldosteronism:** Unlike normal subjects, secretion of aldosterone in these patients is regulated completely by corticotropin. As an autosomal dominant trait, hypertension tends to occur early in life.

   c. **Pheochromocytoma:** Although an uncommon cause of hypertension, pheochromocytoma is an important diagnostic consideration. Besides the usual symptoms that would alert attention to this diagnosis (e.g., headache, palpitation, pallor, perspiration), it is important to consider pheochromocytoma in any patient diagnosed with hyperparathyroidism. The majority of patients with pheochromocytoma release norepinephrine.

IV. Evaluation (Figure 1–1). Hypertension is a **chronic condition.** As such, the evaluation is usually performed in stages over time.

A. History

1. Note **duration and severity of hypertension,** and **any previous evaluations.**

2. Note **previous therapy** and **compliance with medications.**

3. Check for **atherosclerosis** by assessing for chest pain, discomfort, dyspnea, claudication, coronary artery disease (CAD), congestive heart failure (CHF), rhythm disturbance, and cerebrovascular disease.

4. Check for an **endocrinopathy** by assessing for paroxysms of headache, palpitations, pallor and diaphoresis, weight loss or gain, tremor, hair loss, cramping, and weakness.

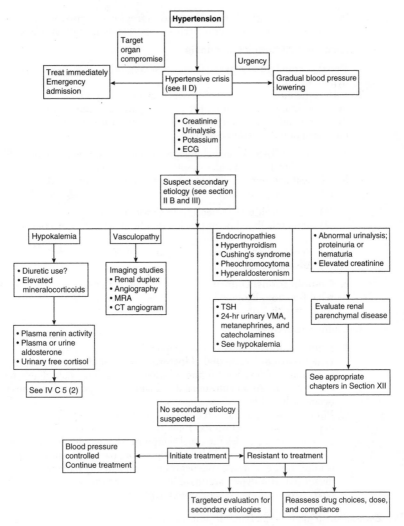

FIGURE 1–1. Algorithm for the workup of a patient with hypertension. *CT* = computed tomography; *ECG* = electrocardiogram; *MRA* = magnetic resonance angiography; *TSH* = thyroid-stimulating hormone; *VMA* = vanillylmandelic acid.

5. Note **past medical history** of renal insufficiency, diabetes, and dyslipidemia.
6. Note **use of medications,** such as antidepressants (especially tyramine use concurrent with monoamine oxidase inhibitors), decongestants or sympathomimetics, oral contraceptives, cyclosporine, erythropoietin, NSAIDs, and steroids.

7. Ascertain **social habits** such as alcohol use, exercise habits, tobacco use, sodium use, and illicit and over-the-counter drug use.
8. Note **family history** of hypertension, renal disease, CAD, cerebrovascular disease, and polycystic kidney disease.
9. Complete a **review of symptoms,** noting essential tremor, migraine headaches, osteoporosis, prostatism, asthma, gout, hepatic disease, and pregnancy.

B. Physical examination

1. **Funduscopic examination:** Assess for hypertensive retinopathy (arteriolar narrowing, arteriovenous nicking, hemorrhage, exudates, or papilledema).
2. **Cardiac assessment:** Assess for lateral displacement of the apical impulse, a forceful or sustained apical impulse, the presence of a fourth heart sound (S_4), or evidence of left ventricular dysfunction [e.g., rales, jugular venous distention (JVD), a third heart sound (S_3)].
3. **Pulmonary:** Note presence of rales or bronchospasm.
4. **Renal palpation:** Note any masses (e.g., a tumor, polycystic kidney disease).
5. **Vascular assessment:** Check for peripheral pulses, aneurysmal dilation, and bruits (especially of the carotid, renal, and femoral arteries).
6. **Endocrine assessment:** Palpate the thyroid; assess for hyperreflexia, tachycardia, skin texture, striae, buffalo hump, moon facies, and central obesity.
7. **Neurologic assessment:** Assess neurologic status, especially in patients who have symptoms, stage III hypertension, or a known history of cerebrovascular disease.

C. Diagnostic tests. The full spectrum of available studies is not pursued in every patient with hypertension. Judicious application is governed by signs, symptoms, and response to therapy.

1. **Initial assessment** (indicated for all patients newly diagnosed with hypertension)
   a. Complete blood count (CBC)
   b. Serum creatinine
   c. Urinalysis
   d. Serum potassium
      (1) The laboratory picture of unprovoked hypokalemia in the setting of metabolic alkalosis and a serum sodium level at the high range of normal should suggest mineralocorticoid-related causes of hypertension.
      (2) It is important to note, however, that 20% of patients with hyperaldosteronism will have normal potassium.
2. **24-Hour ambulatory blood pressure monitoring** (ABPM)
   a. The commonly cited **indications for ABPM** include:
      (1) Patients with "white coat" hypertension (discrepancy between office-based readings and those obtained outside of the medical environment)

(a) When assessed by ABPM, 21% of borderline patients and 5% of established hypertensive patients show evidence of "white coat" hypertension.

(b) The true prevalence of this disorder is unknown. One community-based study found that nearly 25% of patients newly diagnosed with hypertension had daytime ambulatory diastolic blood pressure of less than 90 mm Hg.

(2) Patients with borderline hypertension who are being considered for treatment or who are reluctant to accept treatment

(3) Patients with target organ damage [e.g., left ventricular hypertrophy (LVH), cerebral microvascular disease, retinopathy, microalbuminuria] and normal office-based blood pressure measurements

(a) Evidence suggests a closer correlation between ambulatory blood pressure measurements than office-based measurements when assessing target organ damage.

(b) In patients with elevated office-based blood pressure measurements, ABPM may identify a group at relatively low risk of morbidity.

(4) Patients who are resistant to drug therapy

b. Results are conventionally reported as average 24-hour readings, average daytime and nighttime readings, as well as a percentage of elevated readings.

3. Risk factor assessment

a. Lipid profile determination
b. Serum glucose

4. Target-organ disease assessment

a. Serum creatinine
b. Urinalysis
c. Electrocardiogram (ECG)

(1) This is the standard method for detecting ischemic heart disease and LVH.

(2) The presence of LVH in a patient with hypertension is proof of target-organ damage.

(3) Left atrial enlargement shown by ECG criteria is highly concordant with a S_4. These signs reflect diastolic dysfunction much earlier in hypertensive heart disease than does ECG evidence of LVH.

d. Echocardiography

(1) Echocardiography has **good sensitivity** for the detection of structural changes in hypertensive heart disease.

(2) Indications for echocardiography in patients with hypertension include:

(a) Patients with borderline hypertension and ECG evidence of LVH

(b) Young athletes with hypertension

    (c) Patients with exercise-induced hypertension

    (d) Hypertensive patients with ECG evidence suggestive, but not diagnostic, of LVH

    (e) The clinician's desire to investigate coexistent valvular and myocardial disease

5. Selected ancillary studies (indicated in the evaluation of patients with secondary hypertension)

    a. Serum calcium

    b. Thyroid-stimulating hormone (TSH)

    c. Chest radiograph

    d. Renin and aldosterone levels

        (1) Indications for measuring renin and aldosterone levels include patients with hypertension who have spontaneous or profound diuretic-induced hypokalemia, patients with adrenal-imaging abnormalities (discovered incidentally), or patients with refractory hypertension. Although influenced by the presence of antihypertensive drugs, levels may be obtained while on drug therapy.

        (2) Results

            (a) Plasma renin activity (PRA) is suppressed in almost all patients with primary hyperaldosteronism. Measurements are ideally obtained under conditions of low sodium consumption (40 mg/day) or in the setting of diuretic use (120 mg of furosemide in split doses). Elevated levels of plasma renin suggest secondary hyperaldosteronism (e.g., CHF, cirrhosis).

            (b) Plasma aldosterone. A high plasma aldosterone level following a sodium load (1.25 liters of normal saline over 2 hours or 2 liters over 4 hours), in association with low renin activity, suggests primary hyperaldosteronism.

            (c) Aldosterone-renin ratio. The plasma aldosterone:renin ratio is the most suitable method of distinguishing patients with essential hypertension from patients with primary aldosteronism. A high ratio (> 30) will reliably distinguish patients with hyperaldosteronism from patients with other forms of hypertension.

    e. Angiography is the gold standard test for diagnosing RAS. As RAS is the most common correctable cause of secondary hypertension, appropriate diagnosis holds particular relevance.

        (1) Although unlikely in mild cases, RAS accounts for more than 10% of hypertension in patients with stage III disease.

        (2) RAS can be clinically excluded in patients with normal renal function and patients whose hypertension is easily controlled with one or two drugs.

        (3) Captopril renography has a low diagnostic accuracy with a sensitivity of 65%–77% and a specificity of 90%. It does not perform well in cases of bilateral RAS, unilateral stenosis in a solitary kidney, and renal insufficiency.

  f. **Renal duplex ultrasound scanning:** This test is noninvasive and
requires no contrast. It combines direct visualization of the renal
arteries (B-mode imaging) with measurement of hemodynamic
factors (Doppler) to provide both an anatomic and functional
assessment of renal blood flow.

  (1) When applied to a population of patients with a pretest
likelihood of 70% (by clinical features), renal duplex ultrasound
scanning performs comparably to arteriography.

  (2) The overall sensitivity is 98%, specificity is 99%, positive
predictive value is 99%, and negative predictive value is 97%.

  g. **Renal magnetic resonance angiography:** This test can visualize
most segments of the renal artery.

  (1) Sensitivity is 91%–100%, specificity is 76%–96%, positive
predictive value is 80%, and negative predictive value is
90%–94%.

  (2) Limitations include a limited ability to detect accessory vessels,
high cost, and an overestimation of the degree of stenosis.

  h. **Spiral computed tomography (CT) angiography:** This test
requires contrast injection; sensitivity is 90%–96% and specificity is
97%–99%.

SUGGESTED READING

Dalen J (ed): The Sixth Report of the Joint National Committee on Prevention, Detection,
Evaluation and Treatment of High Blood Pressure. *Arch Intern Med* 157:2413–2446, 1997.

2

Palpitations

Thomas Frates

I. Definition. Palpitation is a subjective sensation of an unduly rapid or irregular heartbeat.

II. Clinical Approach (Figures 2–1, 2–2, and 2–3)

  A. Differential diagnosis. Categorize the mechanisms as resulting from either cardiac or noncardiac causes.

    1. Cardiac causes

      a. Arrhythmias: Any rhythm other than normal sinus may be perceived as palpitations. Frequent causes include:

        (1) Atrial fibrillation
        (2) Atrial flutter
        (3) Supraventricular tachycardia
        (4) Premature atrial or ventricular beats
        (5) Ventricular tachycardia
        (6) Sick sinus syndrome
        (7) Pacemaker malfunction

      b. Valvular disorders

        (1) Regurgitant valvular heart disease
        (2) Stenotic heart valves
        (3) Mitral valve prolapse
        (4) Aortic insufficiency
        (5) Prosthetic heart valves

      c. Structural abnormalities

        (1) Myocardial hypertrophy
        (2) Cardiac and extracardiac shunts
        (3) Atrial myxomas
        (4) Cardiomegaly
        (5) Hyperkinetic heart syndrome

      d. Myocardial ischemia [principally due to coronary artery disease (CAD)]: This may be considered an indirect cause of palpitations, as it may precipitate the development of an arrhythmia.

    2. Noncardiac causes

      a. Psychiatric causes such as panic attacks, anxiety, or somatization
      b. Medications: Those most frequently associated with palpitations include:

        (1) Anticholinergics (e.g., atropine, scopolamine, nicotine, tubocurarine, pancuronium, succinylcholine)
        (2) Vasodilators (e.g., nitrates, minoxidil, hydralazine, propranolol, calcium channel blockers)

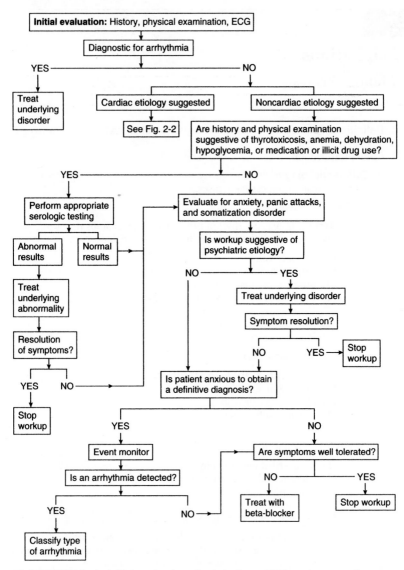

■ **FIGURE 2–1.** Initial evaluation of palpitations. *ECG* = electrocardiogram.

     (3) Sympathomimetics (e.g., epinephrine, norepinephrine,
        isoproterenol, dopamine, dobutamine, theophylline
        ephedrine, amphetamines)

  c. **Habit-forming substances** such as caffeine, nicotine, or cocaine
  d. **Metabolic disorders** such as hypoglycemia and thyrotoxicosis

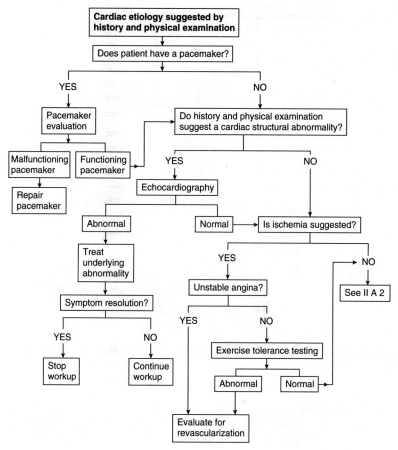

FIGURE 2–2. Evaluation of palpitations when a cardiac etiology is suspected.

  e. **High output states** such as anemia, pregnancy, or fever
  f. **Dehydration** and **orthostatic hypotension**
B. **History.** Important aspects of the history include the symptoms experienced by the patient, the presence of any associated symptoms, the setting in which the palpitations occurred, the past medical history, and a list of any medications taken by the patient.
C. **Physical examination.** A patient with palpitations is usually asymptomatic at the time of the physical examination. Therefore, the clinician should look for evidence of any physical abnormalities that would predispose the patient to palpitations. Although the evaluation of the cardiovascular system is the most important aspect of the physical examination, the clinician should also evaluate for signs of thyrotoxicosis, congestive heart failure (CHF), and dehydration (e.g., dry oral mucosa, tenting of the skin).

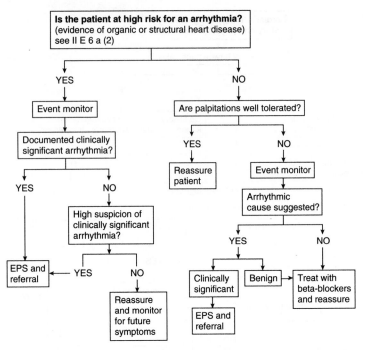

FIGURE 2-3. Evaluation of palpitations in patients at high risk for arrhythmia. *EPS* = electrophysiologic studies.

D. Electrocardiogram (ECG). A 12-lead ECG should be performed on any patient complaining of palpitations. ECG findings often point to the cause. Examples include arrhythmias (see II A 1 a) and other more subtle ECG findings:

1. **Q waves** suggest prior myocardial damage with scar formation. This predisposes the patient to premature ventricular contraction (PVC) or polymorphic ventricular tachycardia.
2. **Complete heart block** predisposes the patient to PVC, polymorphic ventricular tachycardia, or bradyarrhythmias.
3. **Left ventricular hypertrophy** (LVH) suggests hypertrophic obstructive cardiomyopathy.
4. A **short PR interval** and **delta waves** suggest atrioventricular reentrant tachycardia.
5. **Prolonged QT intervals** suggest a familial long QT syndrome, which predisposes the patient to polymorphic ventricular tachycardia.

E. Laboratory studies. Routine laboratory studies are not generally informative. However, the patient history may suggest specific laboratory tests:

1. **Thyroid function tests** (see Chapter 16): Hyperthyroidism is associated with atrial fibrillation, atrial flutter, paroxysmal

supraventricular tachycardia, and CHF. In the elderly, symptoms of hyperthyroidism may be more subtle, with CHF often the main characteristic.

2. **Electrolytic and renal function testing:** Laboratory studies including blood urea nitrogen and creatinine, as well as urine specific gravity, can help confirm a diagnosis of hypovolemia and dehydration. Disturbances of sodium, potassium, magnesium, and calcium balance may all be associated with rhythm disturbances.

3. **Complete blood count (CBC):** Palpitations may occur due to hypoxemia, with or without cardiac ischemia, as well as to the high-output state associated with severe anemia.

4. **Blood glucose:** Hypoglycemia has been associated with palpitations.

5. **Drug levels:** Toxicology tests should be ordered (e.g., for theophylline, amphetamines, cocaine) when indicated by the patient's history.

6. **Ancillary testing**

   a. **Patients in need of further evaluation**

   (1) Patients whose initial evaluation (history, physical examination, ECG) was suggestive but not diagnostic of an arrhythmia

   (2) Patients who are at increased risk for an arrhythmia (i.e., those with organic or structural heart disease)

   (3) Patients whose symptoms place them at a high risk for an arrhythmogenic event (i.e., those with syncope, hypoperfusion, ischemia)

   (4) Patients who have recurrent symptoms with no clear cause

   (5) Patients who are anxious to obtain a definitive diagnosis

   b. **Test options**

   (1) **Exercise tolerance testing** is indicated in patients who are known to have or are suspected of having CAD.

   (2) **Echocardiography** is indicated in patients whose history and physical examination are suggestive of valvular heart disease, CHF, or any structural abnormality.

   (3) **Ambulatory monitoring devices** have proven to be the most effective ambulatory test because of their ability to provide a diagnosis. Two different types of monitors are available, the Holter monitor and the event monitor (which may include a loop recorder).

   (a) The **Holter monitor** is an instrument that continuously records the patient's heart rhythm for a period of 24–48 hours. The rhythm strips are compared to a diary in which the patient has recorded the time of day when symptoms occurred to see if there is any correlation. The main disadvantage of the Holter monitor is that many patients do not experience palpitations on a daily basis.

   (b) The **event monitor** is a patient-activated device. The loop recorder will continuously record the patient's underlying heart rhythm. The data will be saved only if the patient manually activates the monitor. The loop recorder will provide the clinician with rhythm strips generated during the 2 minutes preceding and following the palpitations.

These monitors are generally worn for a period of up to 30 days. Loop monitors have advantages over Holter monitors in that they are more cost-effective and can record information over a longer period, thus increasing the likelihood of the patient being monitored during a symptomatic episode.

(4) Electrophysiologic studies (EPS) are indicated in patients with:

(a) Syncope plus structural heart disease
(b) Defined rhythm disturbances and palpitations with documented rapid pulse

c. Pacemaker evaluation: All patients with pacemakers who complain of palpitations should have the pacemaker evaluated to ensure that it is functioning properly.

SUGGESTED READING

Weber BE, Kapoor WN: Evaluation and outcome of patients with palpitations. *Am J Med* 157:1782–1788, 1997.

Zimetbaum P, Josephson M: Evaluation of patients with palpitations. *N Engl J Med* 338: 1369–1372, 1998.

Zimetbaum P, Kim K, Josephson M, et al: Diagnostic yield and optimal duration of continuous-loop event monitoring for the diagnosis of palpitations. *Ann Intern Med* 128:850–895, 1998.

3

Syncope
Guy T. Napolitana

I. **DEFINITION.** Syncope is a transient decrease in cerebral blood flow associated with a loss of consciousness and postural tone.

II. **ETIOLOGY**

  A. **Cardiac causes** of syncope have the potential for the highest mortality (20%–30%). The two most common causes are pump failure and arrhythmia.

   1. **Pump failure** is most commonly caused by outflow obstruction, seen as in aortic stenosis or hypertrophic cardiomyopathy. Other causes include pulmonary emboli, aortic dissection, atrial myxoma, and pulmonary hypertension.

   2. **Arrhythmia** can be either ventricular, supraventricular, or bradycardic. Patients with abnormal ventricular function from any etiology ranging from prior myocardial infarction (MI) to idiopathic cardiomyopathy are at risk for ventricular tachycardia.

   3. **Cardiac ischemia** rarely causes syncope, unless it is associated with global myocardial ischemia or arrhythmia. In patients who enter the emergency room with syncope but do not have electrocardiogram (ECG) changes or chest pain, it is highly unlikely that ischemia was the cause of their loss of consciousness.

   4. **Ventricular tachycardia** must be pursued aggressively in high-risk patients (i.e., those with known ischemic heart disease or left ventricular dysfunction) because it could be the harbinger of sudden death.

   5. **Supraventricular tachycardia** rarely leads to syncope, unless the patient has a structurally abnormal heart or an accessory bypass tract.

   6. **High-degree atrioventricular (AV) block** and **sinus node disease** are common causes of syncope.

  B. **Neurologic causes**

   1. **Reflex syncope**

      a. **Vasovagal syncope** is the most common type of syncope. Its mechanism involves the activation of C-fibers in the left ventricle by a forceful systolic contraction. With this activation, afferent traffic to the central nervous system (CNS) results in hypotension and/or bradycardia. Catecholamines enhance the activity of C-fibers and beta-blockers inhibit them (and can be used therapeutically).

      b. **Situational syncope** (e.g., micturition, deglutination, pregnancy) is mediated via the same reflex mechanism as a vasovagal event.

   2. **Transient ischemic attacks** can be accepted as the cause of syncope if they involve the vertebrobasilar system and are accompanied by brainstem dysfunction such as diplopia, ataxia, or vertigo.

C. Noncardiovascular causes

1. **Orthostatic hypotension** causes syncope in as many as 10% of cases.
2. **Psychiatric causes** of syncope are common in patients with panic disorder or major depression.
3. **Medications** may result in syncope by many mechanisms including hypotension, conduction system blocks, or by predisposing to ventricular tachycardia.

D. Unknown causes. A diagnosis may not be established in a substantial number of patients who present with syncope.

III. CLINICAL APPROACH

A. History (Figure 3–1)

1. The history is crucial in distinguishing whether a transient loss of consciousness is related to seizure or syncope.

   a. A witness to the event can help determine if seizure activity was present.
   b. The best discriminating historical feature is orientation immediately after the event, with seizure being five times more likely if the patient is disoriented.

2. The **classic prodrome** of a vasovagal event consists of diaphoresis, nausea, graying of vision, and a sense of doom. The presence of these symptoms has a high predictive value and is used as the gold standard in the assessment of complementary testing, such as the tilt table test (see III G).

3. A **prior history of fainting** in response to typically inciting events (e.g., pain, blood drawing) is also helpful in securing a diagnosis of a vasovagal event.

4. A **comprehensive drug history** is crucial in assessing whether medications have contributed to the episode.

5. **Historical features** that suggest a structurally abnormal heart or coronary artery disease (CAD) are important. Patients with a structurally abnormal heart need aggressive evaluation because they are at a higher risk for ventricular tachycardia and sudden death.

B. Physical examination. Key elements include:

1. Assessment of **orthostatic blood pressure** (systolic > 20–30 mm Hg or diastolic > 10–15 mm Hg)
2. A careful **cardiac examination** to assess for outflow obstruction
3. A complete **neurologic examination** to exclude focal deficits
4. Selective application of **carotid sinus massage** to assess for carotid sinus hypersensitivity

C. ECG has a low diagnostic yield, but it can help identify "footprints" of underlying structural heart disease.

D. Echocardiogram. Without a history, physical examination, or baseline ECG suggestive of an abnormal heart, the echocardiogram has less than a 10% positive diagnostic yield.

E. Arrhythmia detection monitors

1. A **24-hour Holter monitor** (see also Chapter 2) is most often used in patients with symptoms that suggest arrhythmia or in patients with

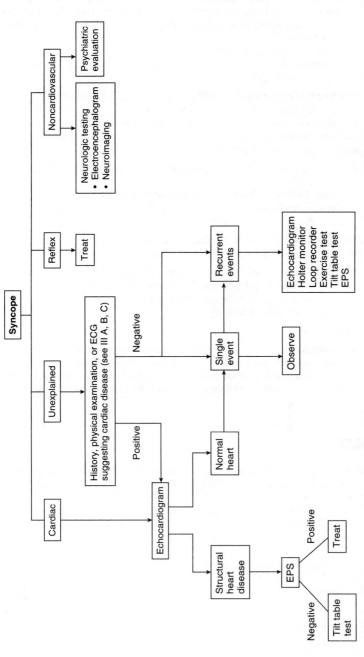

■ **FIGURE 3-1.** Algorithm for the workup of a patient with syncope. *ECG* = electrocardiogram; *EPS* = electrophysiologic studies.

17
▲

unexplained syncope. Because there is a low correlation between a detected arrhythmia and a recorded symptomatic event, the diagnostic yield is only about 20%. A higher diagnostic yield is found in patients with frequent episodes.

2. **Ambulatory loop monitors** allow continuous long-term monitoring in patients with recurrent, unexplained episodes. The diagnostic yield is approximately 35%.

F. **Electrophysiology studies (EPS):** Patients with syncope and a structurally abnormal heart should be strongly considered for EPS. Included are those with prior MI, low ejection fraction, hypertrophic cardiomyopathy, and patients with resting ECG suggesting an accessory bypass tract or intraventricular conduction delay.

1. The most significant finding on EPS is monomorphic ventricular tachycardia.
2. Other findings of high diagnostic yield include specific AV node and sinus node disease, supraventricular tachycardia, atrial fibrillation, and atrial flutter with hypotension.

G. **Tilt table testing** is used to evaluate syncope of unknown etiology and can be diagnostic of neurocardiogenic syncope.

1. A positive test would induce the patient's typical event and would demonstrate a hypotensive and/or bradycardic event.
2. A tilt table test should be used when cardiac causes of syncope have been reasonably excluded.

H. **Other testing**

1. **Neurologic testing** should be performed only if the history or physical examination suggests an event such as seizure or stroke.
2. **Psychiatric evaluation:** Underlying psychiatric illness is most common in young patients with frequent, unexplained episodes of syncope.

SUGGESTED READING

Linzer M, Yang EH, Estes MA, et al: Diagnosing syncope. Part 1: Value of history, physical examination and electrocardiography. The Clinical Efficacy Assessment Project of the American College of Physicians. *Ann Intern Med* 126:989–996, 1997.

Linzer M, Yang EH, Estes MA, et al: Diagnosing syncope. Part 2: Unexplained Syncope. *Ann Intern Med* 127:76–86, 1997.

4

Chest Pain and Coronary Artery Disease
John A. Paraskos and Frederick J. Curley

Nontraumatic Chest Pain and Coronary Artery Disease
John A. Paraskos

I. OVERVIEW. This section will deal with chest pain resulting from **nontraumatic pathology,** with emphasis on chest pain secondary to coronary artery disease (CAD).

    A. Angina pectoris is a diagnosis based on history. The clinician is faced with the task of assessing the likelihood that the patient has coronary disease as well as the likelihood that the patient's pain is cardiac in origin. After a careful initial evaluation, many patients must be treated as if they have myocardial ischemia until further diagnostic tests have eliminated the possibility, since the cardiac cause may be sinister.

    B. CAD is a diagnosis based on **gender, age,** and **character of chest pain.** The likelihood of significant CAD has been estimated at a pooled mean prevalence of 89% for all patients with chest pain typical for angina, 50% for patients with chest pain atypical for angina, and 16% for all other subjects. The prevalence is heavily influenced by age, gender, family history, and other risk factors. The estimate of the prevalence of significant CAD has important implications for the interpretation of noninvasive tests for myocardial ischemia.

II. Clinical Approach

    A. Introduction. When evaluating nontraumatic chest pain, the clinician must determine whether the patient's pain is

        1. Typical for myocardial ischemic pain
        2. Atypical for, but possibly caused by, ischemic pain
        3. Unlikely to be ischemic in origin
        4. Likely to be of a serious nature

    B. Differential diagnosis. Patients suspected of having an acute myocardial infarction (MI) or unstable angina pectoris are admitted for intensive care monitoring because short-term survival is enhanced by early intervention.

        1. Stable angina pectoris is often brought on by exercise and relieved by rest or nitrates. It may be provoked by a large meal and mistaken for indigestion. If the coronary disease is stable, pain episodes are usually short-lived (i.e., 5–15 minutes).

        2. Unstable angina pectoris is characterized by a less predictable course with a higher likelihood of leading to acute MI or sudden death. The instability is usually the result of a complication in the coronary artery (e.g., plaque rupture, thrombosis, spasm). Features that mark instability include:

a. New-onset angina
b. Accelerating angina (occurring more frequently or at lower workloads)
c. Rest angina
d. Angina that wakes the patient from sleep
e. Prolonged anginal episodes
f. Anginal episodes that are not responsive to nitrates
g. Angina associated with severe nausea, weakness, dyspnea, sweating, palpitation, syncope, or pulmonary edema

3. Acute MI is characterized by pain similar to that of angina pectoris; however, it is usually much more severe and longer lasting (an hour or more). The pain of MI usually includes a number of features of instability, and is more often accompanied by nausea and sweating.

4. Other causes. Even typical angina pectoris does not always indicate serious coronary disease.

a. Less threatening causes include conditions such as mitral valve prolapse and nonthreatening, stable coronary disease.
b. Alternatively, chest pain may result from other **life-threatening conditions that require immediate attention,** such as:

(1) Aortic dissection
(2) Critical aortic stenosis
(3) Accelerating hypertension
(4) Pulmonary thromboembolism
(5) Pulmonary hypertension

C. Ischemic versus nonischemic chest pain. A single convincing nonischemic feature cancels several ischemic-like features if it is clearly part of the same chest-pain symptom complex.

1. Location of pain. Nonischemic chest pain syndromes are associated with sharply localized pain, especially in the costochondral or inframammary region, radiating outside the limits of C3 to T6.
2. Patterns of relief are also helpful in assessing the cause of chest pain.

a. Prompt relief within 2 to 10 minutes of rest is most characteristic of effort-induced angina pectoris.
b. A more gradual disappearance over 1 hour or longer is more typical of musculoskeletal pain.
c. Occasionally, effort-induced ischemic pain disappears while the activity continues; this is known as **walkthrough** or **second wind angina.**
d. Relief within several minutes of the administration of sublingual nitrates is characteristic of angina pectoris; however, the pain of spastic gastrointestinal disorders also occasionally responds dramatically to nitrates.
e. Prompt relief with induced bradycardia (as with a Valsalva maneuver or carotid sinus pressure) is also seen in angina pectoris.
f. Relief with food or antacids suggests esophagitis or peptic disease.
g. Partial relief by sitting forward is more typical of pericarditis or

pancreatitis. Occasionally, pericarditis develops as a complication of MI, and these patients can have pericardial chest pain with both pleuritic and positional components.

D. Physical examination is frequently unremarkable during an episode of angina pectoris or an evolving MI. Often, however, a careful physical examination provides useful clues to the diagnosis of a noncardiac cause.

1. **Abnormal physical findings** may be found in cases of chest-wall tenderness, musculoskeletal disease, breast disease, thoracic outlet syndromes, or neurologic syndromes.

2. **Aortic dissection** may be suggested by absent pulses or the inequality of blood pressure in the arms or legs. Suspicion of aortic dissection is heightened if aortic regurgitation or an enlarging pleural effusion exists.

3. **Mitral valve prolapse** may be recognized by the characteristic non-ejection click with or without a mid to late systolic murmur at the apex.

4. **Pericardial or pleural friction rubs** may unmask serosal inflammation, but friction rubs may also be caused by transmural MI or proximal aortic dissection with bleeding into the pericardial sac.

5. **Valvular lesions** or **hypertrophic cardiomyopathy** may coexist with significant and symptomatic coronary disease.

6. **Ventricular dysfunction** is often evident, although it is common for CAD to present without abnormal physical findings.

7. **Severe stenosis of the left main or left anterior descending coronary artery** may be associated with an early to mid-diastolic high-pitched murmur and is a rare physical finding.

III. Diagnostic Evaluation

A. Electrocardiography

1. An **electrocardiogram (ECG) performed at rest** and in the absence of stress or ongoing chest pain is an **insensitive test** for the presence of CAD.

   a. Most patients with CAD have a normal resting ECG.

   b. The presence of abnormal Q waves may indicate previous MI, but their absence is not helpful in excluding significant CAD.

   c. ST-T wave abnormalities, arrhythmias, and conduction abnormalities are nondiagnostic findings.

2. **During chest pain,** however, an **ECG is the most valuable tool** for initial patient assessment (i.e., aside from the history and physical examination).

   a. Evidence for **ischemia** may be in the form of horizontal or downsloping ST-segment depression of at least 1 mm, with or without abnormally inverted T waves.

   b. **Myocardial injury or infarction** usually causes ST-segment elevation with eventual development of abnormal Q waves. Reciprocal changes in the early to mid-precordial leads (V-1 through V-4) suggest true posterior wall infarction.

(1) During the early stages of MI, the ECG may be totally normal. If the history and patient setting are suggestive, the diagnosis must be entertained despite a normal ECG.

(2) While a normal ECG taken during an episode of chest pain is important testimony against ischemic disease, it does not by any means exclude it.

c. **Acute pericarditis** usually causes diffuse ST-segment elevations and possibly PR-segment depressions.

d. Occasionally, the ECG suggests acute right ventricular strain, which in turn suggests a **massive pulmonary embolism.**

e. ECG may uncover **arrhythmias, conduction abnormalities,** or **hypertrophic patterns.**

B. Imaging

1. **Chest radiographs** are likely to be unremarkable during an acute ischemic episode or in an uncomplicated MI.

   a. The heart shadow is usually normal. A large heart shadow during an ischemic episode or in the early stages of an infarct suggests antecedent myocardial damage, valvular disease, or pericardial effusion.

   b. Pulmonary infiltrates, pneumothorax, rib fractures, and metastatic lesions are other sources of chest pain that may be discovered by the chest film.

   c. Although a widened mediastinum on the posteroanterior view is usually seen in aortic dissection, it is nonspecific and often seen in the elderly. However, a normal mediastinal width makes aortic dissection less likely.

2. **Spiral CT** can be useful in making the diagnosis of aortic dissection and pulmonary thromboembolism.

C. Echocardiography may be helpful in delineating the cause of cardiac chest pain.

1. A **transthoracic echocardiogram** may reveal wall-motion abnormalities during an episode of ischemic heart pain and in the early stages of MI, even when the ECG is normal. It may also be useful and accurate in the early diagnosis of aortic dissection.

2. Unsuspected valvular disease, pericardial effusion, widened aortic root, and occasionally dissection of the ascending aorta may be demonstrated.

D. Laboratory studies

1. **Arterial blood gases** and **pulse oximetry** are usually at normal levels in acute ischemic heart disease, unless significant left ventricular congestion or antecedent lung disease coexist. Hypoxia with associated hypocapnia is a nonspecific finding common to pulmonary congestion, pulmonary embolism, and other acute respiratory problems.

2. A **complete blood count** (CBC) may be valuable in the differential diagnosis of chest pain. Severe anemia is occasionally first manifested by angina. MI and pulmonary embolism both may be associated with a modest granulocytosis; however, a markedly elevated leukocyte count (> 15,000/ml) with a shift to the left should raise suspicion of an infectious process.

3. Evaluation of **cardiac enzymes** during the initial patient assessment may be helpful (see Chapter 5).

E. Noninvasive evaluation. If the patient's history of chest pain suggests a stable pattern of angina pectoris, the workup can proceed with the use of noninvasive procedures. Most of these procedures involve repeated evaluation of cardiac enzymes (see Chapter 5) and monitoring of the ECG under either physiologic or pharmacologic stress. Simultaneous use of myocardial imaging techniques greatly improves the sensitivity, specificity, and predictive value of the tests.

1. Test selection. Selection of the most appropriate test depends on the patient's exercise capacity, ability to tolerate pharmacologic intervention, and especially the pretest ratio of significant obstructive coronary disease. Angina pectoris is rare before 35 years of age, especially in women. However, its likelihood increases with each decade. Between 35 and 65 years of age, men have a higher likelihood of CAD; after age 65, it is distributed relatively equally among men and women. Combining these factors, the clinician can arrive at a level of suspicion (low, intermediate, or high) for CAD. Tests for ischemia provide a degree of positive or negative confirmation of that pretest likelihood.

2. Test options

   a. Exercise treadmill test (Figure 4–1)

   (1) The exercise treadmill test has the lowest predictive accuracy and the least ability to quantify the extent of ischemia.

   (a) Exercise treadmill testing is likely to be valuable in those patients with a normal resting ECG, because resting ST-T abnormalities or left bundle branch block (LBBB) interferes with interpretation of the test.

   (b) Exercise treadmill testing is best reserved for those patients with a somewhat moderate or intermediate pretest likelihood of disease, in whom the probability of a false-negative result is also low.

   (c) A positive test carries a chance of being falsely positive and may require further testing with myocardial imaging.

   (2) If a patient develops **angina-like chest pain** associated with horizontal or developing ST-segment depression of more than 1 mm, the likelihood of CAD is high.

   (a) If the test is positive with marked ST depression at a low level of exercise, widespread ischemia is suggested. Other features of widespread ischemia are ischemic changes associated with a drop in blood pressure while exercise continues and prolonged postexercise ischemic changes. For such patients, cardiac catheterization is usually the next step.

   (b) A person with **high pretest likelihood of CAD** and the absence of ischemic changes on exercise treadmill testing still has a moderate possibility of CAD. This person will require more sensitive testing (e.g., myocardial imaging or even coronary arteriography).

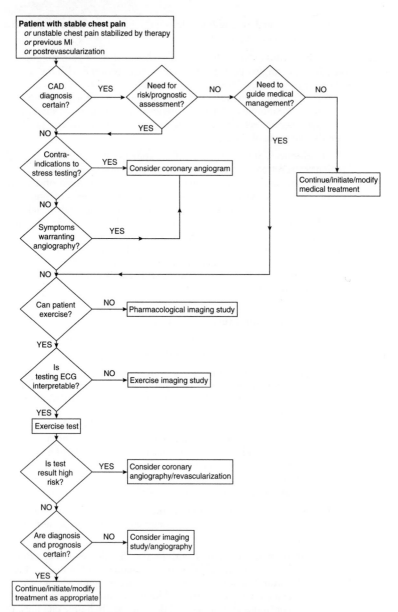

■ **FIGURE 4–1.** Exercise testing guidelines for patients with chest pain of suspected cardiac origin. *CAD* = coronary artery disease; *ECG* = electrocardiogram *MI* = myocardial infarction. (Reprinted with permission. Gibbons RJ, Balady GJ, Beasley JW, et al: ACC/AHA guidelines for exercise testing: executive summary. A Report of the American College of Cardiology/American Heart Association Task Force on Practice Guidelines. *Circulation* 98:345–354, 1997.

    (c) Exercise treadmill testing may offer prognostic information in patients with suspected CAD.

   (3) The **Duke Prognostic Treadmill Score** is an attempt to stratify patients into high-, intermediate-, and low-risk groups, based on their performance on a treadmill test. The prognostic component is not intended to answer the question "Does the patient have ischemic symptoms at this time?" but rather "What is the patient's risk of dying from CAD over the next few years?"

b. **Stress imaging studies** in general have a higher positive and negative predictive value than exercise ECG alone. For patients with abnormal ECG at baseline [ST-segment changes, LBBB, paced rhythms, left ventricular hypertrophy (LVH), use of digoxin or diuretics, and patients with pre-excitation], stress imaging allows a more reliable diagnosis of exercise-induced ischemia than the ECG alone. Stress echocardiography, on the other hand, has a greater specificity and a greater ability to evaluate cardiac anatomy and function. The choice of which test to use will depend on local expertise and availability.

   (1) **Exercise perfusion scintigraphy** with thallium or sestamibi carries a better predictive accuracy than simple exercise treadmill testing. Stress nuclear perfusion studies have a higher technical success rate than stress echocardiography and have a higher sensitivity, especially when multiple wall motion abnormalities are present. A negative test, even in a patient with a high pretest likelihood of disease, decreases the possibility of myocardial ischemia considerably so that other causes of chest pain must be considered. Rarely is the pretest likelihood so compelling that other imaging techniques (stress echocardiography, coronary arteriography) are needed to exclude a false-negative nuclear test.

   (2) **Stress echocardiography** can be accomplished with dipyridamole, dobutamine, or adenosine. Early results suggest excellent predictive accuracy. Treadmill or bicycle echocardiography also can be performed, but the exertion and hyperventilation involved may interfere with adequate transthoracic echocardiographic imaging.

c. **Pharmacological stress imaging studies**

   (1) **Dipyridamole perfusion scintigraphy:** For patients who are unable to exercise, the use of pharmacologic stress with imaging is indicated. (Dipyridamole, adenosine, and dobutamine have all been used.) Dipyridamole perfusion scintigraphy is often useful in those patients who are unable to exercise adequately on a treadmill. Dipyridamole causes maximum dilation of the coronary arteries. In the presence of significant CAD, coronary flow reserve is limited and disparities occur in the distribution of the thallium. Predictive accuracy is equivalent to an exercise scintigram. Patients with severe obstructive lung disease or asthma often cannot tolerate dipyridamole; in such patients, stress may be accomplished with dobutamine.

(2) Other nonstress and noninvasive techniques

    (a) Positron-emission tomography and 24-hour ambulatory ECG (Holter monitoring) are occasionally useful in the evaluation of ischemic chest pain. **Holter monitoring** is too insensitive to be used routinely as a diagnostic test for ischemia, but it may be particularly valuable in patients who experience pain only at rest or who are strongly suspected of having episodes of silent ischemia.

    (b) Esophageal manometry with or without provocation, **24-hour ambulatory esophageal monitoring of pH,** and **psychologic testing** may be in order when the likelihood of a cardiac condition is excluded or considered unlikely. Further workup of recurrent chest pain of obscure origin depends on the special characteristics of the patient and the pain.

F. Invasive evaluation. Coronary arteriography is the most reliable test for determining the diagnosis and extent of coronary disease. Indications for coronary arteriography include chest pain suspicious for CAD undiagnosed by thorough noninvasive evaluation, chest pain thought to result from coronary disease but unresponsive to medical therapy, unstable angina, and postinfarction angina. The more unstable the angina, the more reasonable it is to use coronary arteriography early, even as one of the first diagnostic tests. Coronary arteriography in at least two orthogonal views allows an excellent assessment of the extent of CAD as well as the potential for instability in the form of high-grade proximal stenoses, intraluminal thrombus, and ruptured or complicated plaques. Along with the patient's clinical course, this information is used to select medical therapy, angioplasty, stent, or coronary artery bypass surgery in the management of the patient.

IV. Conclusions. When a patient's chest pain has characteristics suspicious for myocardial ischemia and the patient's age, gender, and other risk factors make coronary disease possible, the clinician should exclude myocardial ischemia as a cause. If the characteristics suggest an unstable pattern of myocardial ischemia, the clinician should exclude acute or recent MI and assess the advisability of urgent antithrombotic therapy or the need for invasive diagnostic procedures. The more carefully the history is taken, the less likely it is that expensive procedures are ordered unnecessarily. After history, physical examination, ECG, and cardiac enzymes are assessed in acutely ill patients, the choice of tests for diagnostic evaluation include exercise treadmill testing, exercise treadmill testing with imaging, and coronary arteriography. Imaging techniques with radionuclide or echocardiography greatly improve diagnostic accuracy. Although expensive, their use could limit the number of coronary arteriograms otherwise required.

Noncardiac Chest Pain
Frederick J. Curley

I. Overview

A. **Definition.** Noncardiac chest pain is pain felt in the thorax not arising from the cardiac structures or from coronary ischemia.

B. **Incidence.** A systematic evaluation of noncardiac chest pain should yield a diagnosis more than 75% of the time. Approximately 11% of patients have an easily recognizable musculoskeletal cause, 20%–30% have anxiety and/or hyperventilation syndrome, at least 30% have an esophageal abnormality, and at least 10% have easily recognized syndromes of herpes zoster, aortic dissection, trauma, pneumothorax, or breast or kidney disease.

1. **Acute noncardiac chest pain** is most frequently caused by benign overuse syndrome, trauma, cocaine use, costochondral syndromes, gallbladder disease, gastroesophageal reflux disease (GERD), irritable esophagus, herpes zoster, pectoral girdle syndrome, pleurisy, pneumonia, or renal calculi.

2. **Chronic noncardiac chest pain** is most frequently caused by benign overuse syndrome, asthma, breast cancer, drug use, fibrocystic breast disease, GERD, irritable esophagus, anxiety, and/or hyperventilation syndrome, or pectoral girdle syndrome.

II. Clinical Approach

A. **Introduction.** In order to ensure that potential causes of pain are not overlooked, clinicians should employ an anatomic approach to assessing thoracic pain.

1. In many cases, **history and physical examination alone are adequate to establishing a diagnosis.** This is especially true with trauma, breast, neck, musculoskeletal, neurologic, or skin disease. Classic presentations of diseases, such as pulmonary embolism or pneumothorax, should be evaluated in a traditional fashion.

2. Figure 4–2 displays a suggested approach to diagnosis when the history and physical examination do not suggest a clear diagnosis.

B. **Differential diagnosis**

1. **Pain in the thorax** may arise from the structures in the thorax or be referred from adjacent structures. Pain may arise from the lungs and pleura, the gastrointestinal tract, muscles and skeletal structures, skin, breasts, mediastinal structures, the neck, nerves, kidneys, and from drug use.

2. **Pleurisy,** a sharp, superficial chest pain aggravated by inspiration, cough, or change in position, most commonly results from **viral inflammation** or **idiopathic** causes (46%–53% of cases), **pneumonia** (8%–18% of cases), and **pulmonary embolism** (21% of cases). Other causes accounting for 8%–25% of cases include pneumothorax, empyema, cervical or thoracic disk disease, costochondritis, or trauma. Asthma, radiation pneumonitis, sarcoidosis, mediastinitis or mediastinal tumors, and sickle cell disease may also cause pleurisy.

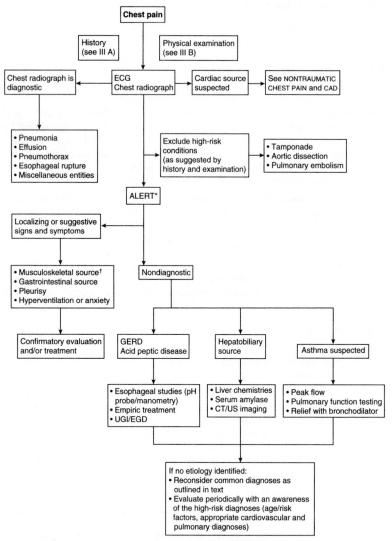

■ **FIGURE 4–2.** Algorithm for the diagnosis of chest pain. *CT* = computed tomography; *ECG* = electrocardiogram; *EGD* = esophagogastroduodenoscopy; *GERD* = gastroesophageal reflux disease; *UGI* = upper gastrointestinal series; *US* = ultrasound.

*This algorithm is intended to direct the workup in patients with chest pain of unclear etiology.

†Many of these patients will be discovered to have musculoskeletal syndromes that are diagnosed through a detailed history and physical examination. Musculoskeletal diagnoses to specifically consider include overuse syndromes, costochondritis, pectoral girdle syndrome, and xyphodynia.

3. **Mediastinitis or pneumomediastinum** may result as a consequence of deep infections of the neck or pharynx, rupture of mediastinal structures, cardiac surgery, tracheostomy, mechanical ventilation, or dental work with a high-speed drill.

4. **Panic, anxiety, or hyperventilation syndrome** occurs in 13% of patients seeking medical care, and 60% of these patients have chest pain. Up to 55% of patients with noncardiac chest pain have some component of this disorder. Due to the high prevalence of anxiety and hyperventilation in the general population, these conditions may be present but not be the cause of the pain. This is considered a diagnosis of exclusion.

   (a) The diagnosis of **panic** can be established primarily by interview, asking about sensations of smothering, palpitations, sweating, lightheadedness, flushing, trembling, fear of dying or going crazy, nausea, numbness, or depersonalization.

   (b) Signs and symptoms of **hyperventilation syndrome** include headache, numbness and tingling of the extremities, impaired thinking, sighing, yawning, aerophagia, muscle stiffness or cramps, carpopedal spasm, and irritability.

5. **Irritable esophagus** is a term used to encompass GERD and motility disorders that result in chest pain. Many of these patients have other gastrointestinal symptoms in addition to chest pain, although it is important to note that chest pain may be the only manifestation. Most patients complain of a dull aching that lasts hours and may radiate to the neck or shoulders. Other gastrointestinal etiologies, which may result in chest pain, include esophageal rupture, incarcerated diaphragmatic hernia, pancreatitis, biliary colic, ulcer disease, aerophagia, and gas entrapment.

6. **Thoracic muscles and bones** are frequently overlooked causes of pain. Overuse or pressure trauma to the pectoral muscles (carrying objects, unsupported arm work, sewing, knitting, prolonged flexion of the neck, and tight brassiere straps) may produce the **pectoral girdle syndrome;** 50% of those with this syndrome have tenderness in the serratus anterior muscle. **Benign overuse syndrome** may result from repetitive activities. Other rheumatologic causes include sternoclavicular joint disease or xyphoidynia-xyphoidalgia, ankylosing spondylitis, and rib, spine, or shoulder disease. **Fibromyalgia** involving the chest frequently has trigger points in trapezius, deltoid, pectoralis, rotator cuff, and posterior cervical muscles. The **thoracic outlet syndromes** cause pain due to compression of the subclavian artery, vein, and brachial plexus at the root of the neck.

7. **Intercostal nerve injury** may cause pain 4 months to 5 years after internal mammary grafting. Traumatic or postsurgical neuromas usually have point tenderness. Sternal wires in postmedian sternotomy have caused pain due to nickel hypersensitivity or entrapment of nerves.

8. **Skin infections, subcutaneous neuromas, and herpes zoster** may cause pain.

9. **Breast pain** may arise from mastitis, gynecomastia, fibrocystic disease, cancer, trauma, or breast implants. Mammary duct ectasia occurs in elderly women with atrophic breasts and presents as intermittent infra-areolar pain, bloody nipple discharge, swelling, and erythema.

10. **Pyelonephritis, renal infarct, and renal calculi** may all present with lower lateral thoracic pain and associated typical symptoms.

11. **Medications:** 5-fluorouracil, bleomycin, methotrexate, ranitidine, ondansetron, cocaine, 100% oxygen, vancomycin, ergotamines/triptans, and sertraline have all been associated with specific chest pain syndromes.

III. Evaluation

A. Historical features.
It is extremely important for the clinician to avoid anchoring to inappropriate diagnoses in the face of compelling historic information. For example, if a young patient presents with classic anginal symptoms, the clinician must resist the temptation of dismissing a cardiac diagnosis because of the patient's age. Thus, the history must be obtained with an open mind.

1. **Medical history** should focus on the timing, duration, character, and provocative factors of the pain.

2. **Cardiac risk factors** should always be assessed, and heart disease should be considered.

3. **Specific items** that should always be asked include history of cancer or radiation therapy, trauma, tobacco use, HIV status, known pneumocystis pneumonia infection, prior deep venous thrombosis or pulmonary embolism, bedrest/immobility, recent surgery, fever, sputum production, asthma, wheezing, heartburn, dysphagia, prior renal calculi or infection, and hematuria.

4. **Occupation and hobbies:** A clear description of occupation and hobbies should be obtained to evaluate for pectoral girdle syndrome and benign overuse syndrome.

B. Physical examination

1. **Inspection** is helpful in detecting scoliosis, kyphosis, pectus excavatum, trauma, skin rashes (herpes zoster), deformities of the acromioclavicular or costochondral joints, Horner's syndrome, tracheal deviation, jugular venous distention (JVD), and cyanosis.

2. **Palpation** should include examination of the major bones (acromioclavicular joints, ribs, spine, sternum, costochondral junctions, scapula, and xyphoid) and major muscle groups (sternocleidomastoid, trapezius, rotator cuff, deltoid, biceps, and paraspinal muscles).

3. The **abdomen** should be checked for hepatosplenomegaly, right upper quadrant tenderness, flank pain, and pregnancy.

4. **Breasts** should be examined for masses and cysts, superficial thromboses, nipple discharge, and implants.

5. **Auscultation** may help identify carotid or renal bruits, pleural rubs, absent bowel sounds, or decreased breath sounds.

6. **Musculoskeletal causes** are almost always detected by examination.

   a. Range of motion of the shoulder and neck, and cervical compression help detect **cervical spine disease.**

   b. Pain from **rotator cuff injury** is aggravated by a downward pull on the relaxed arm and is relieved by allowing the weight of the arm to fall away from the acromium. This can be accomplished by allowing the arm to dangle when the hip and trunk are flexed.

    c. **Adson's maneuver** (extension of the neck toward the side opposite the lesion and deep inspiration) and the **costoclavicular maneuver** (standing in an exaggerated military attention posture) narrow the thoracic outlet and may reproduce pain or cause a diminution of pulse.

    d. **Spurling's maneuver** (traction of an adducted arm with head rotation to the same side) and **crowing rooster maneuvers** (extension of the cervical spine while applying posterior traction to extended arms) may be helpful in detecting **costo-chondritis.**

    e. Fingers should be hooked under the lower ribs and pulled to determine if there is a **slipping rib syndrome.**

C. Laboratory assessment

1. **Chest radiography** should be a mandatory examination in virtually all patients. Chest radiographs provide valuable information about pneumothorax, pulmonary hypertension, pneumonia, trauma, aerophagia, aortic dissection, mediastinal disease, shoulder disease, and spine disease. The chest radiograph influences clinical judgment in approximately 23% of cases.

2. **Pulmonary embolism:** There is no national consensus on the best evaluation for venous thromboembolism, and the best diagnostic algorithm varies with what testing is available at each hospital. Most clinicians agree that normal ELISA-based d-dimer levels rule out deep-vein thrombosis and pulmonary embolus in patients with a low clinical probability.

    a. A **ventilation perfusion scan** is the first-line test for pulmonary embolism in institutions without d-dimer testing. Although a normal or high probability scan is extremely helpful in ruling in or ruling out pulmonary embolism, this pattern occurs in only about 27% of patients being screened.

    b. **Pulmonary angiography,** where available, is the most specific test for pulmonary embolism. Although spiral CT scans with intravenous contrast are now routinely used, many troublesome issues remain such as the best technique to use, the reliability of interpretation, and the sensitivity and specificity of the test in routine hands. The safety of withholding treatment on the basis of a "negative" CT angiogram is not known at this time.

3. **Irritable esophagus:** Most major studies now recommend ambulatory esophageal pressure and pH monitoring studies as the single best screening test for esophageal disease suspected of causing chest pain. Where this testing is available, it has replaced acid infusion, balloon distention, and cholinergic stimulation tests.

4. **Hyperventilation provocation tests** with voluntary hyperventilation, infusion of lactate, or CO_2 breathing are typically sensitive but not specific. This leaves anxiety or hyperventilation syndrome as a diagnosis of exclusion. Cardiopulmonary exercise testing may be helpful in that patients with only a hyperventilation anxiety syndrome have a normal physiologic response to exercise but an abnormal pattern of hypocapnia.

SUGGESTED READING

Constant J: The clinical diagnosis of non-anginal chest pain: the differentiation of angina from non-anginal chest pain by history. *Clin Cardiol* 6:11–16, 1983.

Epstein SE: Implications of probability analysis on the strategy used for noninvasive detection of coronary artery disease: role of single or combined use of exercise electrocardiographic testing, radionuclide cineangiography and myocardial perfusion imaging. *Am J Cardiol* 46:491–499, 1980.

Kuntz KM, Fleischmann KE, Hunink MG, Douglas PS: Cost-effectiveness of diagnostic strategies for patients with chest pain. *Ann Intern Med* 130:709–718, 1999.

Shaw LJ, Peterson ED, Shaw LK, Kesler KL, DeLong ER, Harrell FE Jr, Muhlbaier LH, Mark DB: Use of prognostic treadmill score in identifying diagnostic coronary disease subgroups. *Circulation* 98:1622–1630, 1998.

5

Cardiac Markers

Fauzia Khan, John A. Paraskos,
and L. Michael Snyder

I. Overview. Cardiac markers are an important component in the diagnosis of acute myocardial infarction (MI) mainly because the other two clinical indicators—chest pain and electrocardiogram (ECG)—may be inconclusive in many cases. The testing is based on the observation that at the time of infarction, certain enzymes and troponin, a protein, are released into the bloodstream.

   A. Traditional approach. Figure 5–1 presents the cardiac markers as they are traditionally used.

   B. Cost-effective approach. A more specific and certainly more cost-effective approach is outlined in Figure 5–2.

II. Individual Cardiac Markers

   A. Creatinine kinase (CK). Total CK can be separated into three fractions or isoenzymes: CK-MB is found predominantly in cardiac muscle, CK-MM in skeletal muscle, and CK-BB in brain and lung muscle.

      1. CK-MB levels begin to rise 3 to 6 hours after the onset of MI, peak at 12 to 24 hours, and return to normal in 24 to 48 hours.

      2. Testing recommendations

         a. It is recommended that 2 to 3 **sequential samples** be obtained: the first immediately at presentation and subsequent at about 8-hour intervals during the first 24 hours.

         b. Immunochemical techniques using monoclonal or polyclonal antibodies are very sensitive and specific for CK-MB. Turnaround time is around 15 minutes. For CK-MB to be 95%–100% sensitive, samples must be obtained about 8 hours after the onset of symptoms.

      3. Results

         a. The **CK-MB index** is calculated as CK-MB/total creatinine phosphokinase × 100. A CK-MB index greater than 4% is diagnostic of MI.

         b. Falsely elevated results may occur when total CK values are low to start, such as in patients with small muscle mass.

   B. Troponin I and T. Troponin I and T are regulatory proteins found in skeletal and cardiac muscle fibers. Cardiac isoforms are specific for troponin I and T, and are completely specific to the myocardium in adults.

      1. The **rate of change** of troponin is more important than the absolute

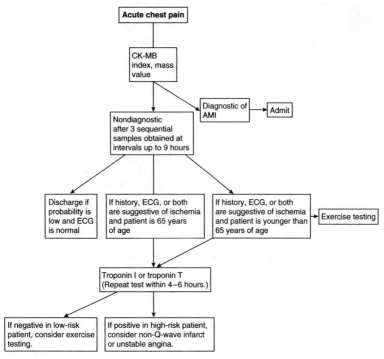

■ **FIGURE 5–1.** Diagnostic workup of patients with acute chest pain. *AMI* = acute myocardial infarction; *CK-MB* = creatinine kinase, myocardial bound; *ECG* = electrocardiogram.

value. Elevated levels without a rate change may be seen in congestive heart failure (CHF), or unstable angina.

a. Troponin I and T behave much like CK-MB in that they rise in about 4 to 6 hours following the acute event and peak at about 12 hours.

(1) Unlike CK-MB, however, troponin T remains elevated for about 10 days before it normalizes. Troponin T, therefore, gives a cumulative patient history in that it reflects the events of the previous week or so.

(2) Troponin I returns to reference range in about 4 days.

b. Troponin I and T are raised on an average 3.8 hours after the onset of symptoms compared with 4.8 hours for CK-MB. Therefore, they play a role in the early diagnosis of MI.

2. Troponin is most useful in patients who do not have raised CK-MB or ST elevation but have an ECG suggestive of ischemia. If patients are positive for cardiac troponin I (cTn-I), they have a 26% greater chance of having a combined event than those patients who are negative for cTn-I.

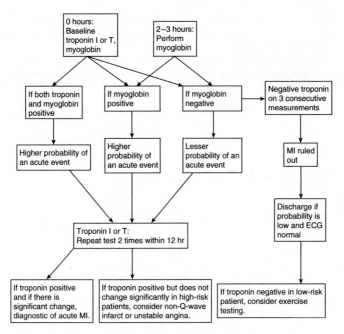

■ FIGURE 5–2. Cost-effective workup for acute chest pain. *ECG* = electrocardiogram; *MI* = myocardial infarction.

3. Presently, there is **no clear advantage** for choosing between troponin I and T.

   a. A normal value for troponin T is in the range of 0.1 to 0.2 ng/ml.
   b. The normal values for troponin I vary with each assay used.

4. **Results.** Patients who have elevated troponin levels should be considered high risk even in the absence of other high-risk criteria. Conversely, the absence of elevated troponin levels does not by itself rule out MI.

C. Myoglobin. Myoglobin is another marker that doubles within 2 hours of presentation with MI, and peaks at about 4 hours. Serial measurements of myoglobin are more sensitive than CK-MB for MI, but they are less specific.

SUGGESTED READING

American College of Emergency Physicians: Serum marker analysis in acute myocardial infarction. American College of Emergency Physicians. *Ann Emerg Med* 35(5): 534–539, 2000.

Antman EM, Fox MK: Acute ischemic heart disease. Guidelines for the diagnosis and management of unstable angina and non-Q wave myocardial infarction: Proposed revisions. *Am Heart J* 139:461–475, 2000.

Polanczyk CA, Kuntz KM, Sacks DB, et al: Emergency department triage strategies for acute chest pain using creatine kinase-MB and troponin assays: a cost-effective analysis. *Ann Intern Med* 131:909–918, 1999.

6

Hyperlipidemia

Howard Sachs and Ira Ockene

I. **Overview.** Cardiovascular disease is the leading cause of mortality in the United States, accounting for over 500,000 deaths annually.

II. **Clinical Approach**

A. **Risk factors.** As hyperlipidemia is only one risk factor for the development of coronary heart disease (CHD), evaluation should include a comprehensive investigation of all risk factors.

1. **Hypertriglyceridemia** has been correlated with the risk of developing CHD in univariate analysis, but the ability to predict CHD is diminished in multivariate analysis. It is a more potent predictor of risk in women.

2. **Cholesterol levels.** Table 6–1 details the current classification scheme established by the **National Cholesterol Education Program (NCEP).**

a. Elevations of **total serum cholesterol** and **low-density lipoproteins** (LDLs) are directly correlated with the risk of developing CHD.

b. **High density lipoproteins** (HDLs), on the other hand, are inversely correlated with CHD risk.

(1) A low HDL cholesterol level (< 40 mg/dl) is classified as a major risk factor for CHD.

(2) Conversely, a high HDL cholesterol level (> 60 mg/dl) appears to be protective against CHD.

(3) It should be recognized that HDL is a continuous variable, and that classifying HDL into above and below 40 mg/dl is artificial. A level of 32 mg/dl defines the lowest tenth percentile for men, whereas an HDL of 37 mg/dl defines the lowest tenth percentile for women.

c. **Lowering cholesterol** by diet, medication, or surgery reduces the risk of CHD.

3. **Genetic disorders.** Important genetic disorders of lipoprotein metabolism include:

a. **Familial hypercholesterolemia:** This is an autosomal dominant disease with both homozygous (rare) and heterozygous forms. The heterozygous form is present in approximately 1:500 people. It results in a defective LDL receptor and is characterized by an LDL level > 260 mg/dl, xanthomas, and the frequent presence of premature CHD.

b. **Familial combined hyperlipidemia** is characterized by elevations of both cholesterol and triglyceride levels. Multiple family members may be affected. It is present in approximately 1% of the population

---

TABLE 6–1. Initial Classification Based on Total Cholesterol and HDL Cholesterol

Total cholesterol

< 200 mg/dl	Desirable blood cholesterol
200–239 mg/dl	Borderline high blood cholesterol
≥ 240 mg/dl	High blood cholesterol

HDL cholesterol

< 40 mg/dl	Undesirably low HDL cholesterol

National Cholesterol Education Program: Second report of the Expert Panel on Detection, Evaluation, and Treatment for High Blood Cholesterol in Adults. National Institutes of Health; National Heart, Lung, and Blood Institute; NIH Publication No. 93–3095, September 1993.

HDL = high-density lipoprotein.

and is associated with a predisposition to CHD. Family history is key, as this genetic disorder is mimicked by the metabolic disorder seen in diabetes and hypothyroidism, and is also often seen with excessive alcohol intake.

4. **Lipoprotein(a)** is a modified form of LDL cholesterol, which has been associated with an increased risk of CHD in patients with hypercholesterolemia. The level appears to be genetically determined. Postulated mechanisms that account for the associated increase in atherosclerosis include:

a. The presence of a sequence homologous to plasminogen, which competitively inhibits the fibrinolytic system

b. Lipoprotein(a) has a high affinity for tissue macrophage receptors and promotes foam cell formation and the deposition of cholesterol into atherosclerotic plaques

B. **Differential diagnosis.** There is no differential diagnosis per se regarding the hyperlipidemic states. However, patients should be assessed for secondary and exacerbating conditions including:

1. Hypothyroidism
2. Diabetes mellitus
3. Obstructive liver disease
4. Nephrotic syndrome
5. Chronic renal failure
6. Alcohol abuse
7. Medications

III. **Evaluation**

A. **Screening.** All adults should be screened at 18 to 21 years of age, with repeat screenings at a minimum of 5-year intervals thereafter. Patients should be aware of their lipid values so as to make appropriate decisions regarding lifestyle modification.

1. The **NCEP** recommends that screening include total cholesterol and HDL levels. In clinical practice, a full "lipid profile" (lipoprotein analysis) is usually obtained, which generally includes total cholesterol, triglycerides, HDL, and LDL cholesterol.

2. The **LDL cholesterol** has historically been a calculated value. The formula for calculating LDL assumes a triglyceride level below 400 ng/dl.

LDL cholesterol = total cholesterol − HDL cholesterol − (triglycerides/5)

   More recently, the direct measurement of LDL has become available.

3. Measurements of total cholesterol and HDL cholesterol may be obtained in the nonfasting state, as they do not change appreciably after a meal. However, as LDL is a calculated value, estimated from measurements that include triglycerides, **a fasting specimen for lipoprotein analysis is preferred,** because triglycerides can fluctuate with meals.

B. **History.** In the patient with hyperlipidemia, the medical history should focus on cardiovascular symptoms and prior events, family history of cardiovascular disease, lifestyle issues (e.g., diet, exercise, alcohol use), present and past treatments, signs and symptoms of secondary causes (see II B), and comorbid conditions that will influence treatment.

C. **Physical examination.** It is important to identify evidence of end organ damage with a focus on the cardiovascular system. The clinician should pay particular attention to the presence of distal pulses, bruits, and the heart examination itself. In the high-risk patient, xanthomas should be sought (periorbital and extensor surfaces).

D. **Lipoprotein measurements** can vary among laboratories, have considerable innate biological variation, and be influenced by factors such as stress, posture, and season. Thus, it is prudent to repeat values on more than one occasion before making treatment decisions.

SUGGESTED READING

Expert Panel on Detection, Evaluation, and Treatment of High Blood Cholesterol in Adults: Summary of the second report of the National Cholesterol Education Program (NCEP) Expert Panel on Detection Evaluation and Treatment of High Blood Cholesterol in Adults (Adult Treatment Panel II). *JAMA* 269:3015–3023, 1993.

Third Report of the Expert Panel on Detection, Evaluation, and Treatment of High Blood Cholesterol in Adults (Adult Treatment Panel III). Bethesda, MD: National Institutes of Health, National Heart, Lung, and Blood Institute; NIH Publication No. 01–3095, 2001.

7

Pericardial Disease

John A. Paraskos

I. Types of Pericardial Disease

A. **Acute pericarditis** refers to inflammation of the pericardium.

B. **Cardiac tamponade.** Any cause of pericarditis may cause pericardial effusion and eventual tamponade.

   1. Large effusions are caused, in general, by neoplasm, infection, autoimmune diseases, and radiation (Table 7–1).
   2. The most common causes of cardiac tamponade are neoplastic, uremic, traumatic, or ventricular rupture, or proximal dissection of the aorta. **Rapid accumulation** (as with stab wounds, or myocardial or aortic rupture) may lead to considerable pressure increase with even smaller volumes of fluid.

C. **Constrictive pericarditis.** Any cause of acute pericarditis may cause constriction. As left ventricular filling is compromised, stroke volume, cardiac output, and blood pressure are limited or diminished. Eventually, cardiac cirrhosis may develop with a small contracted liver. Elevated systemic venous pressure may eventually cause portal hypertension and even a protein-losing enteropathy with hypoalbuminemia and anasarca.

II. Clinical Diagnosis

A. History and physical examination

   1. **A sharp, very distinct precordial pain** is diagnostic. It is worsened by inspiration or cough, and somewhat lessened by leaning forward. The pain often radiates to the left trapezius ridge, and may worsen with each heartbeat.
   2. **Fever** and **chills** suggest an infectious etiology.
   3. **Symptoms of acute pericarditis** may be present in patients with cardiac tamponade. In addition, dyspnea, fatigue, confusion, and agitation are common.
   4. A **pericardial friction rub** may be revealed on physical examination. This is a scratchy precordial noise. If a significant effusion has developed, the rub often disappears.
   5. **Fatigue, hypotension, and reflex tachycardia** are common in constrictive pericarditis.
   6. **Distended jugular veins that do not drop on inspiration** (Kussmaul's venous sign) also indicate **constrictive pericarditis.** Elevated systemic venous pressure may lead to tender hepatomegaly, peripheral edema, and ascites.
   7. **Pulsus paradoxus** is characterized by a greater than 10 mm Hg drop in systolic blood pressure with inspiration. It is caused by filling of the right ventricle on inspiration impinging on the already restricted left

TABLE 7–1. Causes of Acute Pericarditis

Infectious agents	Noninfectious agents
Viral, especially echovirus, Coxsackie B, and HIV	Uremia
Tuberculosis, with the incidence increasing in AIDS patients and other immunosuppressed individuals	Post-MI pericarditis, with early inflammation caused by irritation of necrotic tissue and Dressler's syndrome caused by autoimmune response weeks to months after the event
Other bacterial agents, especially pneumococcus and staphylococcus, although other organisms may be causative	Postpericardiotomy syndrome, which is similar to Dressler's syndrome after open heart surgery
	Neoplastic disease, including metastatic or local spread, especially to the lung, breast, and lymphoma
	Radiation-induced, especially if cumulative dose to thorax exceeds 4000 rads
	Autoimmune and connective tissue diseases, such as SLE, rheumatic diseases, scleroderma, and drug-induced conditions
	Idiopathic; many cases are likely to be viral in origin but are so limited that viral titers are not measurable

MI = myocardial infarction; SLE = systemic lupus erythematosus.

ventricular filling. This finding may be found in patients with cardiac tamponade, but it is not specific and may also be seen in patients with bronchospasm and artificial ventilation (especially with positive end-expiratory pressure).

B. Electrocardiogram (ECG)

1. During the **acute stage of inflammation,** the ECG will show ST-segment elevation in almost all leads except the aVR (which will show ST depression). In the subacute and chronic phase of continued inflammation, ST and PR segments return to baseline and T waves flatten and then invert.

2. In **cardiac tamponade,** the ECG may show signs of pericarditis. Swinging of the heart will be noted as an alternating shift in axis known as electrical alternans.

C. Imaging studies

1. The **chest radiograph** in constrictive pericarditis may be normal with a small cardiac silhouette. Approximately 50% of cases will demonstrate calcification of the pericardium.
2. **Computed tomography (CT) scan or magnetic resonance imaging (MRI)** demonstrates evidence of a thickened pericardium. Normal pericardial thickness by either technique excludes constriction.

D. Echocardiogram

1. **Acute pericarditis.** The echocardiogram is often normal in acute pericarditis. If present, pericardial effusion will be noted.
2. **Cardiac tamponade.** The echocardiogram in cardiac tamponade will demonstrate the effusion.
3. **Constrictive pericarditis.** The echocardiogram in constrictive pericarditis shows brisk ventricular filling that terminates abruptly in early diastole.

E. Cardiac catheterization may be indicated in patients with constrictive pericarditis.

1. Diastolic pressure tracings are elevated in all chambers and are "equalized."
2. Ventricular pressure tracings demonstrate an early diastolic dip with rapid rise and plateau.
3. Atrial pressure tracings show a prominent early diastolic drop (y descent).

F. Additional studies. In those patients where the diagnosis of acute pericarditis remains uncertain, **pericardiocentesis** or **pericardial biopsy** may be of benefit. However, the diagnostic yield is relatively low.

SUGGESTED READING

Gintzton LE, Laks MM: The differential diagnosis of acute pericarditis. *Circulation* 65:1004–1009, 1982.

Dermatology

8

Pruritus

Caroline Baltimore

I. Overview. Itching is the most common presenting dermatological complaint.

  A. Definition

    1. **Pruritus** refers to any form of itching.

    2. **Generalized pruritus of undetermined origin** (GPUO) is defined as continuous itching for 3 weeks duration that is unresponsive to 2 weeks of conservative management (i.e., emollients and antihistamines) and not associated with a primary dermatologic condition. GPUO warrants further investigation, particularly to look for internal and potentially serious causes.

  B. Types. Pruritus may be localized or generalized, and it may be associated with a primary skin disorder or manifest as a symptom of an internal disease process.

  C. Etiologies

    1. **Common skin conditions** causing itch are **xerosis** and **atopic dermatitis.** Other causes include dermatitis (contact, asteatotic), psoriasis, lichen planus/simplex, urticaria, dermatitis herpetiformis, sunburn, insect bites, and some skin infections (e.g., folliculitis, scabies).

    2. **Constant scratching** may produce secondary lesions (e.g., lichenification, neurotic excoriations), which may make it difficult to identify the primary cause.

    3. **Environmental factors,** such as the climate, bathing, soaps, and medications, may cause pruritus.

    4. **Systemic illness** is associated with 14% to 50% of cases (Table 8–1). Pruritus may precede overt manifestations of **internal illness** by even a year.

    5. **Psychogenic causes** should also be considered, and may be as simple as a self-perpetuating scratch-itch cycle.

II. Clinical Approach (Figure 8–1)

  A. History. The history must be meticulously obtained and should include the following information:

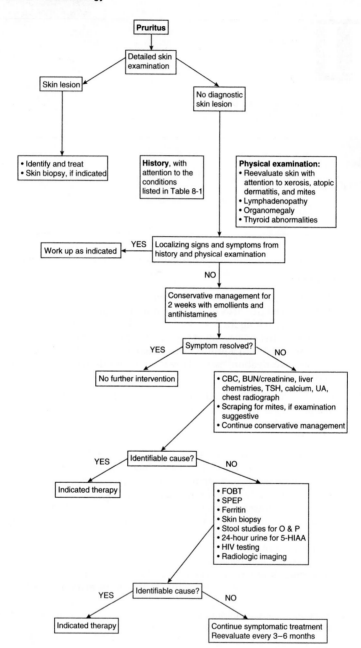

■ **FIGURE 8–1.** Algorithm for the workup of patients with pruritus. *5-HIAA* = 5-hydroxyindoleacetic acid; *BUN* = blood urea nitrogen; *CBC* = complete blood count; *FOBT* = fecal occult blood test; *O&P* = ova and parasites; *SPEP* = serum protein electrophoresis; *TSH* = thyroid-stimulating hormone; *UA* = urinalysis.

1. **Onset, duration, and location of itching**
   a. If itching worsens in the evening, it may be associated with scabies.
   b. If itching awakens the patient at night, it may represent systemic disease.
2. **Precipitants and environmental factors** (e.g., frequency and temperature of bathing, seasonal associations, association with menstrual cycle)
3. **History of atopy** (hay fever, eczema, asthma), as well as family history of atopy and general illness
4. **Social history** (e.g., occupational exposures, pets, travel, sexual history)
5. **Review of systems** (see Table 8–1). Inquire about age-appropriate health maintenance screening. Keep in mind that xerosis may be worse just after bathing. It tends to occur on the anterior legs and lateral arms.

TABLE 8–1. Medical Illnesses Associated with Pruritus

System	Definite association	Probable association
Renal	Uremia	
Hepatic	Primary biliary cirrhosis Extrahepatic obstruction Cholestasis of pregnancy	
Hematologic	Polycythemia vera Lymphoma (Hodgkin's and non-Hodgkin's)	Iron-deficiency anemia Multiple myeloma and other paraproteinemias* Mastocytosis* Hemochromatosis Mycosis fungoides Leukemia
Endocrine	Hyperthyroidism Hypothyroidism Diabetes	
Neurologic		Cerebrovascular accident Abscess* Multiple sclerosis* Tumor*
Miscellaneous		Other disseminated malignancies Carcinoid syndrome* AIDS* Sjögren's syndrome* Dumping syndrome* Giardia infection

*Case reports indicate an association.

B. Physical examination

1. **Skin examination.** Special scrutiny must be given to the skin.

   a. If no obvious lesions are present, it is important to look carefully for fine scaling, which may represent **xerosis.**

   b. **Scabies infestation** is frequently subtle. It is important to carefully inspect the skin for burrows and to consider skin scrapings to identify the mites or eggs.

2. The **"butterfly sign,"** while not pathognomonic, may suggest local versus systemic disease. Because the upper mid-back is difficult to reach, it may be spared in systemic processes while lesions in this area suggest primary dermatoses.

3. Particular attention should be paid to identifying the presence of **lymphadenopathy** and **organomegaly.**

C. Diagnostic testing. The yield of **specific tests** in the population of patients with generalized pruritus cannot be definitively stated. The indications for extensive laboratory evaluation and radiologic imaging are governed by patient-related factors (e.g., duration and persistence of pruritus, associated symptoms, response to therapy, anxiety regarding symptoms).

SUGGESTED READING

Kantor G, Bernhard J: Investigation of the pruritic patient in daily practice. *Seminars Dermat* 14:290–296, 1995.

9

Urticaria and Angioedema

Richard Palken

I. Definition

A. Urticaria is a pruritic, edematous, pink or red wheal that can occur anywhere on the surface of the skin. The reaction generally lasts less than 24 hours.

B. Angioedema is a larger swelling that occurs subcutaneously or submucosally, lasts somewhat longer than urticaria, and is generally less pruritic.

II. Clinical Approach (Figure 9–1)

A. History

1. A **detailed history,** elicited best through a standard questionnaire, should focus on the pattern and onset of hives in relation to any physical stimuli, exposure history to any potential ingested allergens, and associated comorbid symptoms.

2. Urticaria is divided arbitrarily into **acute** and **chronic** varieties:

   a. Acute urticaria is self-limited, lasts less than 6 weeks, and does not warrant extensive diagnostic evaluation.

   (1) Ingested foods. Evaluate the ingredients listed in the foods ingested. A variety of nuts, fruits, seafood, and food additives have been linked to urticaria. Benzoates, sulfites, and azo dyes are identified as putative agents.

   (2) Medications are a common cause of urticaria. Drug reactions usually start within 3 weeks of exposure to a new medication. The one exception is angiotensin-converting enzyme (ACE) inhibitors, where urticaria has been reported up to 4 years into medication use.

   b. Chronic urticaria has an extensive differential diagnosis. It is common for no cause to be found.

   (1) Occasionally, causative **food additives** may be identified.

   (2) Urticaria is rarely the sole manifestation of a **systemic disease** (see Table 9–1).

   (3) Physical urticaria

   (a) Cold urticaria often occurs after rewarming of the skin.

   (b) Pressure urticaria usually occurs after several hours of pressure.

   (c) Cholinergic "heat" urticaria can be brought out by exercise, emotional stress, or hot baths.

   (4) Urticarial vasculitis is associated with individual hives that last more than 24 to 48 hours, hives that are minimally pruritic and

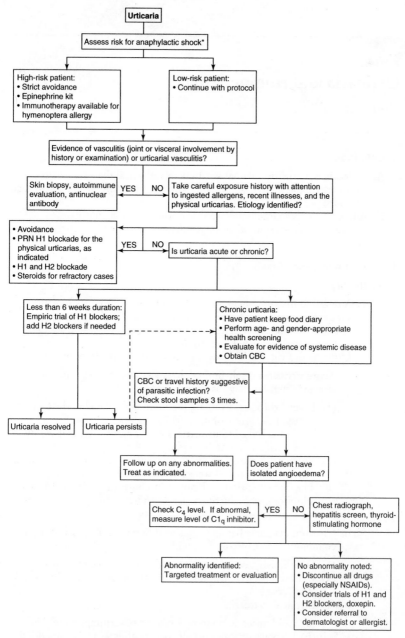

FIGURE 9–1. Algorithm for the workup of urticaria.

*A history of urticarial reaction accompanied by upper or lower respiratory symptoms, urticaria accompanied by hypotension, or a sudden and severe urticarial response to a known venom or ingested antigen all portend the risk of future anaphylaxis.

ANA = antinuclear antibody; *CBC* = complete blood count; *NSAIDs* = nonsteroidal anti-inflammatory drugs.

TABLE 9–1. Differential Diagnoses of Urticaria and Angioedema

Physical urticaria

Dermatographism
Cold
Heat
Solar radiation
Pressure
Vibratory
Aquagenic

Drugs, food, and additives

Almost any medication
Benzoates
Tartrates
Yellow food dye
Nuts
Fruits
Shellfish
Drugs that modulate the breakdown of bradykinin [e.g., angiotensin-converting enzyme
   (ACE) inhibitors]
Drugs that modulate the production of leukotrienes [e.g., nonsteroidal anti-inflammatory
   drugs (NSAIDs)]

Infection

Parasitic gastrointestinal infections
Viral, especially mononucleosis, coxsackievirus, hepatitis B
Fungal (e.g., dermatophytes and candida)
Protozoa (e.g., giardia and trichomonas)
Occult bacterial infections (e.g., sinuses and dental)

Malignancy

Hodgkin's disease
Colon cancer
Lung cancer
Liver cancer
Ovarian cancer

Autoimmune diseases

Vasculitis, primary or associated with other autoimmune diseases
Associated with chronic thyroiditis

tend to scar, hyperpigmentation, lack of response to H1 blockers, and systemic signs such as arthralgias, pain, purpura, nephritis, and fever.

(5) Searching for **occult infection** is rarely rewarding.

B. Physical examination (see Table 9–1)

1. Signs

    a. Hives appear as red, raised wheals, occasionally with central clearing. They can vary in size.

    b. Cholinergic urticaria can present with small hives, 1 to 2 mm in size.

    c. Pigmented skin lesions that urticate on trauma may suggest systemic mastocytosis.

2. Other physical findings

    a. Perform age- and gender-appropriate examination screening for malignancy, including lymph node assessment.

    b. Assess for other dermatologic and rheumatologic findings suggestive of autoimmune disease.

    c. Palpate the thyroid gland.

    d. Assess for stigmata of chronic liver disease.

C. Diagnostic evaluation. Perform laboratory tests in specialized circumstances:

1. Complete blood count (CBC), chest radiographs, liver chemistries, and hepatitis evaluation may be indicated by the history and physical examination.

2. Urinalysis and serum creatinine may be useful if systemic vasculitis is suspected.

3. Tests for thyroid-stimulating hormone (TSH) and thyroid antibodies should be done in all cryptogenic cases, both because of the association with chronic urticaria and because the presence of autoimmune thyroiditis may alter therapy.

4. Intradermal testing can be beneficial.

5. Oral placebo-controlled challenges are useful in limited circumstances.

6. Complement studies: In patients with isolated angioedema alone, measuring C_4 is indicated. The level will be suppressed even between attacks. Further testing for C1q esterase inhibitor should be done if the C_4 level is low.

7. Bone marrow biopsy should be performed if systemic mastocytosis is suspected.

SUGGESTED READING

Beltrani V: Urticaria and angioedema. *Dermatol Clin* 14:171–198, 1996.
Greaves M: Chronic urticaria. *N Engl J Med* 322:1767–1772, 1995.

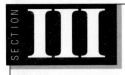

Endocrinology

10

Hypercalcemia
Marjorie Safran

I. **Definition.** Hypercalcemia is an **abnormally high concentration of calcium compounds in the circulating blood.** It can be caused by a number of underlying disorders:

   A. **Primary hyperparathyroidism** accounts for 90% of hypercalcemia in ambulatory patients without evidence of cancer.

   B. In the **hospitalized population,** the majority of patients (65%) with hypercalcemia have an underlying **cancer** as the cause.

II. **Etiologies.** Hypercalcemia can be divided into two categories:

   A. **Disorders with increased calcium absorption**

   1. Increased calcium intake can occur in patients with:

      a. **Chronic renal failure,** who are treated with calcium carbonate or calcium acetate to bind dietary phosphate

      b. **The milk-alkali syndrome,** where excess intake of calcium- and alkali-containing antacids (e.g., calcium carbonate or sodium bicarbonate) leads to hypercalcemia, metabolic alkalosis, and renal failure

   2. **Excessive ingestion of vitamin D or metabolites** can cause hypercalcemia.

   3. **Increased production of 1,25 OH vitamin D** can occur in granulomatous disease, lymphoma, or rarely, in the absence of an underlying disease.

   B. **Disorders with increased bone resorption**

   1. **Primary and tertiary hyperparathyroidism** (see Chapter 16)

   2. **Malignancy** as a result of metastatic resorption or production of parathyroid hormone-related protein (PTHrP)—rarely as a result of ectopic production of PTH

   3. **Hyperthyroidism**

   4. **Immobilization**

   5. **Paget's disease of bone** (which is primarily associated with bed rest)

6. **Tamoxifen,** which is used in patients with breast cancer and skeletal metastases
7. **Hypervitaminosis A**

C. Other causes

1. **Lithium** (which increases the set point for calcium suppression of PTH)
2. **Thiazide diuretics** (which decrease calcium excretion)
3. **Pheochromocytoma** [as part of multiple endocrine neoplasia, type II (MEN-II), or rarely, in isolated cases]
4. **Adrenal insufficiency**
5. **Rhabdomyolysis** and **acute renal failure**
6. **Familial hypocalciuric hypercalcemia** (see Chapter 16, HYPER-PARATHYROIDISM)

TABLE 10–1. Laboratory Results in Common Causes of Hypercalcemia

Disorder	Serum phos	Intact PTH	Urine calcium excretion	Miscellaneous
Primary hyper-parathyroidism	↓	↑	NL or ↑	Metabolic acidosis
Familial hypocalciuric hypercalcemia	Variable	NL or SL ↑	↓	
Humoral hypercalcemia of malignancy	↓	↓	NL or ↑	↑ PTHrP
Granulomatous disease	NL or ↑	↓	↑↑	↑ 1,25-OH vitamin D, ↑ angiotensin-converting enzyme
Vitamin D toxicity	NL or ↑	↓	↑↑	↑ 1,25-OH vitamin D
Milk-alkali syndrome	NL or ↑	↓	↓	Metabolic alkalosis
Metastatic bone disease	NL or ↑	↓	↑	
Thiazide diuretics	NL	↓	↓	
Lithium	NL	↑	↓	

NL = normal level; PTHrP = parathyroid hormone-related protein; SL = _____.

Normal values: Urine calcium: 100–250 mg/24 hr (females) and 100–300 mg/24 hr (males); serum phosphate: 2.5–4.5 mg/dl; PTH (intact): 12–72 pg/ml; 1,25-OH vitamin D: 14–78 pg/ml; angiotensin-converting enzyme: 14–70 units; PTHrP: < 2.8 pmol/L.

III. When to Suspect Hypercalcemia

    A. Signs and symptoms. Patients can present with confusion, lethargy, and weakness, even coma and death. Gastrointestinal complaints include nausea and constipation. Polyuria and polydipsia are secondary to a loss of renal-concentrating ability, with or without nephrocalcinosis.

    B. Laboratory findings include a shortened QT interval and renal failure. In most patients, the cause of hypercalcemia is suggested clinically (see II) and can be confirmed by a minimal number of laboratory tests.

IV. How to Confirm the Diagnosis

    A. Laboratory tests (Table 10–1 and Figure 10–1)

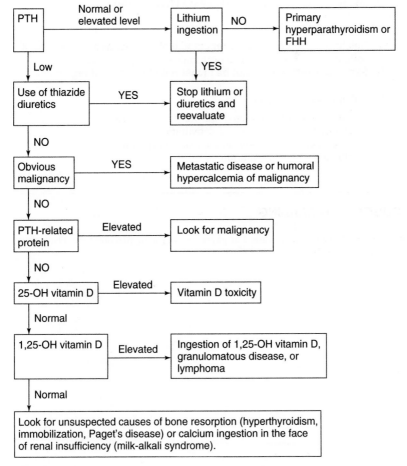

■ **FIGURE 10–1.** Algorithm for the workup of hypercalcemia. *FHH* = familial hypocalciuric hypercalcemic; *PTH* = parathyroid hormone.

1. **Calcium** circulates 40% to 45% protein bound (predominantly to albumin), and only the free calcium (ionized calcium) concentration is physiologically important. Total serum calcium falls 0.8 mg/ml (0.2 mmol/L) for every 1-g/L fall in albumin. If ordering tests for ionized calcium, also obtain a blood pH; ionized calcium is increased in acidosis and decreased in alkalosis.
2. **Parathyroid hormone (PTH)** measurements have become much more sensitive and specific with currently available assays for intact PTH. PTH will be elevated in 80% to 90% of patients with primary hyperparathyroidism.
3. **PTHrP** is the most common tumor product implicated in the hypercalcemia of malignancy. PTHrP is undetectable in 97% of normal subjects and in patients with renal failure. PTH does not cross-react in the PTHrP assay.

B. Imaging (see Chapter 16, HYPERPARATHYROIDISM)

V. Common Pitfalls

A. Calcium results need to be repeated if abnormal. As many as 53% of patients are found to be normocalcemic upon repeat testing.
B. Serum calcium should not be measured after a recent high-calcium meal.
C. Calcium values may be:

1. **Increased** with prolonged tourniquet use, thiazides, hyponatremia, elevated serum protein, and dehydration
2. **Decreased** with hypomagnesemia, hyperphosphatemia, low serum albumin, and hemodilution

---

SUGGESTED READING

Strewler GJ: Mechanisms of disease: The physiology of parathyroid hormone-related protein. *N Engl J Med* 342:177–185, 2000.

11

Gynecomastia
Howard Sachs

I. **Definition.** Gynecomastia is the **excess development of male mammary tissue, usually greater than 0.5 cm in diameter.** It may be present unilaterally or bilaterally. A breast mass, per se, would not be classified as gynecomastia.

   A. **Gynecomastia develops in response to a variety of causes.** They generally share in common an imbalance between the stimulatory effects of estrogens (estradiol, estrone) and the inhibitory effects of androgens (testosterone, androstenedione). Thus, any condition that alters this balance will favor the proliferation of breast tissue.

   B. **Persistent postpubertal gynecomastia, drugs, and idiopathic categories** account for more than half of all cases. Workup is directed at identifying the more sinister, albeit less common, etiologies.

II. **Clinical Approach to Gynecomastia** (Figure 11–1). As gynecomastia may be a normal finding in adults, the workup for **pathologic entities** can be reasonably limited to situations where there is rapid growth, a progressive increase in breast size, or enlargement beyond the physiologic range (> 2 cm). A physiologic approach broadly considers states of estrogen excess, androgen deficiency, or an imbalance between the two. Not all etiologies can be categorized in this manner.

   A. **Differential diagnosis** (see Figure 11–1)

      1. **Physiologic gynecomastia**

         a. Neonatal
         b. Adolescent or persistent postpubertal
         c. Advanced age

      2. **Estrogen excess**

         a. **Increased production:** Testicular neoplasm (nongerm cell tumors), exogenous administration of estrogen or precursors
         b. **Increased aromatase activity or availability of substrate for conversion to estrogens:** Obesity, liver disease, alcohol (especially beer), adrenal sources (congenital adrenal hyperplasia, adrenocortical carcinoma, adenoma)

      3. **Androgen deficiency**

         a. **Primary gonadal failure**
         b. **Secondary hypogonadism** [testicular defects (trauma, torsion, or infection); pituitary failure (infarction or adenoma)]
         c. **Klinefelter's syndrome**
         d. **Androgen resistance or testosterone synthesis defects** (frequently present at birth and associated with ambiguous genitalia or feminization)

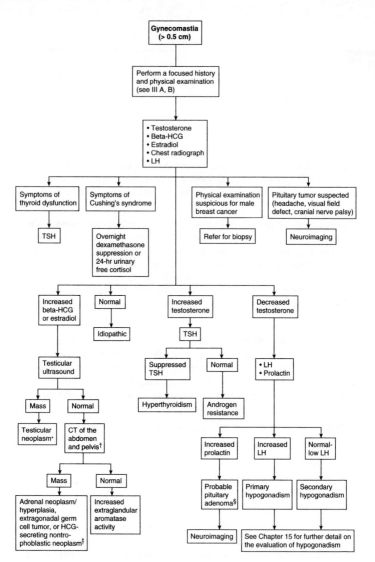

■ FIGURE 11–1. Algorithm for the workup of gynecomastia. *CT* = computed tomography; *HCG* = human chorionic gonadotropin; *LH* = luteinizing hormone; *TSH* = thyroid-stimulating hormone.

*The neoplasm is likely a germ cell tumor if the HCG is elevated, or a nongerm cell tumor if the estradiol is elevated.

†Abdomen and pelvic images are obtained to identify either an extraglandular germ cell tumor or an HCG-secreting nontrophoblastic neoplasm. An adrenal mass or hyperplasia is sought if the estradiol is elevated.

‡Common nontrophoblastic neoplasms include lung and gastrointestinal sources.

§An elevated prolactin level may be seen secondary to hypothyroidism, resulting from an elevated TSH. A number of medications can elevate the prolactin level. Before proceeding with neuroimaging, be certain to exclude these possibilities. A prolactin level > 200 ng/dl is usually indicative of an adenoma.

4. **Estrogen–androgen imbalance:** These disorders share in common a relative excess of estrogen compared to androgen concentrations.

   a. **Hyperprolactinemia**
      (1) Adenoma
      (2) Drugs (e.g., metoclopramide, phenothiazines, tricyclic antidepressants)
      (3) Hypothyroidism
   b. **Renal insufficiency**
   c. **Hypergonadotropic syndromes**
   d. **Beta-human chorionic gonadotropin (HCG) elevation:** Administration or ectopic production [most commonly seen in tumors of the lung, testes (germ cell tumors), and gastrointestinal tract]

5. **Drugs:** The more commonly cited agents include:

   a. **Androgen antagonists and inhibitors** (e.g., spironolactone, cimetidine, marijuana, flutamide, leuprolide, ketoconazole, finasteride, diazepam, tricyclic antidepressants, phenothiazines, alcohol, chemotherapeutic agents)
   b. **Estrogenic effects** (e.g., digitalis, diethylstilbestrol, marijuana, heroin, isoniazid, alcohol)
   c. **Increased availability of substrate or activity of aromatase** (e.g., exogenous administration of gonadotropins, testosterone, or phenytoin)
   d. **Unknown mechanism** {e.g., methyldopa, antihypertensives [angiotensin-converting enzyme (ACE) inhibitors, calcium channel blockers], narcotics, metronidazole, amiodarone, omeprazole}

6. **Miscellaneous**

   a. **Refeeding** is associated with regaining weight following starvation or a chronic illness
   b. **Hyperthyroidism**
   c. **Cushing's syndrome** (diminished testosterone through central and peripheral mechanisms)
   d. **Chronic disease:** Besides renal and hepatic diseases, a number of chronic illnesses (e.g., diabetes) will result in gynecomastia.

B. **Notes on the differential diagnosis**

1. The mechanism of gynecomastia in **liver disease** is twofold.

   a. The damaged hepatocyte has an impaired ability to clear androstenedione, which is then available for peripheral aromatase activity and subsequent conversion to estrogens.
   b. The second mechanism is through induction of sex hormone-binding globulin (SHBG). As SHBG binds testosterone with greater affinity than estrogen, any condition that increases SHBG will alter the estrogen–androgen ratio in favor of estrogen.

2. **Hyperprolactinemia** is rarely a cause for gynecomastia. The principle mechanism appears to be through its indirect effects on gonadotropin-releasing hormone (GRH), luteinizing hormone (LH), and testosterone. Each are diminished, resulting in a shift in the estrogen–testosterone balance favoring estrogen.

3. **Hypothyroidism,** when associated with an elevated level of thyrotropin-releasing hormone, will result in elevated prolactin levels.
4. The mechanism in **renal failure** is multifactorial.

   a. The etiologies include low testosterone levels related to primary testicular dysfunction, and hyperprolactinemia related to decreased clearance.
   b. Renal failure is also associated with an increased LH level, which stimulates the production of estradiol by the Leydig cells.
   c. Increased prolactin levels, linked to secondary hyperparathyroidism, may also contribute.

5. **The hypergonadotropic disorders are defined by a relative deficiency of androgen secretion.** The compensatory increase in LH and follicle-stimulating hormone (FSH) induces a relative rise in estradiol concentration.
6. **Chronic disease:** Although this group of disorders contributes significantly to the prevalence of gynecomastia, they do not obviate the evaluation for other "red flag" etiologies. The most common causes seen in clinical practice include idiopathic (~25%), persistent post-pubertal (25%), drugs (10%–20%), cirrhosis and malnutrition (8%), hypogonadism (10%), testicular tumors (3%), hyperthyroidism (1.5%), and renal disease (1%).

C. **Notes on the red flag etiologies.** Assessing **red flag etiologies** is a primary concern confronting the clinician.

1. **Male breast cancer:** This is an uncommon disease with about 1000 new cases per year. The incidence increases with age. A painless, firm subareolar mass is the most common presenting symptom, occurring in more than 75% of cases. In a patient older than 40 years of age, presenting with a **unilateral** breast mass, breast carcinoma should be considered. In these patients, if the examination is suspicious, then a biopsy needs to be pursued, regardless of other potential explanations (see III B).
2. **Prolactinoma:** The major clinical features in men with hyperprolactinemia are erectile dysfunction and loss of libido. They may present with visual field defect, headache, or cranial nerve palsies (symptoms of tumor enlargement). Because of the indolent nature of hyperprolactinemia in men, macroadenomas tend to be quite large by the time medical attention is sought. Both galactorrhea and gynecomastia may be seen but are uncommon. Prolactin levels > 200 ng/ml are almost always indicative of a pituitary tumor.
3. **Testicular neoplasms:** Testicular neoplasms account for as many as 3% of all gynecomastia. The mechanism is related to elevation of the estrogen level either by direct production from the tumor cells or through stimulation of interstitial cells by beta-HCG. Approximately 20% of Leydig cell tumors and 33% of Sertoli cell tumors are associated with gynecomastia. These nongerm cell tumors cause gynecomastia through increased production of estrogen by the tumor cells. Germ cell tumors, on the other hand, under the influence of beta-HCG, cause a disproportionate increase in the production of estrogen over testosterone.

III. Evaluation. Once the decision is made to evaluate a patient, a focused workup should be initiated.

A. Historical features

1. **Pain:** Gynecomastia tends to present with discomfort, as opposed to breast cancer, which is more typically painless.
2. **Symmetry:** Gynecomastia is often bilateral, albeit asymmetrically, whereas breast cancer is almost always unilateral.
3. **Other historical features** that suggest breast cancer include a positive family history, rapid onset, older age, and breast discharge.
4. A careful **drug history** must be obtained.
5. **Other findings**
   a. Assess for loss of libido and erectile dysfunction (which suggests hypogonadism, primary or secondary).
   b. Check for a history of liver disease, or for risk factors associated with liver disease, chronic renal insufficiency, a pituitary mass, thyroid dysfunction, or Cushing's syndrome.
   c. Check for symptoms of an underlying malignancy, specifically focusing on testicular, lung, and gastrointestinal sources.
   d. Assess weight changes and refeeding.

B. Physical examination features

1. **Breast examination characteristics**
   a. **Breast cancer** usually manifests as a hard nodule that is fixed to the underlying soft tissue. Other characteristics include a unilateral presence, nipple discharge, eccentric positioning, skin ulceration, and axillary adenopathy.
   b. **Gynecomastia,** on the other hand, is usually characterized by firm-rubbery, well-defined masses, discoid in shape and mobile, concentric with origination beneath the nipple or areolar region, frequently bilateral, and tender to palpation. Unilateral gynecomastia may be seen as a stage in the development of bilateral gynecomastia. Asymmetry is a frequent finding in patients with gynecomastia.
2. **Testicular examination:** Assess for signs of hypogonadism or neoplasm.
3. **Neurologic examination:** Assess the visual fields and cranial nerves.
4. Palpate the **thyroid gland** for size and nodularity.
5. Assess for stigmata of **Cushing's syndrome** (strength, striae, fat pad distribution, hirsutism).

C. Laboratory assessment (see Figure 11–1)

1. The **initial evaluation** should include
   a. Beta-HCG (to rule out ectopic production)
   b. Chest radiograph (to rule out pulmonary malignancy)
   c. Testosterone, LH, and estradiol measurements
2. **Supplemental hormonal evaluation,** as determined by clinical judgment:
   a. **Prolactin levels** should be obtained in any patient with suspicion of a mass lesion or erectile dysfunction, or when secondary hypogonadism is identified (i.e., low testosterone or low-to-normal LH).

      b. **Dehydroepiandrosterone sulfate (DHEAS)** assesses for adrenocortical tumor in the setting of elevated estradiol.

      c. **Thyroid-stimulating hormone (TSH)** and **overnight dexamethasone suppression test** (or 24-hour urinary free cortisol)

D. Neuroimaging should be reserved for those cases where a mass lesion is suspected (e.g., headache, visual field defect, cranial nerve palsy) or the hormonal evaluation leads one to suspect a pituitary tumor (i.e., elevated prolactin level or Cushing's disease).

SUGGESTED READING

Braunstein G: Gynecomastia. *N Engl J Med* 328:490–495, 1993.

12

Galactorrhea
Suzanne Blood

I. **Definition.** Galactorrhea is any persistent discharge of milk or milklike secretions from the breasts in the absence of a gestational event or beyond 6 months postpartum in a woman who is not nursing.

II. **Overview**

A. **Estrogen and progesterone**

1. **Estrogen** promotes breast ductal development during pregnancy, but it also inhibits lactation.

2. **Progesterone** promotes lobular-alveolar development and, like estrogen, inhibits lactation.

3. With delivery of the placenta, levels of estrogen and progesterone decline precipitously, thereby triggering lactation.

B. **Prolactin** is necessary in all phases of breast development and milk production.

1. Prolactin promotes lobular-alveolar development and controls milk protein synthesis and milk secretion.

2. Prolactin is secreted in high levels throughout pregnancy and in the first few weeks postpartum. Between the third and seventh week postpartum, once the breast enzyme systems are activated normal, levels of prolactin are necessary to maintain lactation.

III. **Clinical Approach to Galactorrhea**

A. **Distinguishing galactorrhea from other forms of nipple discharge**

1. Green, yellow, bloody, or multicolored fluid should lead the investigator to look for other causes of nipple discharge.

2. When gross inspection does not permit the identification of the nipple discharge, **microscopic examination** can be helpful. Milk is rich in lipid content, and thus a fat stain is highly sensitive in confirming the diagnosis of galactorrhea.

B. **Differential diagnosis.** Conditions causing galactorrhea are myriad, ranging from benign physiologic entities to significant endocrine disorders and tumors. True galactorrhea is rarely associated with breast cancer (Table 12–1).

C. **Notes on the differential diagnosis of galactorrhea**

1. **Physiologic causes**

a. **Galactorrhea from perpetuation or reactivation of lactation:** This accounts for the vast majority of galactorrhea cases. In general, prolactin levels, menses, and fertility are normal. Reactivation of pregnancy-related lactation may occur after a spontaneous first-trimester pregnancy loss, therapeutic abortion, or ectopic pregnancy.

TABLE 12–1. Galactorrhea

PHYSIOLOGIC CAUSES

- Excessive breast stimulation or tight garments
- Perpetuation or reactivation of postpartum lactation
- Stress, surgery, venipuncture
- Coitus
- Pseudocyesis

PATHOLOGIC CAUSES

Pituitary disorders

- Prolactinomas
- Pituitary angiosarcoma
- Acromegaly
- Cushing's disease
- Empty sella syndrome
- Stalk transsection or compression (postsurgical, head trauma, tumor)

Central nervous system (CNS) and hypothalamic disorders

- Craniopharyngioma
- Rathke's pouch cyst
- Ectopic pinealomas
- Encephalitis
- Pseudotumor cerebri
- Infiltrative hypothalamic processes (e.g., glioma, histiocytosis, sarcoidosis, tuberculosis)
- Irradiation

Metabolic and endocrinologic disorders

- Adrenal hyperplasia or carcinoma
- Hypothyroidism or hyperthyroidism
- Liver disease
- Chronic renal failure
- Sheehan's syndrome
- Anovulatory disorders (e.g., polycystic ovarian disease, Chiari-Frommel syndrome)
- Idiopathic galactorrhea and amenorrhea

Chest wall lesions

Ectopic prolactin production

- Bronchogenic carcinoma
- Renal cell carcinoma

PHARMACOLOGIC CAUSES

- Antidepressants (e.g., tricyclics, monoamine oxidase inhibitors, selective serotonin reuptake inhibitors)

continued

TABLE 12–1. Galactorrhea (*Continued*)

- Neuroleptics (e.g., phenothiazines and butyrophenones)
- Opiates and narcotics
- H2-blockers (e.g., cimetidine)
- Oral contraceptive pills
- Calcium channel blockers (e.g., verapamil)
- Benzamines (e.g., metoclopramide)
- Alpha-receptor blockers (e.g., reserpine, methyldopa)
- Cocaine
- Amphetamines

FUNCTIONAL/IDIOPATHIC

b. **Disorders of the chest wall:** Although rare, chest wall injury from surgery such as mastectomy, trauma, infiltrating tumors, and herpes zoster eruptions can produce galactorrhea. Hyperprolactinemia may or may not be present. The mechanism for this milk formation is uncertain, but may be due to chronic neuronal stimulation from the breast to the hypothalamus. Other causes must be ruled out prior to attributing galactorrhea to this cause.

2. **Pathologic causes**

a. **Pituitary tumors** (see also Chapter 16): Foremost in the evaluation of a patient with galactorrhea is the consideration of a pituitary tumor. Serum prolactin levels greater than 100 mg/L should raise clinical suspicion. The higher the serum prolactin, the more likely a tumor will be found.

b. **Idiopathic galactorrhea with amenorrhea:** Generally, this small group of women has elevated prolactin levels and normal imaging. Possible mechanisms for this disorder include interference of luteinizing hormone–releasing hormone (LHRH), release in the hypothalamus by prolactin, alteration of pituitary sensitivity to LHRH, or interference with steroidogenic action of gonadotropins at the level of the ovary.

c. **Anovulatory syndromes**

(1) **Chiari-Frommel syndrome** is characterized by galactorrhea and amenorrhea that occur more than 6 months postpartum in the absence of nursing and in the absence of a pituitary tumor. About half of these women will resume normal menses over the next few months. A small minority may have occult micro-adenomas, which may become clinically apparent with time.

(2) **Polycystic ovary syndrome (PCOS)** is characterized by obesity, oligomenorrhea, infertility, and hirsutism. Elevated prolactin levels may accompany this syndrome, thus producing galactorrhea (see also Chapter 13).

d. Endocrinopathies

(1) Hypothyroidism is a rare cause of galactorrhea. Prolactin levels may be normal or slightly elevated. The galactorrhea is corrected with restoration of euthyroidism.

(2) Galactorrhea is a frequent finding in women with thyrotoxicosis. Serum prolactin is normal, and the mechanism of galactorrhea is unknown.

(3) Cushing's syndrome and acromegaly can be associated with galactorrhea. Workup for these conditions should be undertaken only if specific signs and symptoms are present.

e. Ectopic prolactin production is a very rare cause of galactorrhea, and other causes should be excluded first. Tumors that have been associated with ectopic production include renal cell and bronchogenic carcinomas.

3. Pharmacologic causes

a. Galactorrhea associated with elevated prolactin levels. Most pharmacologic agents that cause prolactin release either block dopamine receptors (e.g., neuroleptics) or deplete dopamine in the tuberoinfundibular neurons (e.g., centrally acting alpha-blockers). All types of antidepressants can cause galactorrhea, but selective serotonin reuptake inhibitors (SSRIs) do so more commonly than other antidepressants.

b. Galactorrhea associated with oral contraceptive pills (OCPs): Both usage and discontinuation of OCPs can cause galactorrhea. The exact mechanisms are unknown. The abrupt cessation of estrogen and progesterone mimics their withdrawal at the time of delivery and can trigger milk production. A minority of these patients may harbor occult microadenomas. Estrogen at postmenopausal replacement doses is not associated with galactorrhea.

IV. Evaluation (Figure 12–1). The differential diagnosis of galactorrhea is broad (see Table 12–1). First and foremost, the investigator must exclude pituitary adenoma or other space-occupying lesions as the cause of galactorrhea.

A. History

1. **Menstrual and reproductive history:** Hyperprolactinemia can lead to hypoestrogenemia, with amenorrhea and infertility. Higher levels of prolactin are associated with more significant menstrual derangements. Galactorrhea can be seen during pregnancy, including ectopic pregnancy and in the immediate postpartum period.

2. **Drug history** (see III C 3)

3. Assess for **symptoms of hypothalamic or pituitary disease.** These include cranial neuropathies (nerves 3, 4, or 6), visual field deficits (bitemporal hemianopsia, optic chiasm, or optic nerve compression), or headache (a nonspecific finding, but when coupled with galactorrhea and amenorrhea is suggestive of a pituitary tumor). Abnormalities of temperature, thirst, and appetite regulation suggest hypothalamic disease.

4. Assess for **symptoms of other endocrinopathies,** such as thyroid dysfunction (hyper- or hypo-), glucocorticoid excess, and acromegaly.

5. Assess for a history of **chest wall surgery, trauma, or zoster eruption**

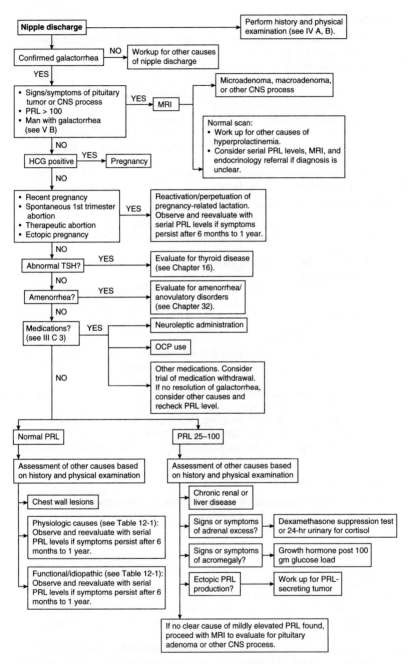

FIGURE 12–1. Algorithm for the workup of galactorrhea. *CNS* = central nervous system; *HCG* = human chorionic gonadotropin; *MRI* = magnetic resonance imaging; *OCP* = oral contraceptive pill; *PRL* = prolactin; *TSH* = thyroid-stimulating hormone.

B. Physical examination

1. **Eye examination:** Check visual acuity and visual fields, and examine the cranial nerves.
2. **Breast and chest wall examination:** Confirm galactorrhea; palpate for masses, scars, and eruptions.
3. **Skin examination:** Note abnormal skin texture (e.g., myxedema), striae, pigmentation, or hirsutism (which are suggestive of anovulatory disorder, Cushing's syndrome, or thyroid dysfunction).
4. **Endocrine examination:** Assess for thyroid dysfunction, stigmata of Cushing's disease (striae, buffalo hump, central obesity), and acromegaly.
5. **Pelvic examination:** Check ovarian and uterine size for causes of amenorrhea and anovulation.

C. Laboratory evaluation

1. **Serum prolactin level** (preferably in a fasting, nonstressed state)
2. **Beta-human chorionic gonadotropin (beta-HCG) level** to exclude pregnancy
3. **Serum thyroid-stimulating hormone** (TSH) to exclude hyper- and hypothyroidism
4. Consider a workup for **less common endocrinopathies** (e.g., Cushing's syndrome and acromegaly) after excluding more common causes, and only if history and physical findings raise clinical suspicion.

D. Diagnostic imaging

1. **High-resolution computed tomography (CT) scanning** is more sensitive and specific for localization of pituitary tumors than plain films. Limitations of CT scanning include use of contrast dye and imaging that can only be performed in the coronal plane. CT is good for detecting bony erosions in the floor of the sella.
2. **Magnetic resonance imaging (MRI)** is slightly more sensitive than high-resolution CT in identifying microadenomas (85%–90% sensitivity for MRI with contrast versus 70%–85% for high-resolution CT).

V. Pitfalls and Caveats

A. Women with significant hyperprolactinemia are unlikely to get pregnant. However, if symptoms or signs of pituitary tumor are present in a pregnant woman, neuroimaging should be performed to search for a tumor.
B. Galactorrhea in men suggests a pathological process and should always have an aggressive workup assessing for a pituitary adenoma and hypogonadism.
C. Mildly elevated prolactin levels (25–100 ng/ml) should prompt investigation for a tumor, even if no other clear cause for the hyperprolactinemia is identified or if symptoms and signs of pituitary and central nervous system (CNS) processes are present.
D. Medication-induced hyperprolactinemia should be a diagnosis of exclusion. Workup is based upon symptomatology and prolactin level. In patients on medications (e.g., neuroleptics) with prolactin levels less than

100 ng/ml and no signs or symptoms of CNS processes, imaging for a pituitary tumor does not need to be done. Levels greater than 100 ng/ml, however, should prompt neuroimaging.

E. The clinician must **balance the necessity of a medication with the benefit of cessation.** Galactorrhea secondary to medication use is not generally of serious consequence. The primary concern lies in eliminating the more sinister diagnoses.

SUGGESTED READING

Yazigi R, Quintero C, Salameh W: Prolactin disorders. *Fertility Sterility* 67:215–225, 1997.

13

Hirsutism
Marjorie Safran

I. **Definition.** Hirsutism is the **presence of excess terminal hair in androgen-dependent areas in women** (see II B). This condition needs to be differentiated from hypertrichosis, which is excess terminal hair throughout the body, and increased vellus hair, which is the soft, unpigmented hair that covers the whole body.

II. **How to Confirm the Diagnosis of Hirsutism** (Figure 13–1). The clinical approach to a patient with hirsutism includes assessing the degree of androgen excess and its cause (Table 13–1).

   A. **History**

      1. The presence of hirsutism alone is usually a **benign condition.**

      2. Hirsutism occurring at a later age, with rapid onset, associated with the abrupt cessation of menses, or the presence of other features of virilization (see B 2), is more often associated with **potentially serious disorders, such as adrenal or ovarian tumors.**

      3. Assess **menstrual history** and the **presence of galactorrhea.**

      4. Note **use of drugs** associated with hirsutism and hypertrichosis.

      5. Inquire about **family history** of hirsutism and polycystic ovary syndrome (PCOS).

   B. **Physical examination**

      1. **Look for and quantify increased hair in androgen-dependent regions,** such as the face, chest, areola, linea alba, lower back, buttock, inner thigh, and external genitalia.

      2. **Look for evidence of virilization,** such as clitoral enlargement, deepening of voice, frontal balding, increased musculature, and loss of female body contour.

      3. **Look for evidence of Cushing's syndrome.**

      4. **Other physical findings** may include acne, acanthosis nigricans, breast discharge, and an abdominal or pelvic mass.

   C. **Laboratory testing** (see Figure 13–1). **Total serum testosterone** is adequate to exclude testosterone-secreting tumors, but **free testosterone** may be necessary to identify smaller increases in testosterone, especially since sex hormone binding globulin (SHBG) is decreased by hyperandrogenism and hyperinsulinemia (in patients with PCOS).

III. **Special Notes**

   A. **Free testosterone** may be elevated even with a normal total testosterone because of decreased serum binding.

   B. **Dehydroepiandrosterone sulfate (DHEAS)** is not a good marker for adrenal overproduction because it is secreted in a pulsatile manner.

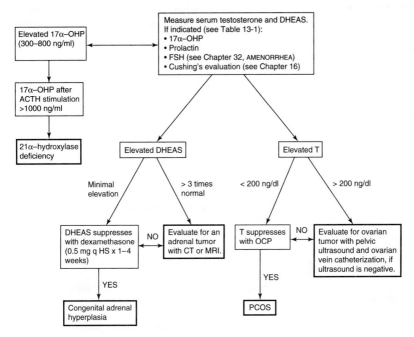

■ **FIGURE 13–1.** Diagnostic algorithm for hirsutism. *17α-OHP* = 17α-hydroxy-progesterone; *ACTH* = adrenocorticotropic hormone; *CT* = computed tomography; *DHEAS* = dehydroepiandrosterone sulfate; *FSH* = follicle-stimulating hormone; *MRI* = magnetic resonance imaging; *OCP* = oral contraceptive pill; *PCOS* = polycystic ovary syndrome; *T* = testosterone.

TABLE 13–1. Differential Diagnosis of Conditions Accompanied by Hirsutism and Their Specific Features

Differential diagnosis	Specific features
Idiopathic hirsutism	Hirsutism accompanied by no other clinical or biochemical abnormalities
Polycystic ovary syndrome (PCOS)	Onset of hirsutism around the time of puberty, gradual increase in hair growth, menstrual irregularity, obesity, glucose intolerance
Hyperprolactinemia	Galactorrhea, amenorrhea, or both may be present
Drugs	Danazol, androgenic progestins, phenothiazines, phenytoin, diazoxide, minoxidil; cyclosporin can cause hypertrichosis

(continued)

TABLE 13–1. Differential Diagnosis of Conditions Accompanied by Hirsutism and Their Specific Features (*Continued*)

Differential diagnosis	Specific features
Late-onset congenital adrenal hyperplasia	Usually presents at birth or in infancy, but the nonclassical form of 21α-hydroxylase deficiency can present prepubertally; 17α-hydroxyprogesterone > 1000 ng/dl after administration of adrenocorticotropic hormone; less common form is 11β-hydroxylase deficiency
Hyperthecosis	Increased ovarian testosterone production by luteinized stromal theca cells
Ovarian tumors	Usually occur later in life, serum testosterone usually greater than 150–200 ng/ml
Adrenal tumors	More often carcinomas, can be with or without evidence for Cushing's syndrome, DHEAS usually 800 μg/dl
Insulin resistant syndromes	Frequently associated with acanthosis nigricans
Menopause	Secondary to altered estrogen-androgen ratios

DHEAS = dehydroepiandrosterone sulfate.

C. **17α-hydroxyprogesterone (17a-OHP)** varies with menstrual cycle and increases with ovulation.

SUGGESTED READING

Waggoner W, Boots LR, Azziz R: Total testosterone and DHEAS levels as predictors of androgen-secreting neoplasms: a population study. *Gynecol Enocrinol* 13:394–400, 1999.

14

Osteoporosis
Marjorie Safran

I. **Definition.** The World Health Organization defines osteoporosis as **bone mineral density (BMD) more than 2.5 standard deviations below the mean of young normal controls (T-score).**

A. A patient has osteoporosis if the BMD is diagnostic, or if spontaneous, nontraumatic fractures are present (e.g., of the wrist, spine, or hip).

B. Patients with osteoporosis have normal bone composition, but too little bone. This is in contrast to patients with osteomalacia, in whom there is failure of normal mineralization of bone matrix. Osteopenia is a decrease in bone mass.

C. Osteoporosis is generally a disease found in **women. Men may also be affected,** particularly those with hypogonadism, or those taking medications that increase the risk of osteoporosis (see II G).

D. **Osteoporotic fractures** (especially of the hip) are a significant cause of morbidity and mortality, particularly in the elderly.

II. **Risk factors** (for bone loss and osteoporotic fractures)

A. Caucasian and Asian races

B. Women older than 55 years of age and men older than 65 years of age

C. Postmenopausal state (i.e., women not on estrogens) or hypogonadism

D. Patients with a history of falls

E. Glucocorticoid use (> 3 months of 7.5 mg prednisone, or equivalent, daily)

F. Acquired osteopenia secondary to disorders such as anorexia nervosa, exercise-associated amenorrhea, delayed puberty, cystic fibrosis

G. Drug use

1. **Anticonvulsants** (cause decreased bone mass secondary to vitamin D deficiency)
2. Prolonged administration of **heparin**
3. Excessive doses of **thyroxine**
4. High doses of **methotrexate**

H. Sedentary lifestyle

I. Cigarette smoking and alcohol abuse

III. **Diagnostic Evaluation** (Figure 14–1)

A. **Laboratory evaluation** (Table 14–1)

B. **Bone densitometry.** Multiple techniques have been developed for the measurement of bone mass, and usage depends mainly on local availability.

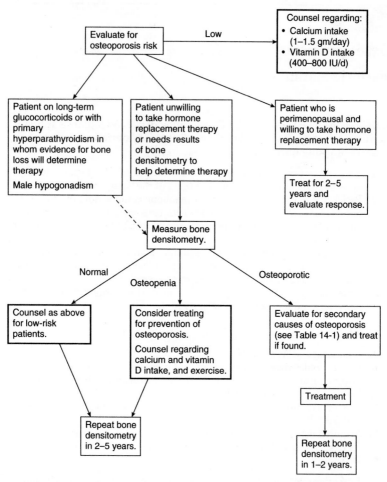

FIGURE 14–1. Algorithm for the evaluation of a patient with suspected osteoporosis.

TABLE 14–1. Laboratory Evaluation of Patients with Osteoporosis

Evaluation	Indication	Considerations
Complete blood count	Routine	When abnormal, rule out an underlying malignancy

continued

TABLE 14–1. Laboratory Evaluation of Patients with Osteoporosis (*Continued*)

Evaluation	Indication	Considerations
Bicarbonate	Routine	When low, consider metabolic acidosis
Calcium	Routine	When high, consider primary hyperparathyroidism, metastatic cancer, or multiple myeloma When low, consider osteomalacia or renal failure
Alkaline phosphatase	Routine	When high, consider osteomalacia or another bone disease*
Creatinine	Routine	When high, consider renal failure
TSH	Routine	When low, consider hyperthyroidism
Testosterone	Routine in men	When low, consider hypogonadism
Serum protein electrophoresis	Low Z-score,† hypercalcemia, or anemia	When abnormal, consider multiple myeloma
Serum 25-hydroxy vitamin D	Elderly with poor intake, history of GI disease, liver disease, or anticonvulsants	When low, consider vitamin D deficiency
Spine radiograph	Significant kyphosis	When the solitary fracture is above T-7, look for an alternative diagnosis
Intact parathyroid hormone	Hypercalcemia, history of renal stones, predominantly cortical osteopenia	When high, consider hyperparathyroidism
Urinary free cortisol or overnight dexamethasone suppression test	Cushing's syndrome suspected	When high, consider Cushing's syndrome

GI = gastrointestinal; TSH = thyroid-stimulating hormone.

*Alkaline phosphatase can be transiently elevated with fracture.

†Bone mineral density is greater than 2.5 standard deviations below the mean of age-matched controls.

IV. Special Notes

A. Since BMD varies between sites, **evaluation at more than one site is recommended.**

B. **Decreased BMD** is only one risk factor for fractures.

SUGGESTED READING

Cummings SR, Nevitt MC, Brownner WS: Risk factors for hip fracture in white women. *N Engl J Med* 332:767–773, 1995.

15

Male Hypogonadism
Marjorie Safran

I. **Definition.** Male hypogonadism reflects **abnormal testicular function of the seminiferous tubules and/or the Leydig cells, resulting in decreased sperm production and/or testosterone production, respectively.** Seminiferous tubule dysfunction is manifested by infertility and decreased testicular size.

II. **Overview.** The consequences of testosterone deficiency vary according to the age of onset (Table 15–1)).

III. **Causes.** The causes of male hypogonadism can be separated into primary and secondary (Table 15–2). Prognosis depends upon the cause of hypogonadism.

   A. **Klinefelter's syndrome** is the most common cause of primary gonadal failure. It occurs in 1:1000 live births and is associated with an abnormal genotype, most commonly 47 XXY, although other karyotypes can be seen.

   B. **Kallmann's syndrome** is a hypogonadotropic hypogonadism that is associated with anosmia and secondary to Xp22.3 deletion. Its prevalence is one-tenth that of Klinefelter's syndrome.

   C. **Pituitary or hypothalamic mass lesions** can be benign or malignant tumors (e.g., pituitary adenoma, craniopharyngioma), infiltrative diseases (e.g., sarcoidosis, eosinophilic granuloma, hemochromatosis), or infectious tuberculosis.

   1. With large lesions, hypogonadism may be secondary to compression of normal tissue, and there may also be evidence of adrenal or thyroid deficiency.

   2. If the patient has a functional pituitary adenoma [i.e., producing adrenocorticotropic hormone, growth hormone, thyroid-stimulating hormone (TSH), or prolactin], specific signs of hypersecretion of these hormones may be present.

   3. A prolactin-secreting pituitary adenoma suppresses gonadotropin secretion directly.

   D. **Idiopathic hypogonadotropic hypogonadism (IHH)** can be congenital or acquired, and is essentially a diagnosis of exclusion when other known causes of hypogonadotropic hypogonadism are ruled out.

IV. **Diagnostic Evaluation** (Figure 15–1)

   A. **Physical examination.** The **lack of findings on examination** is not helpful since it takes years for secondary sex characteristics, such as loss of body hair and muscle mass, to regress in the absence of testosterone.

   B. **Laboratory testing** is usually necessary to confirm hypogonadism by demonstrating **decreased spermatogenesis and/or testosterone production.**

TABLE 15–1. Manifestations of Testosterone Deficiency

Age of onset	Manifestations
First trimester	Abnormal sexual differentiation varying from female external genitalia to partial virilization
Third trimester	Micropenis, cryptorchidism
Prepubertal	Absent or incomplete puberty, eunuchism
Postpubertal	Early: decreased energy and libido Late: decreased androgen-dependent hair, muscle mass, and bone mineral density (BMD)

TABLE 15–2. Causes of Hypogonadism

Primary hypogonadism*	Secondary hypogonadism†
Congenital	
Klinefelter's syndrome and variants	Kallmann's syndrome
Cryptorchidism‡	Hypopituitarism
Disorders of androgen synthesis	Idiopathic hypogonadotropic hypogonadism (IHH)
Myotonic dystrophy‡	IHH with mental retardation (e.g., Prader-Willi syndrome)
FSH receptor gene mutation	Abnormal luteinizing hormone β (LHβ) subunit
Acquired	
Chemotherapy, radiation therapy	Mass lesions in pituitary or hypothalamus
Infection (e.g., mumps, orchitis)	Hyperprolactinemia
Drugs (e.g., ketoconazole, glucocorticoids§)	Pituitary apoplexy
Trauma	Trauma to the base of the skull
Testicular torsion	Chronic disease (e.g., hepatitis, chronic renal failure, AIDS)
Autoimmune damage	High-dose glucocorticoids

continued

TABLE 15–2. Causes of Hypogonadism (*Continued*)

Primary hypogonadism*	Secondary hypogonadism†
Liver cirrhosis§, chronic renal failure§	Hemochromatosis
	Adult onset IHH

FSH = follicle-stimulating hormone.

  *Primary hypogonadism refers to intrinsic testicular dysfunction, which results in absent pituitary-hypothalamic feedback and thus elevated gonadotropins (i.e., hypergonadotropic hypogonadism).

  †Secondary hypogonadism refers to inadequate testicular function secondary to pituitary or hypothalamic dysfunction.

  ‡Patients may present with normal testosterone and subnormal sperm count only.

  §These conditions have multifactorial etiologies.

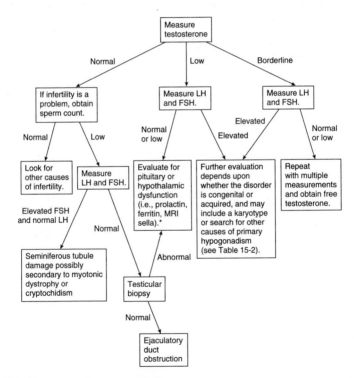

■ **FIGURE 15–1.** Algorithm for the workup of male hypogonadism. *FSH* = follicle-stimulating hormone; *LH* = luteinizing hormone; *MRI* = magnetic resonance imaging.
  *An exception would be in adolescents when delayed puberty is suggested by history, constitutional short stature, delayed dental maturation, or family history of delayed puberty. Alternatively, the presence of other hormonal defects, evidence of lesions affecting the optic chiasm, or midline defects suggests pituitary disease, and the presence of anosmia suggests Kallmann's syndrome.

V. Special Notes

  A. Free testosterone measurement is needed when sex hormone binding
  globulin (SHBG) is abnormal; it decreases in obesity, or increases with age,
  hyperthyroidism, liver cirrhosis, and estrogen therapy.
  B. A **subnormal or borderline testosterone level** needs to be repeated with
  concomitant testing for luteinizing hormone (LH) and follicle-stimulating
  hormone (FSH).
  C. Acute illness may result in temporary hypogonadotropic hypogonadism.

SUGGESTED READING

Nachtigall LB, Boepple PA, Pralong FP, Crowley WF Jr: Adult-onset idiopathic hypogo-
    nadotropic hypogonadism—A treatable form of male infertility. *N Engl J Med*
    336:410–415, 1997.
Smyth CM, Bremner WJ: Klinefelter syndrome. *Arch Intern Med* 158:1309–1314, 1998.

16

Diagnostic Approach to Other Endocrine Disorders

Marjorie Safran, Mira Sofia Torres,
and Christopher Sorli

Disorders of the Thyroid Gland

Marjorie Safran

Hyperthyroidism

I. **Definition.** Hyperthyroidism is the result of **excess circulating thyroid hormone concentrations, leading to clinical manifestations.**

II. **Overview.** The prevalence of overt hyperthyroidism is approximately 0.6%. The most common form is Graves' disease (70%–80%).

III. **Types**

A. **Diffuse toxic goiter (Graves' disease)** is the prototypic autoimmune hyperthyroid condition. Patients will frequently have a family history of hyper- and/or hypothyroidism and may report previous episodes of hyperthyroidism. It can be associated with autoimmune ophthalmopathy and occasionally with other autoimmune disorders such as diabetes mellitus (DM). The radioactive iodine uptake (RAIU) is typically elevated unless the patient has been exposed to excess iodine or acutely to large doses of glucocorticoids.

B. **Toxic multinodular goiter (MNG)** and **solitary toxic nodule (Plummer's disease)** are more common in areas of iodine deficiency. Patients present with nodular enlargement of the thyroid gland with many or an **individual nodule producing excess thyroid hormone.**

C. **Silent thyroiditis** must be considered in any patient who presents with a fairly rapid evolution of hyperthyroid symptoms or who is in the postpartum state. The RAIU is low. The hyperthyroid phase of this disorder is self-limited. Patients need to be followed for the subsequent development of hypothyroidism, which may be transient or permanent.

D. **Subacute thyroiditis** is an acute inflammatory disorder of the thyroid gland, most likely induced by a viral infection. The symptoms of fever, malaise, and neck soreness frequently overshadow the symptoms of hyperthyroidism. Major findings are of a tender thyroid gland, an elevated erythrocyte sedimentation rate (ESR), and a low RAIU.

E. **Excess thyroid hormone ingestion** can be either iatrogenic or factitious. The former is usually easily determined. The finding of a low serum thyroglobulin in a patient with biochemical evidence of hyperthyroidism and a low RAIU is very suspicious for factitious hyperthyroidism.

F. **Thyroid storm** represents exaggerated manifestations of hyperthyroidism, including fever, tachycardia, cardiac arrhythmias, and altered mental status. It can be life threatening, with a mortality of 10%–75%.

IV. **When to Suspect Hyperthyroidism.** The signs and symptoms of hyperthyroidism include:

A. Increased anxiety, nervousness, and irritability

B. Increased perspiration and heat intolerance

C. Weight loss despite a good appetite

D. Palpitations, tachycardia, tremor, goiter, proximal muscle weakness, and exophthalmos

E. In women, a light and less frequently occurring menses

V. **How to Confirm Clinical Suspicion of Hyperthyroidism** (Figure 16–1 and the Thyroid Function Tests section of this chapter).

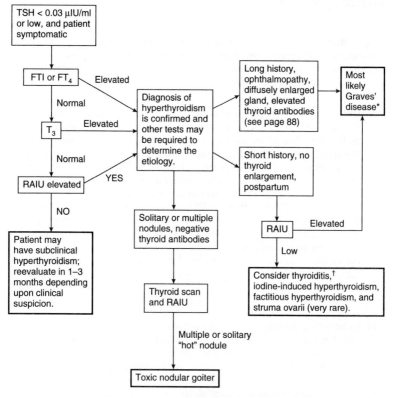

■ **FIGURE 16–1.** Algorithm for the diagnosis of hyperthyroidism.

*Graves' disease can be confirmed by measuring thyroid antibodies.

†Suspect postpartum thyroiditis if within 6 months of delivery, subacute thyroiditis if associated with tender gland and constitutional symptoms, and silent thyroiditis if neither.

T_4 = thyroxine; *FTI* = free thyroxine index; *RAIU* = radioactive iodine uptake; T_3 = triiodothyronine; *TSH* = thyroid-stimulating hormone.

Hypothyroidism

I. **Definition.** Hypothyroidism refers to a **condition in which the amount of thyroid hormones in the body is below normal.** This is the most common thyroid function abnormality.

II. **Overview**

  A. **Incidence**

   1. One **woman** in 10 older than 65 years of age has evidence of subclinical hypothyroidism. Incidence in **men** is 1 in 1000.
   2. **Hypothyroidism** is far more common than hyperthyroidism.

  B. **Prognosis.** Hypothyroidism is usually easily treated with thyroid hormone replacement. However, the uncommon complication of **myxedema coma** [i.e., severe prolonged hypothyroidism manifested by bradycardia, congestive heart failure (CHF), hypothermia, hypoventilation, and paralytic ileus] is a life-threatening condition if not detected and treated promptly.

III. **Types**

  A. **Hashimoto's thyroiditis** (chronic lymphocytic thyroiditis) is the most common cause of hypothyroidism. It usually presents with goiter, hypothyroidism, or both (Table 16–1). Patients will frequently report a family history of hypo- or hyperthyroidism.

  B. **Secondary hypothyroidism**

   1. Previous exposure to **radioactive iodine,** or **surgical treatment** for hyperthyroidism or goiter
   2. Previous episode of **silent, postpartum,** or **subacute thyroiditis**
   3. **Irradiation** for head or neck tumors
   4. **Mantle irradiation** for Hodgkin's disease
   5. **Drugs** (e.g., lithium, amiodarone, interferon)
   6. **Inherited defect** in thyroid hormone biosynthesis
   7. **Pituitary or hypothalamic dysfunction** [Serum thyroxine (T_4) levels are needed in any patient with known pituitary or hypothalamic disease or with evidence for other endocrine end-organ failure, such as gonadal or adrenal insufficiency.]

TABLE 16–1. Presenting Symptoms, Signs, and Risk Factors for Hypothyroidism

Symptoms	Signs	Risk factors
Fatigue, weight gain, depression, cold intolerance, dry skin, brittle hair, constipation, muscle cramps, hypermenorrhea	Thyroid enlargement (goiter), puffy face and hands, slow reflexes	Presence of autoantibodies in the patient and relatives; women older than 50 years of age; previous neck surgery or radioactive therapy; neck or mantle irradiation; lithium, amiodarone, or interferon therapy

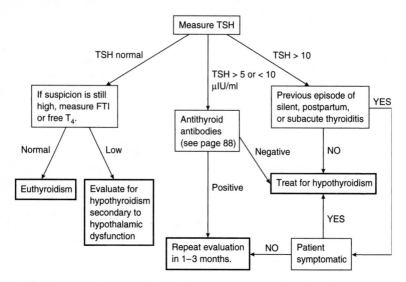

FIGURE 16–2. Algorithm for the diagnosis of hypothyroidism. FT_4 = free thyroxine; *FTI* = free thyroxine index; *TSH* = thyroid-stimulating hormone.

IV. **How to Confirm the Diagnosis** (see Table 16–1 and Figure 16–2)
 V. **Special Notes**

   A. **Hospitalized patients** may have transient elevation of thyroid-stimulating hormone (TSH) during recovery from an acute illness.
   B. Patients can have **significant symptoms** of hypothyroidism even when thyroid hormone levels are within the normal range.

Goiter and Thyroid Nodules

 I. **Definition.** Goiter and thyroid nodules present as **diffuse or nodular enlargement of the thyroid gland.**
II. **Overview.** Thyroid enlargement can be identified during a routine physical examination, discovered by the patient, or found incidentally during an imaging procedure.

   A. **Incidence**

      1. **Thyroid nodules are common,** being clinically detected in 5% of normal persons and identified by ultrasound in as many as 50%.
      2. **Fewer than 10% of thyroid nodules are malignant,** and the diagnostic goal is to efficiently identify those patients who require surgical intervention. A solitary nodule should be evaluated for malignancy no matter what the underlying thyroid disorder.

B. **Prognosis** depends on the identification and therapy of thyroid dysfunction and malignancy. The risk factors for malignancy in patients with thyroid nodules include:

1. Development of **hoarseness, progressive dysphagia,** or **shortness of breath**
2. History of prior **head or neck irradiation**
3. **Family history** of thyroid cancer
4. **Male sex**
5. **Younger than 20 years** or **older than 60 years**
6. **Fixed mass, extrathyroidal extension,** or **cervical lymphadenopathy**

III. Common Causes

A. **Diffuse enlargement** of the thyroid gland is seen **in the following conditions:**

1. **Hashimoto's thyroiditis**
2. **Hyperthyroidism** secondary to Graves' disease or thyroiditis
3. **Simple goiter**
4. **Organification defect** (abnormality in the incorporation of iodine into thyroid hormone precursors)

B. **Nodular enlargement** of the thyroid gland can be found in the following situations:

1. **Benign solid nodule**

   a. Colloid nodule
   b. Follicular adenoma (may be hypofunctioning, autonomous, or toxic) [see also the HYPERTHYROIDISM section of this chapter]

2. **Malignancy**

   a. Differentiated thyroid carcinoma of the papillary or follicular, medullary or anaplastic variants
   b. Non-Hodgkin's and Hodgkin's lymphomas

3. **MNG** can present with or without thyrotoxicosis
4. **Simple cyst**

IV. When to Suspect the Presence of Goiter or Thyroid Nodules

A. Pain, pressure, or fullness in the neck
B. Hoarseness or change in the voice
C. Trouble swallowing

V. How to Confirm the Diagnosis (Figure 16–3)

A. **Fine-needle aspiration (FNA)** biopsy of the nodule is the most time- and cost-efficient evaluation. FNA biopsy should be performed in any patient with a solitary or predominant nodule in a multinodular gland, unless the TSH is suppressed, implying autonomous function and, therefore, a low likelihood of malignancy.
B. **TSH determination** (see Figure 16–3)
C. **Thyroid scintigraphy.** Radionuclide scans can be performed with either iodine-123 or technetium-99m pertechnetate.

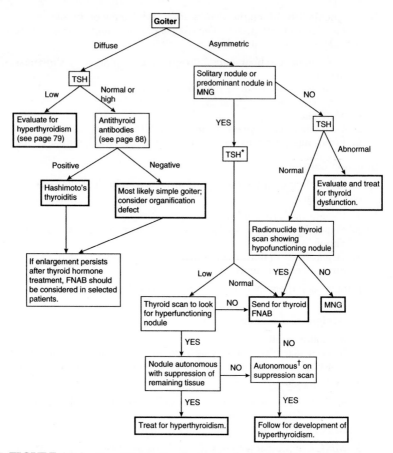

■ **FIGURE 16–3.** Algorithm for the diagnosis of goiter and thyroid nodules.
*Include measurement of serum calcitonin if there is a family history of medullary cancer or multiple endocrine neoplasm, type 2 (MEN2).
†Autonomy is defined as the ability to concentrate radioactive iodine despite TSH suppression.
FNAB = fine-needle aspiration biopsy; *MNG* = multinodular goiter; *TSH* = thyroid-stimulating hormone.

   1. Because 90% of nodules are either hypofunctioning or functioning well, scans are not useful to differentiate between benign and malignant lesions.
   2. Radionuclide scans can be useful to determine the anatomic and functional status of a nodule. They may also be useful to clarify questions of multinodularity, thyroid gland irregularity, or substernal extension.
   D. **Ultrasonography,** like scintigraphy, cannot distinguish between benign and malignant nodules. The technique plays a limited role in the workup of thyroid nodules:

1. **Nonpalpable single or multiple nodules smaller than 1 cm,** if detected solely by ultrasound, usually do not require further evaluation.
2. Ultrasonography may be useful to follow a nodule that is **difficult to palpate** or to **direct an FNA** biopsy in selected patients.

VI. Special Notes. Approximately 20% of FNA biopsies are classified as suspicious or indeterminate, requiring further workup, such as surgical biopsy.

SUGGESTED READING

Helford M, Redfern CC: Screening for thyroid disease: An update. *Ann Intern Med* 129:144–158, 1998.
Roth RN, McAuliffe MJ: Hyperthyroidism and thyroid storm. *Emerg Med Clin North Am* 7:873–883, 1989.

Thyroid Function Tests

Marjorie Safran

I. Overview. The thyroid is controlled by a typical endocrine feedback loop. TSH is secreted by the pituitary and stimulates the thyroid gland to produce **both** the prohormone T_4 and the active hormone triiodothyronine (T_3). T_4, in turn, is metabolized by peripheral tissues to T_3, and both hormones feed back to the pituitary to inhibit TSH secretion. This feedback loop is very sensitive to changes in circulating thyroid hormone concentration: A twofold change induces a tenfold change in TSH, in both directions. Thus, when the hypothalamic-pituitary axis is intact, TSH is the most sensitive marker of thyroid hormone action and is, thereby, used as a screening test for thyroid status.

A. **Indications** (see the HYPERTHYROIDISM, HYPOTHYROIDISM, and Goiter and Thyroid nodules sections in this chapter)

B. **Techniques and interpretations**

1. **Hormone assays:** Most hormones are measured by immunoradiometric assay or, more commonly, chemoluminescence immunometric assay.

   a. **The normal range for TSH** is approximately 0.35–5.00 U/ml. Eighty percent of normal people have a TSH of less than 3.0 U/ml. An assay with functional sensitivity < 0.05 U/ml is attained with so-called "third generation" or "ultrasensitive" TSH assays.

      (1) In **hyperthyroidism,** serum TSH is below normal and frequently < 0.1 U/ml. TSH may remain decreased for many months in treated—formerly hyperthyroid—patients; therefore, thyroid hormone levels more accurately reflect the clinical situation.

(2) Primary **hypothyroidism** is easily diagnosed by an elevated TSH. However, when hypothyroidism is caused by hypothalamic-pituitary dysfunction (secondary hypothyroidism), TSH is no longer a good marker for hypothyroidism, and circulating thyroid hormone concentrations need to be obtained. During treatment for hypothyroidism, as many as 6 weeks are needed to reach a new steady thyroid state.

b. **T_4 and T_3** circulate tightly bound to serum proteins [thyroxine-binding globulin (TBG), transthyretin (TTR), and albumin], and only the free hormone (0.03% for T_4 and 0.3% for T_3) is available to initiate thyroid hormone action. Changes in binding protein concentrations and hormone affinity can alter total thyroid hormone levels **without affecting free hormone concentrations** (Table 16–2). Total serum T_4 and T_3 concentrations are usually measured by immunoassays, which include both bound and free hormone. A number of alternative methods have been developed to estimate free hormone concentrations.

c. **Free T_4 index** (FTI or FT_4I) is a calculated value that uses the total T_4 and the T_3 resin uptake test to estimate free hormone indices.

(1) The T_3 resin uptake test is performed by incubating the patient's serum with radioactive T_3, then adding a resin, which traps all of the unbound radiolabeled T_3. It can be expressed directly as the percent of total counts bound to the insoluble resin (**T_3RU**) or as a ratio of the patient's T_3 resin uptake to that of a pool of normal patients (**THBR**) processed identically. The ratio is by definition 1 or 100%. The resin uptake is inversely proportional to the available free binding sites on the patient's thyroid hormone binding proteins (Figure 16–4).

TABLE 16–2. Clinical Conditions and Drugs That Alter Thyroid Hormone Binding

Decrease thyroid hormone binding	Decrease TBG	Increase TBG
Carbamazepine Phenytoin	Testosterone	Estrogens (OCPs, pregnancy, hormone-replacement therapy)
Rifampin	Corticosteroids	Infectious hepatitis
Salicylates	Severe illness	Neonatal
Euthyroid sick	Cirrhosis	Acute intermittent porphyria
Heparin (acutely)	Nephrotic syndrome Inherited	Inherited

OCPs = oral contraceptive pills; TBG = thyroxine-binding globulin.

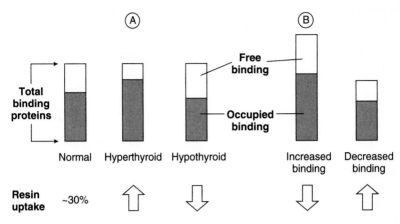

■ **FIGURE 16–4.** Changes in the resin uptake test as determined by binding protein levels and circulating hormone concentrations. *A* shows normal levels of total binding proteins. *B* shows high and low levels of total binding proteins.

      (a) For example, when thyroid hormone secretion is increased in hyperthyroidism, the binding equilibrium is shifted such that more of the binding sites are occupied by the patient's thyroid hormone, there are fewer sites available to bind the radiolabeled T_3, and more of the available radiolabeled T_3 binds to the resin.

      (b) On the other hand, if there is an increase in the concentration of binding proteins (such as the increase in TBG induced by estrogens), the binding equilibrium is unchanged but the number of unoccupied binding sites is increased and less radiolabeled T_3 binds to the resin.

   (2) The FTI or FT_4I is calculated as the product of the total T_4 and the T_3RU or THBR respectively, and corrects for binding abnormalities as shown in Table 16–3.

  d. Free T_4 measurement assays are quite good under conditions of normal-binding proteins, but can be misleading when binding abnormalities are present. If the free T_4 measurement is at odds with the clinical impression, it may be necessary to obtain an FTI or even free T_4 by dialysis.

  e. T_3 is usually elevated with hyperthyroidism. Assessment of T_3 levels is important to determine the severity of the hyperthyroidism and to monitor the response to treatment. Measurement of T_3 is wasteful in patients with hypothyroidism since it is low only in severe hypothyroidism and is also decreased in patients with nonthyroidal illness in the absence of hypothyroidism.

  f. Thyroglobulin is a large glycoprotein that is secreted by thyroid follicular cells. It can be detected in normal serum and is increased with increased thyroid cell mass (e.g., with Graves' disease, toxic MNG, thyroid cancer) and injury (e.g., biopsy, surgery, radioactive

TABLE 16–3. Thyroid Function Test Results in Various Abnormalities of the Thyroid Gland

Clinical Status	Total T4	Resin Uptake	FTI
Hyperthyroidism	High	High	High
Excess TBG	High	Low	Normal
Hypothyroidism	Low	Low	Low
TBG deficiency	Low	High	Normal

FTI = free thyroxine index; TBG = thyroxine-binding globulin.

iodine treatment, external irradiation, inflammation). Its main uses are in distinguishing factitious hyperthyroidism from other causes of low-RAIU hyperthyroidism (values are low to undetectable in the former and measurable or increased in the latter) and in identifying recurrences in patients with thyroid cancer. Normal values vary.

2. **Antithyroid antibodies** are of two types: Those that are **markers** of autoimmune thyroid disease [antithyroperoxidase and antithyroglobulin antibodies and those that are **mediators** of autoimmune thyroid disease (anti-TSH receptor antibodies).

   a. **Antithyroperoxidase** (and to a much lesser degree, antithyroglobulin) is detected in almost all patients with Hashimoto's disease and its variants, in 70% of patients with Graves' disease, and in a smaller number of patients with various other thyroid disorders such as MNG, nontoxic goiter, and thyroid carcinoma. Both are assayed by solid-phase, two-step chemoluminescence immunometric assay.

   b. **Anti-TSH receptor** antibodies are of two types: stimulating and blocking. They can be identified by measuring thyroid-stimulating immunoglobulin (TSI), which will pick up only the stimulating antibodies, or TSH-binding inhibitory immunoglobulin (TBII), which will pick up both types of TSH receptor antibodies. While TSI is present in 70%–100% of patients with Graves' disease, its measurement is not usually necessary for diagnosis, but it may be helpful in prognosis because patients who have very high TSI titers that do not decrease with antithyroid drug treatment are unlikely to go into remission. Measurement of TSI is important in pregnancy, because a high titer at the end of pregnancy correlates with an increased risk of neonatal hyperthyroidism.

II. Special Notes

A. **Drugs may decrease TSH.** These include glucocorticoids and dopamine.
B. TSH may also be **suppressed during illness and increased during recovery** (to as high as 20 U/ml).

C. Total T_4 and T_3 can be affected by alterations in **hormone binding.**

D. In patients with **"T_3-toxicosis,"** T_3 (but not T_4) concentrations are increased.

E. **T_3 levels are decreased by drugs** such as glucocorticoids, propranolol, amiodarone, and cholecystographic agents (e.g., iopanoic acid, sodium ipodate).

F. The **presence of antithyroperoxidase antibodies will falsely decrease or increase** thyroglobulin measurements when analyzed by immunometric assays or radioimmunoassay, respectively, and will confound the usefulness of the test.

G. Titers of antithyroglobulin antibodies **do not correlate with disease severity.**

H. **Commercial assays of TSI are very variable,** and therefore when indicated, it is recommended to measure TBII, which is more sensitive, although less specific.

SUGGESTED READING

Danese MD, Powe NR, Sawin CT, et al: Screening for mild thyroid failure at the periodic health examination. A decision and cost-effectiveness analysis. *JAMA* 276:285–292, 1996.

Surks MI, Chopra IJ, Mariash CN, et al: American Thyroid Association guidelines for the use of laboratory tests in thyroid disease. *JAMA* 263:1529–1532, 1990.

Disorders of the Adrenal Gland

Marjorie Safran

Adrenal Insufficiency

I. **Definition.** Adrenal insufficiency is defined as a **deficiency of hormones synthesized by the adrenal cortex.**

II. **Etiologies**

A. **Primary adrenal insufficiency** (due to intrinsic diseases of the adrenal gland)

1. **Autoimmune adrenalitis (Addison's disease)** [70%–79% of cases]: One-half of patients have other autoimmune disorders, such as hypoparathyroidism, type I DM, Hashimoto's thyroiditis, Graves' disease, or pernicious anemia.

2. **Infectious causes:** Microbial (tuberculosis, meningococcemia, and pseudomonas aeruginosa) or fungal agents (histoplasmosis, paracoccidioidomycosis) constitute 7%–20% of cases.

3. **Adrenal hemorrhage or infarction:** As many as one-third of patients with adrenal hemorrhage are on anticoagulants.

   4. **Metastatic disease** can come from disseminated lung, breast, stomach, or colon cancer; lymphoma; and melanoma (12%–60%).
   5. **Drugs** (e.g., ketoconazole, aminoglutethimide, etomidate)
   6. **The antiphospholipid syndrome**
   7. **Other risk factors** include thromboembolic disease, trauma and stress, adrenoleukodystrophy, and abetalipoproteinemia.

B. Secondary adrenal insufficiency [due to inadequate adrenocorticotropic hormone (ACTH) secretion by the pituitary]

   1. **Panhypopituitarism** (see the HYPOPITUITARISM and PITUITARY TUMORS sections of this chapter): Symptoms are due to a decrease in all pituitary hormones, resulting in hypoadrenalism.
   2. **Isolated ACTH deficiency**
   3. **Megestrol, used as an appetite stimulant,** interacts with the glucocorticoid receptor and suppresses the hypothalamic-pituitary-adrenal axis.

C. Tertiary adrenal insufficiency [most common type; due to inadequate corticotropin-releasing hormone (CRH) from the hypothalamus]

   1. Following **cessation of high-dose glucocorticoid therapy**
   2. Following **correction of Cushing's syndrome**

III. When to Suspect Adrenal Insufficiency

A. Patients with **gradual onset of adrenal insufficiency** may do fine until stressed (i.e., by infection, trauma, or surgery), at which time **adrenal crisis** can occur. This condition consists of shock, anorexia, lethargy, confusion, or coma.

B. Most patients with **chronic adrenal insufficiency** will complain of anorexia, nausea, vomiting, and generalized weakness.

C. Patients with **long-standing primary adrenal insufficiency** may present with hyperpigmentation. Other frequent signs are hypotension or orthostatic hypotension. Calcification of the auricular cartilage occurs in men.

D. Dehydration and hypotension do not occur in **secondary adrenal insufficiency** because mineralocorticoid function is intact.

IV. How to Confirm the Diagnosis (Figure 16–5)

A. Laboratory testing

   1. **An elevated morning ACTH plasma level** in the presence of low cortisol is diagnostic of primary adrenal insufficiency, assuming that no other glucocorticoid is being given to the patient.
   2. **ACTH stimulation test** (see Figure 16–5)
   3. **Antiadrenal antibodies:** Antibodies against the adrenal enzyme 2-hydroxylase (p450c21) are found in 60%–75% of patients with autoimmune adrenal insufficiency. They frequently precede the onset of disease. They are also present in 20% of patients with hypoparathyroidism.

B. Imaging studies. When primary adrenal insufficiency is identified, an abdominal computed tomography (CT) scan or magnetic resonance

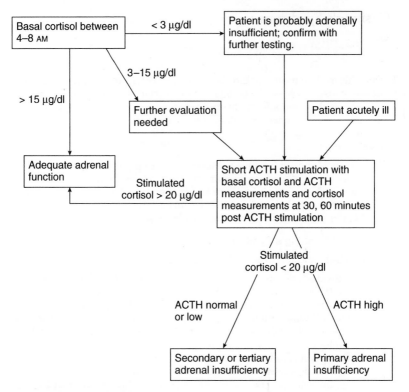

■ **FIGURE 16–5.** Algorithm for the diagnosis of adrenal insufficiency. *ACTH* = adrenocorticotropic hormone.

image (MRI) with specific attention to the adrenals should be obtained to identify a tumor or hemorrhage. Enlarged adrenals suggest infectious, hemorrhagic, or metastatic disease. Conversely, if adrenal hemorrhage is identified by imaging studies, patients should be evaluated for adrenal insufficiency. If secondary adrenal insufficiency is identified, then a pituitary CT scan or MRI should be done to look for masses.

   C. Adrenal biopsy is indicated to identify the etiology of adrenal masses if not otherwise evident.

V. **Special Notes**

   A. Cortisol is secreted in a diurnal pattern with highest levels in the morning. Levels measured later in the day are unreliable.

   B. Patients suspected of having an **adrenal crisis** should be treated immediately with a glucocorticoid that does not cross-react in the cortisol assay (i.e., dexamethasone), and confirmatory tests should be performed within 1–2 days.

Cushing's Syndrome

Marjorie Safran

I. **Definition.** The term **Cushing's syndrome refers to hypercortisolism of any cause.** Its presence is suggested by certain symptoms and signs, but none are pathognomonic and many are common and nonspecific. **Cushing's disease** refers to hypercortisolism due to an ACTH-producing pituitary adenoma.

II. **Overview**

   A. The **incidence** of Cushing's disease is 5 to 25 per million patients per year. Other causes of Cushing's syndrome are much less common.

   B. **Cushing's disease** and **benign and malignant adrenal tumors occur more frequently in women** (female:male ratio equals 3–8:1), but **ectopic ACTH secretion is more common in men.**

III. **Causes of Cushing's Syndrome**

   A. **ACTH-dependent Cushing's syndrome**

   1. **Cushing's disease** is the most common cause of Cushing's syndrome (~70%). The adenomas are frequently small, and even a gadolinium-enhanced, high-resolution MRI of the sella identifies only 50% of them. Pituitary tumors are partially autonomous with a higher set point of feedback inhibition, a feature that is exploited in determining the etiology of Cushing's syndrome.

   2. **Ectopic ACTH secretion** accounts for about 20% of the cases of ACTH-dependent Cushing's syndrome. The most common causes are bronchial or thymic carcinoids, small cell lung cancers, islet cell tumors, and rarely, an ACTH-producing pheochromocytoma.

   3. **Ectopic CRH syndrome** is a rare form of Cushing's syndrome and has been described secondary to a bronchial tumor.

   B. **ACTH-independent Cushing's syndrome**

   1. **Adrenal tumors** account for about 20% of the cases of Cushing's syndrome. It is important to be sure of the biochemical diagnosis prior to performing any adrenal imaging since 4% of patients have an adrenal incidentaloma.

   2. **Pseudo-Cushing's syndrome** may be secondary to excess production of CRH. It is often difficult to distinguish from Cushing's disease. The hormonal abnormalities resolve with remission of the underlying cause, such as depression or alcoholism.

   3. **Iatrogenic or fictitious Cushing's syndrome:** While the most common cause of iatrogenic hypercortisolism is the use of prednisone, it may also be caused by potent inhaled, injected, and topical gluco-corticoids, such as beclomethasone and fluocinolone. Both ACTH and cortisol may be low, confusing the evaluation. Urine high-performance liquid chromatography (HPLC) may be necessary to look for synthetic glucocorticoids.

IV. **Diagnostic Evaluation**

A. **Symptoms and signs**

1. Hypertension
2. Type II DM
3. Menstrual and psychiatric disorders

B. **Physical examination findings**

1. Central obesity
2. Proximal muscle weakness
3. Wide, purple striae
4. Spontaneous ecchymoses
5. Facial plethora (i.e., moon face)

C. **Laboratory investigation** (Figure 16–6). The first step in evaluation is to confirm the presence of excess cortisol production by biochemical testing. The second step is to determine if the hypercortisolism is ACTH dependent, and if so, the source of the ACTH.

1. **Tests used to establish the diagnosis of Cushing's syndrome** (Table 16–4).
2. **Tests used to localize the source of hormone excess** (see Figure 16–6). Once the diagnosis of Cushing's syndrome is confirmed, the next step is to distinguish among the three most common causes: (1) a pituitary tumor, (2) ectopic ACTH secretion, and (3) an adrenal tumor. Determining whether elevated cortisol is ACTH-dependent (due to an ACTH-secreting tumor) or whether it is ACTH-independent (due to a primary adrenal disorder) is based primarily on measuring plasma ACTH levels.

D. **Imaging studies**

1. **Adrenal imaging** is indicated when plasma ACTH levels are < 5pg/ml. Thin section CT or MRI is the next step in evaluating the adrenals. Bilateral adrenal hyperplasia may be present in ACTH-dependent disease.
2. **Somatostatin scanning:** Ectopic sources of ACTH are notoriously difficult to identify. Because many of these tumors are carcinoids and have somatostatin receptors, scintigraphy with the somatostatin analogue indium-111 (^{111}In)-pentreotide can sometimes localize tumors not found by conventional techniques.

E. **Petrosal sinus sampling** is used when the anatomical localization fails to identify an unequivocal lesion as suggested by the biochemical testing. This test allows confirmation of the pituitary source of ACTH and identifies the side of the ACTH-secreting lesion. ACTH is measured simultaneously in samples from catheters placed in the left and right inferior petrosal sinuses and compared to peripheral levels. A gradient of two- to threefold is consistent with a pituitary source of ACTH. CRH can also be given during the procedure to enhance its accuracy.

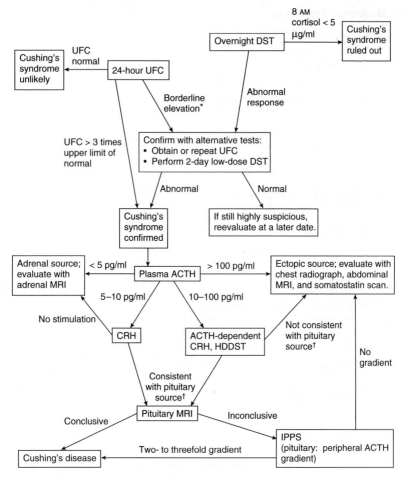

■ **FIGURE 16–6.** Algorithm for the evaluation of Cushing's syndrome.

*Patients with alcoholism or depression may have pseudo-Cushing's syndrome and require a CRH test for further evaluation.

†With a pituitary source, ACTH should increase with CRH, and cortisol production should decrease with HDDST.

ACTH = adrenocorticotropic hormone; CRH = corticotropin-releasing hormone; DST = dexamethasone suppression test; HDDST = high-dose dexamethasone suppression test; MRI = magnetic resonance imaging; IPPS = inferior petrosal sinus sampling; UFC = urinary free cortisol.

V. Special Notes

A. The results of **urinary free cortisol (UFC)** are valid only when a complete 24-hour urine collection is obtained and when the laboratory can measure urinary cortisol reliably.

TABLE 16–4. Common Tests Used to Establish the Diagnosis of Cushing's Syndrome

Test	Normal results	Diagnostic
24-hr urinary free cortisol (UFC)	< 90 µg cortisol per 24-hr period	> 3 times the upper limit of normal
1 mg overnight dexamethasone suppression test (DST) given at 11–12 PM	8 AM plasma cortisol < 5 µg/dL	Cushing's syndrome unlikely if cortisol suppresses normally
Low-dose DST (0.5 mg dexamethasone given every 6 hr for 2 days)	UFC < 10 µg and 17-OHS < 2.5 mg in a 24-hr urine collected on second day	UFC > 36 µg/d 17-OHS > 4 mg/d
12 midnight cortisol	< 5.0 µg/dl	> 7.5 µg/dl

    B. Accuracy of **12-midnight cortisol** requires an in-dwelling catheter and is clearly not convenient in an outpatient setting.

    C. Because both incidental pituitary and adrenal tumors are common, **biochemical evaluation** should be completed before any imaging studies.

SUGGESTED READING

Ganguly A: Primary aldosteronism. *N Engl J Med* 339:1828–1834, 1998.
Orth DN: Cushing's syndrome. *N Engl J Med* 332:791–803, 1995.
Young WF: Pheochromocytoma and primary aldosteronism: Diagnostic approaches. *Endocrinol Metab Clin North Am* 26:801–807, 1997.

Primary Hyperaldosteronism

Marjorie Safran

    I. Definition. Primary hyperaldosteronism is a **syndrome characterized by hypertension, hypokalemia, and suppressed plasma renin activity (PRA) associated with increased aldosterone excretion.**

II. Causes

    A. Aldosterone-producing adenoma (APA) accounts for 65% of cases. Patients tend to have more severe hypertension, lower potassiums levels, higher aldosterone secretion, and are of younger age than patients with idiopathic hyperaldosteronism (IHA). Unilateral adrenalectomy is curative. However, in ambiguous cases, adrenal venous sampling may be required to confirm the presence of unilateral aldosterone excretion.

    B. IHA accounts for 20%–30% of patients with primary hyperaldosteronism. IHA is caused by bilateral hyperplasia.

    C. Primary adrenal hyperplasia. Patients demonstrate physiologic changes associated with IHA, but they are found to have unilateral aldosterone secretion.

    D. Aldosterone-producing adrenocortical carcinoma

    E. Aldosterone-producing ovarian tumor

III. How to Confirm Suspicion of Hyperaldosteronism (Figure 16–7)

    A. Screening tests to diagnose primary hyperaldosteronism (Table 16–5) include:

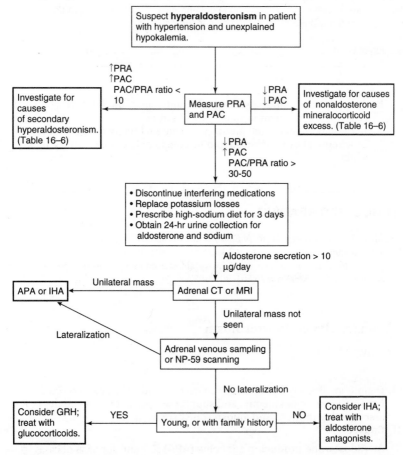

■ **FIGURE 16–7.** Algorithm for the diagnosis of hyperaldosteronism. *APA* = aldosterone-producing adenoma; *CT* = computed tomography; *GRH* = glucocorticoid remediable hyperaldosteronism; *IHA* = idiopathic hyperaldosteronism; *MRI* = magnetic resonance imaging; *PAC* = plasma aldosterone concentration; *PRA* = plasma renin activity.

▲

TABLE 16–5. Summary of Results in Patients with Primary Hyperaldosteronism

Test	Results
Random plasma aldosterone	> 30 ng/dl
24-hour urinary aldosterone	> 15 μg/day
Plasma renin activity	< 1 ng/ml/hr
Plasma aldosterone/renin ratio*	> 30–50
2-liter saline infusion	Plasma aldosterone > 10 ng/dl
3-day salt loading	24-hr urinary aldosterone > 12 μg/day

*A ratio > 30 may represent primary aldosteronism even with a relatively low aldosterone level.

1. Hypokalemia with inappropriate urinary potassium wasting
2. High plasma aldosterone concentration
3. Low PRA

B. Laboratory testing. Once a secondary cause of aldosterone hypersecretion has been ruled out (Table 16–6), the goal of testing is to demonstrate high, nonsuppressible aldosterone secretion in the presence of low PRA. Many antihypertensive agents affect the renin-angiotensin-aldosterone axis and the subsequent evaluation.

1. **Aldosterone measurement:** High plasma aldosterone concentration (more than 30 ng/dl) or an elevated 24-hour urinary aldosterone (more than 15 mcg/dl) is suggestive of hyperaldosteronism.
2. **PRA** is low in primary hyperaldosteronism. Conversely, high PRA can be seen in patients with renovascular or malignant hypertension or secondary to diuretic usage.
3. **Plasma aldosterone/plasma renin ratio:** Because 30% of patients with essential hypertension will have low upright renin levels, an elevated plasma aldosterone is required for diagnosis. Hypokalemia must be corrected and the patient must be off diuretics, angiotensin-converting enzyme (ACE) inhibitors, and high-dose beta-blockers. In patients with essential hypertension, the mean aldosterone/renin ratio is 4:5 as opposed to more than 30:50 in patients with primary aldosteronism.
4. **Aldosterone suppression:** Endogenous aldosterone secretion is normally suppressed to less than 6 ng/dl by sodium loading in normal subjects.

C. Imaging

1. **CT or MRI** is helpful in confirming and locating a unilateral mass, such as adenoma or carcinoma. It will also note adrenal thickening in hyperplasia.

TABLE 16–6. Other Causes of Hypertension Associated with Hypokalemia

Secondary Hyperaldosteronism (high renin and high aldosterone)	Nonaldosterone Mineralocorticoid Excess (low renin and low aldosterone)
Diuretic usage	Congenital adrenal hyperplasia
Renovascular hypertension	Exogenous mineralocorticoids
Renin-secreting tumors	Deoxycorticosterone (DOC)-producing tumor
Coarctation of the aorta	Cushing's syndrome
Malignant hypertension	Liddle's syndrome
Bartter's syndrome	Chronic licorice ingestion

2. **Radionuclide scintigraphy** with iodine-131 (^{131}I)-iodocholesterol may be more accurate in discovering a functional unilateral tumor.

D. **Other causes of hypertension with associated hypokalemia** need to be ruled out (see Table 16–6). These include:

1. **Secondary hyperaldosteronism** (i.e., aldosterone secretion secondary to increased plasma renin)
2. **Nonaldosterone mineralocorticoid excess**

IV. Special Notes

A. Patients should **be off spironolactone** for at least 6 weeks before testing.
B. **ACE inhibitors** can falsely elevate plasma renin.
C. Patients need to be **normokalemic** prior to evaluation of aldosterone because hypokalemia suppresses aldosterone secretion.

Adrenal Masses

Mira Sofia Torres and Marjorie Safran

I. **Definition.** Adrenal masses represent **any enlargement of the adrenal glands.**
II. **Overview**

A. **Adrenal masses** can be found in as many as 4% of abdominal CT scans done on patients without suspected adrenal problems. The majority (about 70%–90%) of adrenal masses found incidentally will be hormonally inactive adenomas that need **not** be removed.
B. While **adrenocortical carcinomas** make up only 10% or less of these masses, most of them are hormonally active.

III. Types/Classification

A. Hormonally active (functional, hypersecretory)

1. Hypersecreting adrenal adenoma
2. Hypersecreting adrenal carcinoma
3. Pheochromocytomas
4. ACTH-dependent Cushing's syndrome with nodular hyperplasia (see the CUSHING'S SYNDROME section of this chapter)
5. Congenital adrenal hyperplasia
6. Primary aldosteronism

B. Hormonally inactive (nonfunctional, nonhypersecretory)

1. Malignant

   a. Primary: Nonhypersecreting adrenal carcinoma
   b. Metastases
   c. Infiltrative: Leukemia, lymphoma

2. Nonmalignant

   a. Nonhypersecreting adrenal adenoma
   b. Granulomatous (e.g., tuberculosis, fungal, sarcoidosis)
   c. Hemorrhage or hematoma
   d. Amyloidosis
   e. Cysts (e.g., simple cysts, parasitic cysts, pseudocysts)
   f. Other benign tumors (e.g., angiomyolipomas, ganglioneuroma, lipoma, hamartoma, teratoma)

IV. How to Confirm the Diagnosis.

The goal of evaluation is to determine which masses are functional (hormonally active) and which ones have the likelihood of being malignant. Benign tumors without hormonal activity need only be followed, while most hormonally active and primary malignant tumors need to be removed.

A. History and physical examination. The presence of signs or symptoms suggestive of hormonal activity warrants further evaluation with appropriate biochemical screening tests.

B. Laboratory testing (Table 16–7 and Figure 16–8)

C. Imaging studies. If the hormonal evaluation reveals a nonfunctional tumor, the next step is to determine the likelihood that the adrenal mass represents a malignancy.

1. **Adrenal scintigraphy** is based on the principle that functioning adrenal cortical tissue will take up the iodinated cholesterol derivative NP-59. Adenomas tend to have normal accumulation of the tracer, while primary and secondary malignancies reveal no or discordant uptake. Although its proponents report high accuracy, this technique is not widely available or well standardized.

2. **CT and MRI:** Size is the most important predictor of the likelihood of malignancy. Lesions larger than 5–6 cm have a 28%–98% likelihood of being primary adrenal carcinomas. Surgical removal is recommended for adrenal masses larger than 4–6 cm, with close follow-up of smaller masses for any change in size.

3. **FNA biopsy** can differentiate adrenal from nonadrenal masses, but not

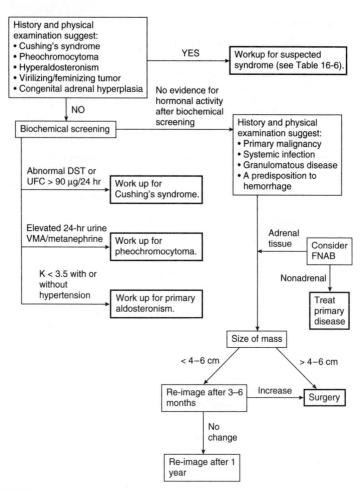

■ **FIGURE 16–8.** Algorithm for the diagnosis of adrenal masses.
Consider both clinical presentation and appearance on imaging in deciding cut-off size.
DST = dexamethasone suppression test; *FNAB* = fine-needle aspiration biopsy;
PE = physical examination; *UFC* = urinary free cortisol; *VMA* = vanillylmandelic acid.

benign from malignant adrenal tissue. It is most useful for patients with a known or suspected primary malignancy when it will impact on the management of the disease. It may also be useful when infectious or granulomatous diseases are highly suspected.

V. Special Notes. In patients with no apparent signs or symptoms, a basic biochemical screening is necessary because as many as 11% of cases will have unsuspected abnormal adrenal function.

TABLE 16–7. Clinical Presentations of Hormonal Hypersecretion and Recommended Screening Test

Disease	Suggestive Clinical Findings	Screening Recommendations
Pheochromocytoma	Hypertension, paroxysms of headaches, sweating, palpitations, tachycardia, orthostasis, glucose intolerance	24-hr urine for vanillylmandelic acid, metanephrines, and catecholamines*
Cushing's syndrome	Cushingoid habitus, hypertension, thin skin, muscle weakness, facial plethora, purplish striae	Overnight 1 mg dexamethasone suppression test or 24-hr urinary free cortisol*
Primary aldosteronism	Hypertension with hypokalemia, metabolic alkalosis	Blood pressure and serum potassium (in salt-replete state)*
		Upright plasma renin activity and plasma aldosterone concentration
		24-hr urine aldosterone
Sex hormone-secreting tumor	Virilization: hirsutism, amenorrhea, frontal balding, acne, clitoromegaly, male secondary sexual characteristics	DHEAS, testosterone, urinary 17-ketosteroid for virilizing tumors, estradiol for feminizing tumors
	Feminization (very rare): gynecomastia, penile or testicular atrophy	
Congenital adrenal hyperplasia (especially late-onset 21-hydroxylase deficiency)	In women: acne, hirsutism, amenorrhea, infertility	ACTH stimulation test for 17-OHP (to be considered in patients 21 years of age or younger in the presence of suspicious clinical features)
	May have suggestive family history	

*Screen in all patients with an incidental adrenal mass.

ACTH = adrenocorticotropic hormone; DHEAS = dehydroepiandrosterone sulfate; 17-OHP = 17-hydroxyprogesterone.

Pheochromocytoma

Marjorie Safran

I. **Definition.** Pheochromocytomas are **catecholamine-producing tumors arising from the chromaffin cells of the adrenal medulla or the sympathetic ganglia (extra-adrenal).** These tumors are curable when diagnosed and treated properly, and they are potentially fatal if missed.

II. **Overview**

　A. **Annual incidence** is 2 to 8 cases/10^6 population.

　B. Patients usually **present with hypertension,** either sustained or episodic. Even with sustained hypertension, symptoms tend to appear in paroxysms, ranging from daily to monthly, and lasting 10–60 minutes.

III. **Types. The 10% rule**—10% of pheochromocytomas are extra-adrenal, 10% are seen in children, 10% are bilateral, 10% represent recurrence, 10% are malignant, and 10% are familial.

　A. **Familial syndromes**

　　1. **Familial pheochromocytomas**
　　2. Associated with **multiple endocrine neoplasia (MEN)**

　　　a. MEN, type 2A (MEN2A) [with medullary carcinoma of the thyroid, hyperparathyroidism]
　　　b. MEN, type 2B (MEN2B) [with medullary carcinoma of the thyroid, mucosal neuromas, marfanoid body habitus]

　　3. **Neurofibromatosis 1**

　B. **Other causes** of sympathetic overactivity should be considered:

　　1. **Abrupt discontinuation of a short-acting sympathetic antagonist** (e.g., clonidine, propranolol)
　　2. **Autonomic dysfunction** (seen with Guillain-Barré syndrome or spinal cord injury)
　　3. **Stress response** after cardiac surgery
　　4. **Panic reaction** (particularly if on a tricyclic antidepressant)
　　5. Use of **sympathomimetic drugs** (e.g., phenylpropanolamine, cocaine, amphetamines)
　　6. **Combination** of monoamine oxidase (MAO) inhibitor and tyramine-containing foods

IV. **How to Confirm the Diagnosis** (Figure 16–9)

　A. **Laboratory testing.** Biochemical documentation of catecholamine hypersecretion is needed prior to any imaging studies, because the incidence of asymptomatic adrenal masses is much higher than the incidence of pheochromocytoma. Evaluation includes analysis of blood or urinary catecholamines and their metabolites.

　B. **Imaging studies**

　　1. **Localization studies:** Ninety percent of tumors are within the adrenal gland. Of the remaining, 5% are intra-abdominal.

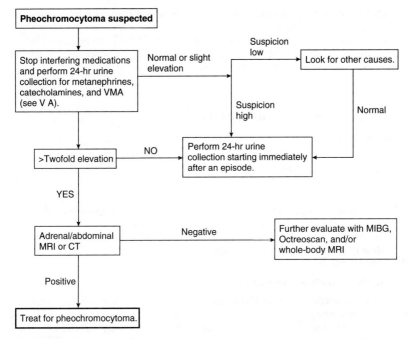

■ **FIGURE 16–9.** Algorithm for the diagnosis of pheochromocytoma. *CT* = computed tomography; *MIBG* = [^{123}I]-metaiodobenzylguanidine; *MRI* = magnetic resonance imaging; *Octreoscan* = [^{111}I]-pentetreotide; *VMA* = vanillylmandelic acid.

    2. CT and MRI of the adrenals and abdomen will detect most sporadic
tumors because they are usually larger than 3 cm in size. MRI has some
advantage since pheochromocytomas have a typical hyperintense
appearance on T2-weighted images.

    **3. Scanning with either [^{123}I]-metaiodobenzylguanidine (MIBG) or
[^{111}In]-pentetreotide (Octreoscan),** which are taken up by adrenergic
tissue, is useful in patients with negative CT or MRI and can help
identify multiple tumors.

V. Special Notes

  A. Patients must be off all interfering drugs before urine or plasma catecholamines can be measured.

    1. Levels are increased by tricyclic antidepressants, labetalol, levodopa (L-
dopa), decongestants, amphetamines, ethanol, and benzodiazepines.

    2. Levels are decreased by metyrosine and methylglucamine, which are
present in contrast media.

  B. In a 24-hour urine test for catecholamines and metabolites, values two
times normal are diagnostic.

  C. Plasma catecholamines can be two to three times elevated in patients with
renal failure. Total catecholamines > 2000 pg/ml is diagnostic of pheochromocytoma.

D. Rare patients with **epinephrine-only secreting tumors** can present with episodic hypertension.

E. As many as 25% of **tumors in patients with MEN2** can be missed by imaging, probably because many of these patients are discovered early and because the frequency of extra-adrenal tumors is higher.

Disorders of the Pituitary Gland

Marjorie Safran

Pituitary Tumors

I. Definition. Pituitary tumors are represented by **any new growth of the pituitary gland, independent of size or symptoms.**

II. Overview. Pituitary adenomas account for 90% of sellar or parasellar masses. Most tumors are considered benign.

III. Classification

  A. Hormonally active tumors

    1. Growth hormone (GH)-secreting tumors present with symptoms of **acromegaly.** Diagnosis is made by demonstrating nonsuppressible GH secretion after glucose administration (nadir > 1 ng/ml) and elevated levels of insulin-like growth factor-I (IGF-I). It is not unusual for GH-secreting tumors to also secrete prolactin.

    2. Prolactin-secreting tumors are the most common pituitary tumors (55%) [see Chapters 12 and 32].

      a. A prolactin of greater than 200 ng/ml almost always indicates a macroadenoma, although other causes should be considered, such as pregnancy, lactation, stress, dopamine receptor antagonists (e.g., neuroleptics, metoclopramide), primary hypothyroidism, and renal failure.

      b. A prolactin of less than 100 ng/ml can be seen with microadenomas.

    3. ACTH-secreting tumors present with symptoms of Cushing's syndrome (see the CUSHING'S SYNDROME section in this chapter).

  B. Hormonally inactive tumors

    1. Nonsecreting pituitary adenoma

    2. Metastatic tumor (breast and lung are the most common sites)

    3. Other brain tumors (e.g., craniopharyngioma, meningioma, glioma)

IV. Diagnostic Evaluation

  A. Symptoms

    1. Hormonally active tumors can be symptomatic even when the size is small.

    2. Nonsecreting tumors do not become symptomatic until their size becomes large enough to cause either pituitary hormone insufficiency (e.g., gonadal dysfunction, secondary hypothyroidism, adrenal insufficiency, growth failure, delayed puberty in children), hyperprolactinemia, or other neurologic symptoms (e.g., headache, visual field defects, diabetes insipidus, other cranial nerve defects).

B. Signs. Occasionally, hemorrhage into a tumor may cause **pituitary apoplexy** (i.e., gross hemorrhage into the pituitary gland).

1. **Incidental microadenomas** (Figure 16–10) rule out prolactin excess, acromegaly, and Cushing's syndrome.
2. When a **macroadenoma** is identified, evidence for hormonal excess should be sought and assessment of overall pituitary function and formal visual fields is required.

V. Special Notes

A. The finding of a large tumor with only minimally elevated prolactin indicates that the tumor is not a prolactinoma but is causing **pituitary stalk compression** and **loss of dopamine inhibition of prolactin secretion.**

B. IGF-I levels need to be corrected for age and sex. Random GH measurements are not reliable since GH is secreted episodically and may be elevated with anxiety, exercise, acute illness, chronic renal failure, and diabetes.

C. Diabetes insipidus is rare with pituitary adenomas and usually indicates an extrasellar lesion.

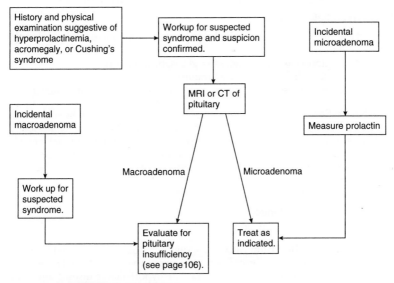

■ **FIGURE 16–10.** Pituitary tumor algorithm. *CT* = computed tomography; *MRI* = magnetic resonance imaging.

Hypopituitarism

Marjorie Safran

I. **Definition.** Hypopituitarism is the **deficiency of one or more pituitary hormones resulting from either pituitary or hypothalamic dysfunction.** The term **panhypopituitarism** is used when all the anterior pituitary hormones are absent. When hypothalamic disease is also present, vasopressin deficiency may occur.

II. **Causes.** Pituitary tumors and other neoplastic processes are the most common cause of acquired hypopituitarism.

A. Pituitary disease

1. Mass lesions
2. Following surgical or radiation treatment
3. Infiltrative diseases (e.g., hemochromatosis, lymphocytic hypophysitis)
4. Pituitary apoplexy, which is manifested by sudden onset of headache, cranial nerve defects, visual defects, and hypotension resulting from infarction or hemorrhage into the pituitary gland
5. Internal-carotid-artery aneurysm
6. Empty sella syndrome, either primary (e.g., a congenital defect in the sellar diaphragm) or secondary to surgery, radiation treatment, or tumor infarction
7. Genetic defects, such as mutations in genes encoding transcription factors necessary for differentiation of anterior pituitary cells, resulting in congenital deficiency of one or more pituitary hormones

B. Hypothalamic disease

1. Tumors [primary (craniopharyngiomas) or metastatic (lung, breast)]
2. Radiation
3. Infiltrative diseases (e.g., sarcoidosis, histiocytosis)
4. Basal skull fracture or head trauma
5. Infections, the most common of which is tuberculous meningitis

III. **When to Suspect Hypopituitarism.** Hypopituitarism should be suspected in any patient with midline defects or pituitary and/or hypothalamic masses. Symptoms are mainly secondary to end-organ (i.e., thyroid, adrenal, gonads) dysfunction, but can also be related to local symptoms if a mass is present (i.e., headache, visual disturbances). In pituitary apoplexy, symptoms can be dramatic.

IV. **How to Confirm the Diagnosis**

A. Laboratory evaluation

1. **ACTH and cortisol**

   a. **Basal function:** Measure serum cortisol between 8 and 9 AM. Cortisol ≤ 3 μg/dl is strongly suggestive of cortisol deficiency, and in a patient with pituitary or hypothalamic disease indicates ACTH deficiency. Basal cortisol ≥ 10 μg/dl is consistent with normal basal function and ≥ 18 μg/dl indicates a likely normal response to stress.

b. **ACTH reserve:** When basal cortisol is between 3 and 10 μg/dl, ACTH reserve may need to be evaluated.

c. **ACTH stimulation test:** Patients should be administered cosyntropin (0.25 mg intravenously), and cortisol and aldosterone should be measured at 0, 30, and 60 minutes. A normal response is cortisol > 20 μg/dl and aldosterone > 4 ng/dl. A normal response does not rule out secondary adrenal insufficiency of recent onset.

d. **CRH test:** Patients should be given bovine CRH (1 μg/kg intravenously at 8 AM), and ACTH and cortisol should be measured at 0, 15, 30, 60, 90, and 120 minutes. ACTH should increase two- to fourfold to 20–100 pg/ml, and cortisol should be 20–25 μg/dl.

e. **Insulin tolerance test:** Patient should be given regular insulin (0.05–0.15 U/kg intravenously), and glucose and cortisol should be measured at 0, 30, 45, 60, and 90 minutes. If glucose falls < 40 mg/dl, cortisol should increase by > 7 μg/dl or to > 20 μg/dl. The test requires close observation for hypoglycemia and is risky in patients with cardiac or neurologic dysfunction.

f. **Metyrapone test:** Patients should be administered metyrapone [30 mg/kg (max 2 g) at 12 midnight]. Cortisol and 11-deoxycortisol should be measured at 8 AM. 11-deoxycortisol should increase to > 7.5 μg/dL and cortisol to < 4 μg/dL. Adequate metyrapone should be given.

2. **TSH**

a. **Basal function:** Low FTI or free T_4 in the absence of appropriately elevated TSH is suggestive of secondary hypothyroidism. Rule out medications that decrease thyroid hormone binding such as phenytoin, salsalate, or high-dose aspirin.

b. **Thyrotropin-releasing hormone (TRH) test:** Patients should be given TRH (500 μg intravenously), and TSH should be measured at 0, 20, and 60 minutes. An increase of > 5 mU/L is normal. A delayed peak is suggestive of hypothalamic rather than pituitary dysfunction, but is relatively nonspecific.

3. **Gonadotropins:** Low levels of follicle-stimulating hormone (FSH) and luteinizing hormone (LH) in postmenopausal women or in men with low testosterone are suggestive of gonadotropin deficiency.

4. **Gonadotropin-releasing hormone (GnRH) test:** Patients should be given GnRH (100 μg intravenously), and LH and FSH should be measured at 0, 30, and 60 minutes. LH should increase by 10 IU/L and FSH by 2 IU/L.

5. **GH**

a. Basal GH and IGF-I levels are nonspecific.

b. Provocative tests with insulin, L-arginine, vasopressin, glucagon, or L-dopa should be used. Peak GH should be > 5–10 ng/ml.

6. **Vasopressin**

a. **Basal serum sodium, osmolality, and urine osmolality:** Hypotonic urine in the presence of increased serum sodium and serum osmolality is suggestive of diabetes insipidus.

b. **Water deprivation test:** The inability to concentrate urine with a response to exogenous vasopressin is diagnostic of central diabetes insipidus (see Chapters 68 and 71).

B. Imaging studies

1. An MRI scan with gadolinium is the first choice to evaluate the pituitary gland, hypothalamus, and pituitary stalk.
2. A high-resolution CT with thin sections through the pituitary fossa is a reasonable alternative.

SUGGESTED READING

Consensus guidelines for the diagnosis and treatment of adults with growth hormone deficiency: summary statement of the growth hormone research society workshop on adult growth hormone deficiency. *J Clin Endocrinol Metab* 83:379–381, 1998.

Freda PU, Post KD: Differential diagnosis of sellar masses. *Endocrinol Metab Clin North Am* 28:81–117, 1999.

Freda PU, Wardlaw SL: Clinical review 110: Diagnosis and treatment of pituitary tumors. *J Clin Endocrinol Metab* 84:3859–3866, 1999.

Parks JS, Brown MR, Hurley DL, Phelps CJ, Wajnrajch MP: Heritable disorders of pituitary development. *J Clin Endocrinol Metab* 84:4362–4370, 1999.

Vance ML: Hypopituitarism. *N Engl J Med* 330: 1651–1662, 1994.

Hyperparathyroidism

Marjorie Safran

I. **Definition.** Primary hyperthyroidism is **autonomous hypersecretion of parathyroid hormone (PTH) from the parathyroid glands.**

II. **Overview.** Primary hyperparathyroidism is frequently identified in asymptomatic patients after routine blood tests. It is estimated to have a prevalence of 1:1000.

III. **Causes.** Primary hyperparathyroidism can usually be differentiated from other causes of hypercalcemia by the demonstration of an elevated serum PTH concentration (see Chapter 10, HYPERCALCEMIA). In hypercalcemia of malignancy, PTH secretion is appropriately suppressed and hypercalcemia is mediated by parathyroid hormone-related protein (PTHrP).

   A. **Parathyroid adenoma** is the most common cause of hyperparathyroidism (> 80%). Most patients have a single enlarged gland with the remaining glands being normal.

   B. **Parathyroid hyperplasia** involves all four glands and can occur either as isolated or as part of a syndrome such as MEN1, MEN2, or familial hyperparathyroidism. It accounts for 15% of patients with primary hyperparathyroidism.

   C. **Parathyroid carcinoma** is a rare cause of hyperparathyroidism and accounts for 1%–2% of cases. It should be suspected in patients with a palpable parathyroid gland, and markedly elevated serum calcium (> 14 mg/dl) and PTH concentrations.

D. Familial hypocalciuric hypercalcemia is characterized by a family history of hypercalcemia, a young age of onset, lack of symptoms or complications, and specifically by a low urine calcium excretion (Ca/Cr clearance ratio < 0.01 in 90% of patients). These patients have a defect in the calcium-sensing receptor, normal or only very slightly elevated PTH concentrations, and are not cured by surgery.

IV. When to Suspect Hyperparathyroidism

   A. Elevated serum calcium levels especially if present over a number of years
   B. Nephrolithiasis
   C. Metabolic acidosis
   D. Unexplained osteoporosis, bone pain, or pathologic fractures

V. How to Confirm the Diagnosis (Figure 16–11)

   A. Laboratory evaluation. The diagnosis of primary hyperparathyroidism depends upon demonstrating elevated **serum calcium** in the presence of increased PTH. A **24-hour urine calcium quantitation** should be measured if FHH is suspected. The differential between adenoma, hyperplasia, and carcinoma is usually made at the time of surgery, although

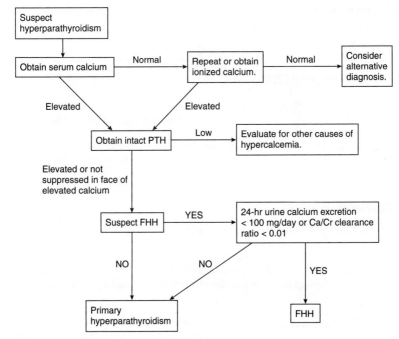

■ **FIGURE 16–11.** Hyperparathyroidism algorithm. *Ca/Cr* = calcium/creatinine; *FHH* = familial hypocalciuric calcemia; *PTH* = parathyroid hormone.

preoperative tumor localization is frequently used to direct the surgeon appropriately (see V B). Patients who are suspected of having hyperpara-thyroidism in the context of MEN1 or MEN2 should also be evaluated for associated disorders, particularly for pheochromocytoma and medullary carcinoma of the thyroid in the latter.

1. **PTH measurements** are elevated in 80%–90% of patients with primary hyperparathyroidism. In most of the remaining patients, "normal" PTH is inappropriate in the setting of an elevated serum calcium. In patients with nonparathyroid-mediated hypercalcemia, intact PTH is < 25 pg/ml. PTHrP, which is the humoral cause of cancer-related hypercalcemia, is not picked up in the intact PTH assay.
2. **Urinary calcium excretion:** Forty percent of patients with primary hyperparathyroidism will be hypercalciuric (excretion > 250 mg/day), and the finding of significant hypercalciuria may be an indication for surgical intervention. However, the main use of urine calcium excretion is to identify patients with familial hypocalciuric hypercalcemia.

B. Imaging studies for tumor localization include high-resolution ultrasonog-raphy or technetium-99m sestamibi scanning, which can correctly identify the location of a solitary adenoma in as many as 80% of cases.

C. Ancillary studies. Selective venous sampling may be required to correctly localize abnormal parathyroid tissue in patients with persistent hyperparathyroidism before reoperation.

VI. Special Notes. An isolated PTH increase in the absence of hypercalcemia may be secondary to vitamin D deficiency.

SUGGESTED READING

Kebebew E, Clark OH: Parathyroid adenoma, hyperplasia, and carcinoma: Localization, tech-nical details of primary neck exploration, and treatment of hypercalcemic crisis. *Surg Oncol Clin North Am* 7:721–748, 1998.

Marx SJ, Stock JL, Attie MF, et al: Familial hypocalciuric hypercalcemia: Recognition among pa-tients referred after unsuccessful parathyroid exploration. *Ann Intern Med* 92:351–356, 1980.

Diabetes Mellitus

Christopher Sorli and Marjorie Safran

I. Definition. The term "diabetes mellitus" collectively represents a **group of disorders sharing in common the clinical finding of hyperglycemia.**

II. Overview

A. Incidence

1. Five percent of world population; 7% of the United States population
2. Fourth leading cause of death in the United States
3. Of the estimated 18 million persons with primary DM in the United States, 90%–95% have type II DM.

B. **Screening in the absence of specific symptoms**

  1. **Obesity:** Sixty percent of obese individuals (> 20% over ideal body weight) will eventually develop diabetes.
  2. **Family history.** Anyone with a first-degree relative with type II DM should be evaluated and followed closely.
  3. **Race:** DM is more common in African-Americans, Hispanic-Americans, Native Americans, Asian-Americans, and Pacific Islanders.
  4. **Age:** Patients 45 years of age or older should receive DM screening.
  5. **Women** between the 24th and 28th weeks of gestation or who have a history of gestational DM or macrosomia (> 9 lb) may be at risk.
  6. **Hypertension** ($\geq$ 140/90 mm Hg)
  7. **Lipid abnormality** [high-density lipoproteins (HDL) < 35 mg/dl or triglycerides > 250 mg/dl, or LDL > 130 mg/dl

III. **Types and Classification**

  A. **Rationale and limitations.** The recent classification focuses on the underlying pathophysiologic processes. The age of onset (juvenile versus adult) is no longer relevant.
  B. **Primary DM** (> 90%)

  1. **Type I: Insulin-dependent diabetes mellitus (IDDM)**

    a. Immune mediated; results in an absolute insulin deficiency
    b. Idiopathic

  2. **Type II: Non-insulin-dependent diabetes mellitus (NIDDM)**

    a. **Relative insulin deficiency** due to abnormalities of both insulin secretion and insulin action
    b. Insulin levels are sufficient to prevent lipid mobilization and ketosis.

  3. **Gestational diabetes**

    a. Only 2% of patients with gestational diabetes remain diabetic after delivery.
    b. Forty percent will develop overt diabetes within 15 years, mostly those with type II DM, but occasionally those with type I DM.

  C. **Specific types of diabetes**

  1. Genetic defects of the beta cell function
  2. Genetic defects in insulin action
  3. Diseases of the exocrine pancreas

    a. Pancreatitis, trauma, pancreatectomy, neoplasia
    b. Cystic fibrosis
    c. Hemochromatosis
    d. Fibrocalculous pancreatopathy

  4. Associated with endocrinopathies (i.e., Cushing's syndrome), drugs (i.e., corticosteroids), or chemicals

IV. **When to Suspect DM**

  A. **History.** The clinical onset of diabetes can be acute or insidious, depending both on the degree of insulin deficiency as well as on the intercurrent level of physiologic stress. Very high levels of suspicion should accompany patients with:

1. Classic symptoms of hyperglycemia (e.g., thirst, polyuria, weight loss, visual blurring)
2. Serendipitous finding of hyperglycemia or known impaired glucose tolerance
3. Complications of diabetes, such as proteinuria, neuropathy, cardiovascular complications, and retinopathy

B. **Physical examination.** Patients with evidence of dehydration, orthostatic hypotension, confusion, or coma should be evaluated for diabetes.

V. **How to Confirm the Diagnosis**

A. **Plasma glucose.** Despite the diversity of the pathophysiologic processes that can lead to diabetes, elevated plasma glucose remains the single, pathognomonic diagnostic finding of DM. The Expert Committee on the Diagnosis and Classification of Diabetes Mellitus has formulated the diagnostic criteria listed in Table 16–8.

1. **Oral glucose tolerance testing** is rarely necessary to diagnose diabetes in adults.
2. In **symptomatic patients** with blood glucose $\geq$ 200 mg/dl or patients with ketonuria and clear manifestations of type I DM, the diagnosis is established and further evaluation is not needed.

B. **Glycosylated hemoglobin A_{1c} (HbA$_{1c}$).** Although not part of the diagnostic criteria for diabetes, HbA$_{1c}$ is an extremely valuable clinical tool useful both in the diagnosis and in the management of diabetic patients.

1. **HbA$_{1c}$** represents the most abundant minor component of circulating hemoglobin molecules. Its circulating life span is close to that of a red blood cell, about 90 days.
2. **Measurement of glycosylated HbA$_{1c}$** provides information about the level of glycemic control over a 3-month period.
3. **Normal value:** 4.8% to 6.2% with a coefficient of variation within each run of 1.5% (ion-exchange HPLC method, which measures the HbA$_{1c}$ fraction specifically)

VI. **Further Testing.** It is recommended that patients with DM should be evaluated with either serum ferritin or serum iron/transferritin saturation to rule out genetic hemochromatosis. If clinically suspicious, consider Cushing's syndrome.

TABLE 16–8. Laboratory Tests for Diabetes Mellitus

Test	Diabetes mellitus	Impaired glucose tolerance (EGT)
Fasting glucose (on two or more occasions)	$\geq$ 126 mg/dl (7.0 mM)	110–125 mg/dl (6.1–6.9 mM)
Random or OGTT* (2-hr plasma glucose)	$\geq$ 200 mg/dl (11.1 mM)	140–199 mg/dl (7.8–11.0 mM)

*Oral glucose tolerance test (OGTT) using 75-gram glucose load.

VII. Complications

A. Acute. Excessive and prolonged hyperglycemia associated with uncontrolled diabetes can cause fluid and electrolyte imbalance, which may be life threatening.

1. **Diabetic ketoacidosis (type I DM):** Absolute insulin deficiency leads to the unopposed action of the counter-regulatory hormones, including glucagon on the liver, adipose tissue, and muscle, leading to unchecked gluconeogenesis and lipolysis.

   a. **Signs and symptoms**

      (1) Dehydration, orthostatic hypotension, tachypnea, tachycardia, abdominal pain, nausea, vomiting, and confusion

      (2) Antecedent history of viral or bacterial illness, trauma, or emotional stress

   b. **Laboratory findings**

      (1) Hyperglycemia (generally ≥ 300 mg/dL), glucosuria, ketonemia and ketonuria, low bicarbonate, elevated blood urea nitrogen, elevated creatinine, pH usually less than 7.3

      (2) Decreased total body potassium and phosphorous; serum levels may be normal due to acidosis and shifts to the extracellular space

2. **Hyperosmolar hyperglycemic nonketotic coma.** Hyperglycemia in patients with type II DM can lead to hyperosmolar coma. The degree of hyperglycemia and dehydration that develop are often far more severe than in patients with type I DM.

   a. **Signs and symptoms**

      (1) Usually occurs in elderly patients with decreased ability to obtain free water; precipitated by illness or drugs

      (2) Decreased mentation, coma

      (3) Dehydration

   b. **Laboratory findings**

      (1) Blood glucose often greater than 600 mg/dl

      (2) Serum osmolality often greater than 320 mOsm/kg

      (3) Bicarbonate remains greater than 15 mEq/L

      (4) pH remains greater than 7.3

B. Diabetic nephropathy

1. Diabetes is now the most common cause of **end-stage renal disease (ESRD)** in the Western countries.

2. Twenty to thirty percent of patients with DM type I or II will develop **evidence of nephropathy.**

3. Earliest evidence of nephropathy is the appearance of low levels (30 mg/day or 20 μg/min) of albumin in the urine, termed **microalbuminuria.**

4. Eighty percent of patients with type I DM and 20% to 40% of patients with type II DM who develop microalbuminuria will progress to **overt nephropathy** (≥ 300 mg/24 hr or 200 μg/min) over a period of 10–15 years if not treated.

    5. Of those patients who develop overt nephropathy, **ESRD can be expected to develop in 75% of patients with type I DM and 20% of patients with type II DM** over 20 years.

    6. Microalbuminuria is a marker of **greatly increased cardiovascular morbidity and mortality** in patients with both DM types I and II.

  C. Retinopathy, neuropathy, and vascular atherosclerosis leading to cardio-vascular disease will not be considered in this chapter.

VIII. Special Notes

  A. If the patient's red blood count has an abnormal survival time (hemolytic anemias), **the HbA$_{1c}$ will be falsely low;** in polycythemia vera or post-splenectomy, it **may be falsely elevated.**

  B. With **hemoglobin F** (HbF) > 5% but < 30%, **falsely low results may require correction;** with HbF > 30%, **no accurate values** can be obtained.

  C. **Laboratory technical error:** If the sample is not incubated for a full 15 minutes prior to running, HbA$_{1c}$ will be falsely elevated.

SUGGESTED READING

American Diabetes Association: Screening for type 2 diabetes (Committee report). *Diabetes Care* 23 Suppl 1:S20–23, 2000.

The Expert Committee on the Diagnosis and Classification of Diabetes Mellitus: Report of the expert committee on the diagnosis and classification of diabetes mellitus. *Diabetes Care* 23 Suppl 1:S4–19.

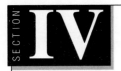

Gastrointestinal, Hepatobiliary, and Pancreatic Disorders

17

Acute Abdomen

W. Christopher Fang and Mark Callery

I. **Definition.** Acute abdomen is defined as **an episode of severe abdominal pain that lasts several hours or longer and requires medical attention.**

    A. The acute abdomen usually, but not necessarily, has a surgical cause. However, the term "acute abdomen" should not be equated with a need for emergency surgery.

    B. The history and physical examination remain the most important aspects of diagnosis.

    C. The key feature in the evaluation of patients with acute abdomen is early diagnosis.

II. **Differential Diagnosis** (Table 17–1)

III. **Notes on the Differential Diagnosis**

    A. **Common gynecologic causes** of lower quadrant pain include mittelschmerz, ovarian cyst, endometriosis, fibroids, ovarian torsion, pelvic inflammatory disease (PID), ovarian tumor, ectopic pregnancy, infection of the uterus, threatened abortion, and round ligament pain secondary to pregnancy.

    B. **Medical causes** that may present as acute abdomen are many. Common examples include lower lobe pneumonias, acute myocardial infarction (MI), diabetic ketoacidosis, acute hepatitis, porphyria, adrenal hemorrhage, and musculoskeletal problems.

    C. **Appendicitis** is a clinical diagnosis. The triad of right lower quadrant pain, anorexia, and leukocytosis is the most sensitive diagnostic tool. Nausea and vomiting usually follow the onset of pain. The patient may have a low-grade fever and mild leukocytosis. Higher fevers or white blood cell (WBC) counts suggest perforation.

        1. Thirty percent of patients with appendicitis have an elevated WBC count, whereas 95% will have a left shift.

        2. The intensity of pain is somewhat in proportion to the degree of irritation to the parietal peritoneum. Thus, a retrocecal appendix (which is the most common location) may cause only a dull ache, given the lack of contact with the parietal peritoneum.

TABLE 17–1. Differential Diagnosis of Acute Abdomen

Right Upper Quadrant Pain

Cholecystitis
Choledocholithiasis
Cholangitis
Hepatitis
Liver tumors
Hepatic abscess
Appendicitis
Peptic ulcer disease (PUD)
Perforated ulcer
Pancreatitis
Gastritis
Pyelonephritis
Nephrolithiasis
Pneumonia

Right Lower Quadrant Pain

Appendicitis
Ruptured ovarian cyst
Meckel's diverticulitis
Cecal diverticulitis
Cholecystitis
Perforated colon
Colon cancer
Urinary tract infection
Small bowel obstruction
Inflammatory bowel disease (IBD)
Nephrolithiasis
Pyelonephritis
Ectopic pregnancy
Bowel incarceration
Pelvic inflammatory disease (PID)

Left Upper Quadrant Pain

PUD
Perforated ulcer
Gastritis
Splenic disease (e.g., infarct,
abscess, or rupture)
Gastroesophageal reflux disease (GERD)
Dissecting aortic aneurysm
Pyelonephritis
Nephrolithiasis
Hiatal hernia
Boerhaave syndrome (i.e., rupture
of the esophagus)
Mallory-Weiss tear
Diverticulitis
Bowel obstruction

Left Lower Quadrant Pain

Diverticulitis
Sigmoid volvulus
Perforated colon
Colon cancer
Urinary tract infection
Small bowel obstruction
IBD
Nephrolithiasis
Pyelonephritis
Ectopic pregnancy
Incarceration
PID

Midepigastric Pain

PUD
Perforated ulcer
Pancreatitis
Abdominal aortic aneurysm
Esophageal varices
Hiatal hernia
Boerhaave syndrome (i.e., rupture
of the esophagus)
Mallory-Weiss tear

The differential diagnosis for an acute abdomen is most appropriately considered by its anatomical location.

IV. Clinical Approach. One of the most important aspects in evaluating an acute abdomen is to first **eliminate the possibility of a surgical emergency** that requires exploration without delay, such as ruptured aortic aneurysm, perforated viscus, ruptured ectopic pregnancy, aortic-enteric fistula, ruptured splenic aneurysm, splenic rupture, ruptured uterus, and ruptured liver hemangioma.

A. History

1. A **thorough history** is the most critical aspect and should include the onset, location, duration (constant, intermittent, postprandial), and intensity (on a scale of 1–10) of the abdominal tenderness.
2. The **quality of the pain** (sharp, dull, colicky, cramping) provides insight into the cause.

   a. Pain that is dull and achy suggests a visceral source (distention).
   b. Pain that is sharp and localized suggests parietal irritation.

3. Other **relevant history** includes the referral pattern of pain, any associated symptoms (e.g., fever, chills, night sweats, anorexia, nausea, vomiting), a change in bowel habits, previous episodes, previous surgery, and relation to meals.
4. A **detailed gynecologic history,** including the timing of the last menstrual period, pregnancy history, and vaginal discharge or dysmenorrhea, should be obtained.
5. A **medication history and assessment of comorbid conditions** should be identified (i.e., pain in the patient with atrial fibrillation or vascular disease) and may suggest mesenteric ischemia.

B. Physical examination. When evaluating a patient with acute abdominal pain, the physical examination is the most important diagnostic tool.

1. **Inspection:** Observe the patient's overall appearance. Note any visual abnormalities such as distention, ascites, ecchymoses, or herniation. A distended abdomen with peristalsis suggests small bowel obstruction.
2. **Auscultation:** The absence of bowel sounds suggests lack of peristalsis, which is frequently seen in peritonitis or prolonged mechanical obstruction. It may also be seen in ileus. High-pitched intermittent bowel sounds are also suggestive of intestinal obstruction.
3. **Percussion:** This frequently confirms the area of maximum tenderness. A hollow tympanitic sound indicates an air collection in the intestine.
4. **Palpation:** The location of tenderness is the key element in examining patients with an acute abdomen. Rebound tenderness, an acute tenderness that occurs when the hand is quickly released from the abdominal wall, is a sign of peritoneal irritation.
5. **Rectal and gynecologic examination:** A rectal examination must be routinely performed on all patients with an acute abdomen. A gynecologic examination must be performed on all female patients presenting with an acute abdomen.
6. **Vascular examination:** Assess for the presence of peripheral pulses and aneurysmal dilatation.

V. Diagnostic Evaluation

A. Laboratory studies are obtained to support a clinical hypothesis. The evaluation generally includes a complete blood count (CBC), liver chemistries, amylase and lipase (see Chapter 24), coagulation profile, urinalysis, and urine pregnancy test.

1. **Lactic acid level** should be obtained on patients with suspected ischemic bowel. An elevated level is associated with tissue hypoperfusion.
2. **Beta-human chorionic gonadotropin (HCG)** levels must be obtained for all women of childbearing age to exclude the possibility of ectopic pregnancy.

B. Radiographic studies

1. **Chest radiograph** should be obtained on all patients with acute abdomen to rule out free air. Pneumonia may present as an acute abdomen.
2. **Abdominal radiograph** is most effective in detecting either bowel obstruction or pneumoperitoneum. An upright and supine view is necessary.

   a. Appendicolith can be seen in 15% of patients with appendicitis, while renal stones may also be visualized up to 85% of the time.
   b. Other radiographic findings of acute appendicitis include right lower quadrant ileus, loss of psoas shadow, deformity of the cecal outline, free air, and soft tissue density.

3. **Abdominal ultrasound** is the study of choice in patients with possible acute cholecystitis or ovarian cyst. A sonographic Murphy's sign is more sensitive than a clinical Murphy's sign for acute cholecystitis. An inflamed appendix can be visualized with compression ultrasound (sensitivity ranges from 80%–90%).
4. **Computed tomography (CT)** can also be used to diagnose appendicitis in patients whose clinical symptoms are ambiguous.

   a. Air in the appendix or a normal-appearing contrast-filled appendix virtually rules out the diagnosis of appendicitis.
   b. CT will give an alternate diagnosis in 15% of patients when assessing for appendicitis.

5. **Arteriography** is the test of choice for patients suspected of mesenteric ischemia.

SUGGESTED READING

Bender JS: Approach to the acute abdomen. *Med Clin North Am* 73(6):1413–1422, 1989.

18

Diarrhea

Richard Lerner

I. **Definition.** Diarrhea is defined as a **stool amount greater than 200 g or an increase in the frequency or fluidity of an individual's normal stools.**

II. **Overview.** Diarrhea can result from any of the following mechanisms:

   A. **Osmosis.** Molecules not normally present in the intestinal lumen increase the osmolality of chyme, drawing water into the lumen (i.e., lactose).

   B. **Secretion.** Substances can cause intestinal cells to secrete sodium and water (i.e., cholera toxin).

   C. **Inflammation** results in denuding of the intestinal lining. This in turn disrupts normal absorption, allowing compounds to leak into the lumen from the lining, which causes increased osmosis.

   D. **Motility.** Hypermotility leads to an increased stool volume. Hypomotility can lead to bacterial overgrowth, which causes diarrhea through several different mechanisms.

   E. **Anal sphincter dysfunction** causes fecal incontinence, which can be interpreted by the patient as diarrhea.

III. **Differential Diagnosis** (Table 18–1)

IV. **Notes on the Differential Diagnosis**

   A. **Laxative abuse** accounts for approximately 15% of all chronic causes. It should be suspected in patients with a mental health disorder.

   B. **Sorbitol** can cause diarrhea. In one study, approximately 17% of people had diarrhea following the ingestion of 4 to 5 mints containing sorbitol.

   C. **Both bile salts and fatty acids** cause secretion of chloride, and thereby water, into the colon. Excess bile salts also lead to a mild degree of fat malabsorption.

   D. **Bacterial overgrowth** can occur secondary to diabetes, blind loop syndrome, amyloidosis, diverticulitis, or scleroderma.

   E. **Irritable bowel syndrome** classically presents with diarrhea alternating with constipation, but it can also occur in a diarrhea-predominant form.

   F. **Gastric surgery syndrome** is secondary to decreased contact time with the luminal surface and decreased digestive juices mixing with the chyme.

   G. **Hyperthyroidism** usually has increased frequency and amount of diarrhea, but not fluidity. Diarrhea is present in approximately 25% of overtly hyperthyroid cases.

   H. **Inflammatory bowel disease** (IBD) [Table 18–2]

      1. **Ulcerative colitis** is a relapsing and remitting disease that leads to acute inflammation of the colorectal mucosa. The rectum is involved in 55% of cases. In severe cases, bloody diarrhea often leads to weight loss, anemia, and electrolyte imbalance.

      2. **Crohn's disease** is a chronic relapsing disorder characterized by transmural, asymmetrical, and segmental inflammation. It typically involves

TABLE 18–1. Differential Diagnosis of Diarrhea

Acute (< 3 weeks):

1. Watery diarrhea indicates a noninflammatory cause (i.e., fecal leukocytes are absent)
   a. Viral: rotavirus, Norwalk virus, adenovirus
   b. Bacterial: *Vibrio cholerae* and *Parahaemolyticus,* toxigenic *Escherichia coli, Bacillus cereus, Staphylococcus aureus, Clostridium perfringens*
   c. Parasitic: *Giardia, Cryptosporidia, Entamoeba histolytica, Cyclospora*
   d. Drugs: Any new drug, particularly laxatives, antibiotics, antacids, NSAIDs
   e. Diet: Alcohol, lactose, sorbitol- or fiber-containing products, caffeine

2. Bloody diarrhea indicates an inflammatory cause (i.e., fecal leukocytes are present)
   a. Bacterial: *Salmonella, Shigella, Campylobacter, Clostridium difficile, Yersinia,* invasive *E. coli, Neisseria gonorrhea*
   b. Parasitic: *Entamoeba histolytica*

Chronic (> 3 weeks):

1. Infection: *Giardia, Entamoeba, Cryptosporidia, Cyclospora.* If the patient is HIV positive, consider also tuberculosis, CMV, *Mycobacterium avium-intracellulare, Microsporidia, and Isospora.*

2. Inflammatory bowel disease (IBD) [see IV H]: Ulcerative colitis, Crohn's disease, and microscopic colitis (collagenous and lymphocytic)

3. Drugs and diet (see IV A, B): Laxative abuse, sorbitol, alcohol, caffeine, fiber

4. Malabsorption (see IV C, D): Small bowel surgery, lactose intolerance (primary or secondary to gastroenteritis), pancreatic insufficiency, bile salts and fatty acids, bacterial overgrowth, sprue, Whipple's disease, infiltrative process (e.g., intestinal lymphoma, scleroderma, amyloidosis)

5. Motility disturbance (see IV E, F): Irritable bowel syndrome, postvagotomy or gastric surgery syndrome, overflow around tumor or impaction

6. Endocrine (see IV G, I, J): Hyperthyroidism, villous adenoma, carcinoid cells, pancreatic cholera (VIPoma), medullary carcinoma of the thyroid, Addison's disease, gastrinoma

CMV = cytomegalovirus; NSAIDs = nonsteroidal anti-inflammatory drugs.

the ileum, colon, or perianal region. Right lower quadrant pain associated with bloody diarrhea is present in as many as 80% of patients.

I. **Neoplasia**

1. Villous adenoma produces prostaglandins, which stimulate chloride and water secretion from the colon.

TABLE 18–2. Ulcerative Colitis and Crohn's Disease

	Ulcerative colitis	Crohn's disease
Distribution	Diffuse inflammation extending from rectum	Skip lesions with rectal sparing
Inflammation	Diffuse and symmetric	Focal and asymmetric
Ulceration	Small, diffuse ulceration	Aphthoid, linear, or serpiginous
Colonic lumen	Often narrow but strictures rare	Strictures common

   2. Serotonin from carcinoid cells stimulates gut motility and increases intestinal secretion.

   3. Tumor-associated calcitonin stimulates gut motility.

   4. Gastrinoma leads to increased gastric acid, which directly causes fluid secretion.

  J. Unclear mechanism. Diarrhea occurs in about 15% of patients with chronic Addison's disease.

V. Clinical Approach

A. History

  1. The duration of symptoms is an important aspect in the assessment of diarrhea.

    a. When symptoms are present less than 3 weeks, infection or adverse effect of a new medication should be suspected.

    b. With persistence of symptoms (> 3 weeks), noninfectious etiologies (except for parasitic illness) become more likely. Even parasites, except for *Entamoeba*, rarely cause diarrhea beyond 3 months.

  2. Pertinent history for acute diarrhea

    a. Fever or bloody stool: More likely to be an invasive organism or IBD

    b. Size and number of stools

      (1) Large volume, small number: Small bowel infection (e.g., *Vibrio cholerae*, toxigenic *Escherichia coli*, *Giardia*)

      (2) Small volume, large number: Large bowel infection (e.g., *Shigella*, *Salmonella*, *Campylobacter*)

    c. Mucus: Small amount more likely indicates irritable bowel; large amount is usually from an invasive organism

    d. Nausea and vomiting: More likely a viral infection, food-borne bacteria, or *Giardia*

    e. Travel: If causative, diarrhea usually starts in the country

(1) Mexico: toxigenic *E. coli* (40% of traveler's diarrhea), *Salmonella*, *Giardia*

(2) Russia: *Giardia*, cryptosporidiosis

(3) Japan: *Vibrio parahaemolyticus*

(4) Southeast Asia and Africa: *Entamoeba* and toxigenic *E. coli*

f. **Domestic animal exposure:** *Campylobacter jejuni, Salmonella*

g. **Drugs and diet:** Recent antibiotics, new medications, dairy products, diet products with sorbitol, antacids with magnesium, caffeine, ethanol

h. **Food types:** Poultry—*Salmonella*; protein product (e.g., ham or salami)—*Staphylococcus aureus* enterotoxin; fried rice—*Bacillus cereus*; contaminated water—*Shigella* or *Giardia*; spoiled milk or dairy—*Staphylococcus, Shigella, Salmonella, C. jejuni, Yersinia*; shellfish—*V. parahaemolyticus, Salmonella*; hamburger meat—*E. coli*; pork—*Yersinia*; berries—*Cyclospora*

i. **Other risk factors**

(1) **Homosexual contact:** *Giardia, Neisseria gonorrhea*, proctitis, *Shigella*

(2) **HIV:** *Cryptosporidiosis, Isospora, Microsporidia*, cytomegalovirus (CMV), *Mycobacterium avium-intracellulare*, tuberculosis

(3) **Day care center:** *Giardia, Cryptosporidia, Shigella*

3. **Pertinent history for chronic diarrhea**

a. **Weight loss:** May indicate an organic process or laxative abuse with anorexia

b. **Alternating diarrhea and constipation:** Often irritable bowel syndrome

c. **Floating stools:** Carbohydrate malabsorption

d. **Greasy, malodorous stools:** Steatorrhea suggestive of malabsorption

e. **Psychiatric history:** Check for laxative abuse

f. **Surgical history:** Gastrectomy and occasionally a vagotomy leads to a dumping syndrome; ileal resection; cholecystectomy

g. **Endocrinopathies:** Assess for symptoms of thyroid, carcinoid, or gastrinoma

h. **Stool on the underwear:** Anal sphincter dysfunction

B. **Physical examination**

1. **Acute diarrhea:** Assess for the following signs and symptoms:

a. Fever

b. Dehydration (e.g., orthostatic hypotension, dry mucous membranes)

c. Abdominal tenderness (isolated left lower quadrant pain suggests large bowel colitis, whereas periumbilical or diffuse pain suggests small bowel involvement)

d. Guarding or rebound

e. Stool for occult or gross blood (rectal examination for occult blood is probably not helpful in mild cases)

2. **Chronic diarrhea:** In addition to the signs and symptoms for acute diarrhea, perform the following:

a. Document weight loss

   b. Examine the thyroid (diffuse goiter or nodule may indicate medullary cancer)

   c. Check for stigmata of bulimia (e.g., poor dentition)

   d. Check the skin for flushing (carcinoid) and hyperpigmentation (Addison's disease, gastrinoma)

   e. Check for stigmata of liver disease (e.g., chronic pancreatitis or insufficiency secondary to chronic alcoholism)

VI. Diagnostic Evaluation

A. Outpatient evaluation

1. Stool cultures

   a. Only one specimen is necessary, unless there is suspicion for *Shigella* (recent travel, bloody diarrhea).

   b. Stool cultures at a hospital lab routinely check for *Salmonella* and *Shigella.*

   c. If suspicious, the clinician will need to specifically order tests for *E. coli, Campylobacter, Vibrio,* and *Yersinia.*

2. Ova and parasite (O&P) wet mount on fresh specimens

   a. There should be three samples, but if the case is very suspicious, six samples may be needed.

   b. The test has a 75%–85% sensitivity.

   c. If *Cryptosporidia, Microsporidia, Isospora,* and *Cyclospora* are suspected, the clinician must specifically request additional samples.

3. Fecal leukocytes

   a. The sensitivity and specificity of fecal leukocytes for predicting a positive *Clostridium difficile* toxin are 28% and 92%, respectively.

   b. For toxigenic-producing strains of *E. coli,* viral agents, *Giardia, Entamoeba,* and *Vibrio,* fecal leukocytes are virtually always negative.

   c. The range of sensitivity is as high as 70% for *Shigella* and 35%–90% for *Salmonella* and *Campylobacter.*

4. *Giardia* antigen detection. One stool specimen yields a 92%–95% sensitivity and a 96%–100% specificity.

5. *C. difficile* toxin. Test yields an 85%–95% sensitivity and a 99% specificity.

6. Endoscopic study

   a. Lower endoscopy: One series has a 20% yield in identifying a pathologic diagnosis. In non-HIV infected patients, the role of sigmoidoscopy versus colonoscopy is unclear. When clinically suspected, even if no gross abnormalities are noted, consider doing blind biopsies looking for lymphocytic and collagenous colitis. The yield of biopsy with no gross abnormalities ranges from 6%–42%.

   b. Upper endoscopy is useful for making the diagnosis of sprue, Whipple's disease, and other small bowel infiltrative processes.

7. Radiologic. An upper gastrointestinal series with small bowel follow-through is most commonly used when evaluating for Crohn's disease.

Enteroclysis is superior, with 100% sensitivity and 98% specificity for small bowel involvement with Crohn's disease.

8. **Nutrition indices.** Complete blood count (CBC), albumin, and potassium (sensitivity of hypokalemia is 100% for pancreatic cholera or VIPoma) are routine studies in the evaluation of chronic diarrhea.

9. **Stool for "cathartic laxative screen."** This test checks for bisacodyl, senna, castor and mineral oils, phenolphthalein (taken off the market), and danthron.

10. **Stool for osmolality gap.** The osmolality gap is calculated by the following formula:

$$290 - 2 \text{ (stool Na + K)}$$

The accuracy is fair in distinguishing between **osmotic (if gap is < 50)** and **secretory (if gap is > 50)** diarrhea.

11. **Stool for pH.** For carbohydrate intolerance (e.g., lactose or sorbitol), one small study found the pH < 5.6. For bile acid-induced diarrhea, the pH is usually over 6.8.

12. **Stool for fecal fat.** This test is used to detect steatorrhea on the basis of malabsorption.

   a. **Qualitative:** Sensitivity is 97%–100%, but the specificity varies from 56%–86%.

   b. **Quantitative:** Based upon a 72-hr collection, the patient should be on a 75- to 100-g fat diet. A nutritional consult is advised to maximize compliance.

13. **Hormonal studies.** Thyroid-stimulating hormone (TSH), fasting serum gastrin level, calcitonin level, and 24-hr urine collection for 5-hydroxyindoleacetic acid (5-HIAA) are recommended.

14. **D-Xylose testing.** This tests for small bowel malabsorption syndromes (e.g., sprue, Crohn's disease, amyloidosis). Twenty-five g of D-xylose are administered. A 5-hr urine collection and a 1-hr serum sample are obtained. A decreased amount of D-xylose in the urine and serum indicates small bowel malabsorption. The test has a 95% sensitivity and specificity for malabsorption. The sensitivity of the test is decreased in the following situations: creatinine clearance of less than 30 mg/dl, portal hypertension, ascites, delayed gastric emptying, fiber supplements, glucose load, aspirin, and glipizide.

15. **Bentiromide** (to test for pancreatic exocrine insufficiency). N-benzoyl-L-tyrosyl para-aminobenzoic acid (NBT PABA) is administered orally. The molecule is cleaved by chymotrypsin, PABA is absorbed, and then measured in a 6-hr urine collection. PABA alone is a somewhat inaccurate measure, so additional markers have been used to increase the accuracy.

B. **Serum immune markers:** There are several serum immune markers performed by enzyme-linked immunosorbent assays (ELISAs), which have been found to be valuable for the diagnosis, stratification, and management of IBD.

   a. **Deoxyribonuclease (DNAse)-sensitive perinuclear anti-neutrophilic cytoplasmic antibody (P-ANCA)** is positive in 60%–80% of adults with ulcerative colitis, and in 83% of children with ulcerative colitis. P-ANCA is positive in 10% of patients with Crohn's disease.

    b. Anti-Saccharomyces cervisiae antibody (ASCA) is present in 70% of patients with Crohn's disease.

    c. Pancreatic antibody may be positive in 30%–40% of patients with Crohn's disease.

    d. Outer membrane porin from _E. coli_ (OmpC) antibody: An immunoglobulin A (IgA) response to OmpC is seen in 55% of patients with Crohn's disease.

C. An **inpatient evaluation** of chronic diarrhea is justifiable when weight loss, malnutrition, or dehydration is present.

    1. Determine secretory versus osmotic diarrhea.

    2. Measure weight of stool for 24 hours.

    3. Check fecal fat for 72 hours.

    4. Observe for laxative abuse.

SUGGESTED READING

Donowitz M, Kokke F, Saidi R: Evaluation of patients with chronic diarrhea. _N Engl J Med_ 332:725–729, 1995.

Stotland RB, Stein BR, Lichtenstein RG: Advances in inflammatory bowel disease. _Med Clin North Am_ 84:291–295, 2000.

19

Dyspepsia and Peptic Ulcer Disease

Gertrude Manchester

I. **Definition.** Dyspepsia encompasses any or all of a great variety of **upper abdominal symptoms,** including upper abdominal pain or discomfort, nausea, bloating, heartburn, early satiety, regurgitation, and belching.

II. **Overview**

    A. **Peptic ulcer disease (PUD).** Epigastric abdominal pain is the most common symptom. Pain is nonradiating and is described as a "gnawing" or "hunger pain." Pain occurs 1–2 hours postprandially and is relieved characteristically by food or antacids.

        1. **Nocturnal pain** is more specific for PUD and is due to the physiologic increase in acid secretion, which occurs in the early morning hours.

        2. **Asymptomatic**

            a. Patients with **PUD induced by nonsteroidal anti-inflammatory drugs** (NSAIDs) are frequently asymptomatic.

            b. As many as 60% of patients who develop **bleeding** as a complication of PUD are also asymptomatic.

    B. **Nonulcerative dyspepsia** is defined as persistent or recurrent abdominal pain or discomfort centered in the upper abdomen without definite structural or biochemical explanation. By definition, nonulcerative dyspepsia is a diagnosis of exclusion. Possible mechanisms include dysmotility of the stomach or small intestine, heightened visceral sensitivity, altered intestinal or gastric reflexes, and psychological distress.

    C. **Dyspepsia** is typically a chronic relapsing condition. Between 65% and 86% of patients with dyspepsia will experience dyspeptic symptoms, at least intermittently, 2 to 3 years after the initial presentation. Long duration of symptoms and intermittent symptoms can also occur in PUD and esophagitis; therefore, these characteristics are not reassuring as to the absence of pathology.

    D. **Gastroesophageal reflux disease (GERD)** and dyspepsia have similar symptoms. Gastroesophageal reflux is a normal physiologic process that occurs daily in all individuals. GERD (expressed clinically as heartburn) occurs when symptoms or tissue injury develop due to the reflux of gastric contents into the esophagus.

    E. ***Helicobacter pylori* infection** is clearly implicated in the etiology of recurrent PUD, yet its role in nonulcerative dyspepsia remains unclear. Between 30% and 60% of patients with nonulcerative dyspepsia have *H. pylori*. However, the background prevalence in the general population is also high.

III. **Differential Diagnosis** (Table 19–1)

IV. **Clinical Approach**

TABLE 19–1. Differential Diagnosis of Dyspepsia

Structural disease involving the stomach or esophagus

Peptic ulcer disease (PUD) [15%–25% of cases]
Reflux esophagitis (5%–15% of cases)
Gastric or esophageal cancer (less than 2% of cases)
Infiltrative disease
Eosinophilic gastritis
Crohn's disease
Sarcoidosis

Other gastrointestinal-related disease

Gallstones
Chronic pancreatitis or pancreatic cancer
Celiac disease
Lactose intolerance
Hepatoma

Medications

Nonsteroidal anti-inflammatory drugs (NSAIDs)
Digitalis
Theophylline
Erythromycin
Alcohol
Caffeine
Nicotine

Other possible causes

Hypothyroidism
Hypercalcemia
Intestinal angina
Pregnancy
Nonulcerative dyspepsia*

***Nonulcerative dyspepsia** occurs in as many as 60% of cases, but the diagnosis requires the exclusion of other diagnostic entities.

 A. History. Even seasoned clinicians achieve diagnostic accuracy of no more than 50% from history alone.

  1. The major focus of history taking is to elicit **red flag symptoms** that suggest a high probability of organic disease. The presence of any of these symptoms would indicate the need for further testing rather than empiric therapy. Indicators of probable organic cause include:

   a. Nocturnal pain
   b. Constant or severe pain

    c. Severe heartburn
    d. Severe regurgitation
    e. Unintended weight loss
    f. Pain relieved by food
    g. Dysphagia
    h. Pain that radiates to the back
    i. Recurrent vomiting
    j. Hematemesis
    k. Melena
    l. Age greater than 45 years

2. History should also include attention to **medications** and temporal relationship to symptoms. It is particularly important to assess NSAID use, including over-the-counter preparations. Alcohol intake, caffeine intake, and smoking behavior should also be assessed.
3. Dyspepsia may be a presenting symptom in **pregnancy** and should be considered in women of child-bearing age.
4. Attention should be focused on **psychosocial stressors,** given the strong correlation of psychosocial stress and nonspecific gastrointestinal symptoms.

B. Physical examination

1. **Vital signs and orthostatics** should be evaluated, particularly if history suggests gastrointestinal bleeding.
2. **Skin examination:** Assess for jaundice and stigmata of chronic liver disease.
3. **Thyroid examination:** Goiter might suggest hypothyroidism.
4. **Abdominal and pelvic examination:** Assess for organomegaly, distension, tenderness, and mass.
5. **Stool guaiac:** Assess for occult bleeding.

V. Diagnostic Testing

A. **Laboratory investigation** may not be necessary in young patients (< 45 years of age) who have a normal examination and no indicators for organic disease.
B. **In older patients and those with red flags,** the minimal lab workup should include a complete blood count (CBC), electrolytes, calcium, and liver chemistries.
C. **Thyroid tests, human chorionic gonadotropin (HCG), amylase, and stool studies** should be ordered if specific features of the history or examination are suggestive.
D. **Additional studies**

1. **Upper endoscopy [i.e., esophagogastroduodenoscopy (EGD)]:** In the majority of cases, this is the study of first choice when further evaluation of dyspepsia is required, including the ability to obtain biopsies. As many as two-thirds of endoscopies are completely normal in younger patients (i.e., < 45 years of age). Thus, it is best applied to older patients and to younger patients with red flag symptoms.
2. **Upper gastrointestinal radiography:** This test is less accurate than upper endoscopy and cannot provide tissue diagnosis. It is best reserved

for situations where endoscopy expertise is unavailable, for patients who refuse endoscopy or have low pretest probability of disease, and in situations where endoscopy might be considered unsafe.

3. *Helicobacter pylori* **testing**

   a. **Serology** is the most commonly used diagnostic test. This assay indicates past or current infection with *H. pylori*. Note that it remains positive even after effective eradication therapy, and thus cannot be used as a test of cure.

   b. **Urea breath test:** It is most commonly used in the research setting to confirm that *H. pylori* has been eradicated by treatment.

   c. **Rapid urease test:** This test requires endoscopic tissue sampling.

   d. **Histologic evaluation:** Histologic detection of *H. pylori* requires gastric tissue specimens and specific staining procedures. It may be most useful where extensive gastric atrophy or recent medication use compromise the ability to detect *H. pylori* by other means.

   e. **Culture of *H. pylori* from gastric tissue:** This approach is tedious, labor-intensive, and expensive.

4. **Gastric emptying studies:** Gastric scintigraphy and gastroduodenal manometry studies generally do not influence medical management and are reserved for patients with normal lab tests and a normal EGD, yet who continue to have frequent or protracted vomiting suggestive of a motility disorder. Even in these cases, empiric treatment with prokinetic agents should probably be tried first.

SUGGESTED READING

American Gastroenterological Association Clinical Practice and Practice Economics Committee: American Gastroenterological Association medical position statement: Evaluation of dyspepsia. *Gastroenterology* 114:579–581, 1998.

Talley NJ, Vakil N, Ballard D, Fennerty B: Absence of benefit of eradicating *Helicobacter pylori* in patients with nonulcer dyspepsia. *N Engl J Med* 341:1106–1111, 1999.

20

Jaundice
Howard Sachs

I. **Definition.** Jaundice is a **yellowish staining of the integument, sclerae, deeper tissues, and excretions with bile pigments, which are increased in the plasma.**

II. **Overview**

   A. **Physiology**

   1. **Serum bilirubin** accumulated when its production from heme exceeds its metabolism and excretion.

   2. An **imbalance between the production and clearance of serum bilirubin** results either from excess release of bilirubin precursors into the bloodstream, or from physiologic processes that impair the hepatic uptake, metabolism, or excretion of this metabolite.

   3. Jaundice is **clinically detectable** when the serum bilirubin exceeds 2.0–2.5 mg/dl. Because elastin has a high affinity for bilirubin, and scleral tissue is rich in elastin, scleral icterus is usually a more sensitive sign than generalized jaundice.

   B. **Bilirubin metabolism**

   1. **Unconjugated bilirubin.** More than 90% of serum bilirubin in normal individuals is in an unconjugated form, circulating as an albumin-bound complex. This is not filtered by the kidneys.

   2. **Conjugated bilirubin.** The remainder is conjugated (primarily as a glucuronide), rendering it water soluble, and thus capable of being filtered and excreted by the kidney.

   3. **Hepatic phase.** Hepatic metabolism has three phases: uptake, conjugation, and excretion.

      a. **Uptake phase:** Unconjugated bilirubin is bound to albumin and is presented to the hepatocyte, where the complex dissociates and bilirubin enters the cell either by diffusion or transport across the membrane.

      b. **Conjugation phase:** Bilirubin is then conjugated in a two-step process. This occurs in the endoplasmic reticulum and is catalyzed by glucuronyl transferase. Bilirubin glucuronide is generated.

      c. **Excretion phase:** In an energy-dependent process occurring in the biliary canaliculi, conjugated bilirubin is excreted into the bile. **It is important to remember that this is the rate-limiting step.** When this phase is impaired, either through obstruction or excretory defects, the conjugated bilirubin is presumed to reflux through the hepatic sinusoids into the bloodstream.

   4. **Intestinal phase.** After excretion into the bile, conjugated bile is transported into the duodenum. It is not reabsorbed by intestinal mucosa. In the intestine, it is either excreted in the feces unchanged or

metabolized by intestinal bacteria to urobilinogen. Urobilinogen is then reabsorbed where a small portion is metabolized in the liver, and the remainder bypasses the liver and is excreted by the kidney.

III. Differential Diagnosis (Table 20–1)
IV. Notes on the Differential Diagnosis

A. **Extrahepatic biliary obstruction**

1. **The history, physical examination, and initial laboratory assessment** have a sensitivity of 90%–95%. The specificity, however, is only 76%. When radiologic imaging is factored in, the specificity rises to 98%.
2. Approximately 40% of patients with this diagnosis present with jaundice.
3. In the setting of **complete obstruction,** acholic stools are seen and no urobilinogen is detected in the urine (given the dependence upon enterohepatic circulation).
4. In patients with extrahepatic biliary obstruction, **alkaline phosphatase** would be expected to rise to levels 2 to 3 times normal. A normal level would be uncommon. Serum transaminases would generally be less than 300 U/L.

B. **Intrahepatic cholestasis.** Consider intrahepatic etiologies in the differential diagnosis because high levels may be seen in patients with primary biliary cirrhosis and granulomatous hepatitis.

1. **This group of disorders is defined by the lack of evidence of mechanical obstruction and cannot be explained on the basis of hepatocellular injury alone.** Among these disorders are those characterized by disordered enzyme function (intrinsic/acquired), infiltrative disorders, and drugs.
2. **A diagnosis of intrahepatic cholestasis made by clinical assessment and supported by negative findings from ultrasound or computed tomography (CT) scan offers 95% specificity.** In a patient in whom extrahepatic obstruction is not strongly suspected, no further investigation of the extrahepatic biliary tree is indicated.

V. **Clinical Approach.** The combination of history and physical examination is useful in directing the initial evaluation.

A. **History**

1. **Seek risk factors for hepatitis and cirrhosis**

a. Drug use [i.e., prescribed or over-the-counter (OTC)]
b. Toxin exposures (alcohol, androgens)
c. Viral exposures (intravenous drug abuse, tattoos, sexual promiscuity, transfusion, travel from endemic areas)

2. **Inquire about changes in stool and urine characteristics**

a. **Stool changes include:**

(1) Acholic (clay-colored) if there is complete biliary obstruction (no conjugated bilirubin entering the intestine)

TABLE 20–1. Differential Diagnosis of Jaundice

1. Unconjugated hyperbilirubinemia
   - Hemolysis
   - Gilbert's syndrome
   - Ineffective erythropoiesis
   - Hematoma resorption

2. Conjugated hyperbilirubinemia
   A. Extrahepatic biliary obstruction
   - Choledocholithiasis
   - Ascending cholangitis
   - Pancreatitis
   - Sclerosing cholangitis
   - HIV cholangiopathy
   - Biliary stricture or cyst
   - Malignancy
     - Pancreas
     - Ampullary carcinoma
     - Cholangiocarcinoma
     - Metastatic
   B. Intrahepatic cholestasis
   - Abscess
   - Tumor
   - Primary biliary cirrhosis
   - Cholestatic jaundice of pregnancy
   - Dubin-Johnson syndrome
   - Rotor's syndrome
   - Benign recurrent intrahepatic cholestasis
   - Sepsis
   - Infiltrative disease
     - Sarcoid
     - Amyloid
   C. Hepatocellular jaundice
   - Hepatitis virus
   - Toxin or drugs (alcohol)
   - Cirrhosis
   - Ischemia

---

    (2) Silver stools (hemoccult-positive and biliary obstruction at the ampulla of Vater)

  b. Urinary pigment changes include:

    (1) No change, suggesting no reflux into serum of conjugated bilirubin (hemolysis, advanced hepatocellular disease)

    (2) Darkening of color suggests reflux of conjugated bilirubin (compatible with, but not diagnostic of, obstructive causes)

3. **Other clinical clues** are sought, which are related to stigmata of liver disease, the presence of hyperbilirubinemia, and associated with the underlying etiologies. These clues include:

   a. Pruritus (in primary biliary cirrhosis, bile salt deposition)
   b. Pain (obstruction)
   c. Fever (cholangitis, abscess)
   d. Weight loss (malignancy)
   e. Prior biliary surgery (recurrent stone, stricture)

B. Physical examination

1. Identify stigmata of chronic liver disease by looking for signs of

   a. Spider angiomata
   b. Palmar erythema
   c. Gynecomastia
   d. Testicular atrophy

2. Seek evidence of portal hypertension (venous congestion, spleno-megaly) and coagulopathy (bruising, bleeding, petechiae), and note characteristics of the liver examination (e.g., the size, texture, bruit/rub, nodularity).

3. Suspect an obstructive or infectious process when pain and fever are present.

4. Identify a primary or metastatic source in patients with asymptomatic jaundice (as neoplasm is a common etiology).

   a. Hemoccult-positive stool suggests a primary gastrointestinal tract tumor.
   b. A palpable, nontender gallbladder suggests the presence of a tumor (e.g., cholangiocarcinoma or adenocarcinoma of the ampulla of Vater or pancreatic head).

5. Look for the presence of scleral icterus, as this is a **key point** in distin-guishing jaundice from hypercarotenemia. Carotene does not deposit in the sclera.

VI. Diagnostic Evaluation (see Appendix A for Jaundice algorithm)

   A. Laboratory evaluation. These studies are of proven benefit in determining the proximate etiologies in the patient presenting with jaundice. With this approach, the clinician can confidently assign probabilities to the major categories that most frequently account for jaundice.

   1. The first step is to determine the **total bilirubin** and the **bilirubin fractions.** This allows the clinician to determine whether the prob-lem is due to excess production or impaired conjugation (indirect/unconjugated predominant) versus impaired excretion (direct/conjugated predominant).

   2. **Alkaline phosphatase elevations** out of proportion to the hepatic transaminases would favor extra- or intrahepatic cholestasis.

   3. **Hepatic transaminase elevations** out of proportion to the alkaline phosphatase favor hepatocellular etiologies.

   4. The **complete blood count** (CBC) can be extremely useful. The most important points include the interpretation of or for:

   a. Anemia (hemolysis, bleeding)
   b. Mean corpuscular volume (microcytosis suggests iron deficiency; round macrocytosis suggests chronic liver disease or ineffective erythropoiesis; gastrointestinal malignancy)
   c. Thrombocytopenia [sequestration in portal hypertension, sepsis, autoimmune disease, bone marrow suppression (alcohol)]
   d. Reticulocytosis (hemolysis)

5. **Urinalysis** provides information about bilirubinuria and urobilinogen. In reality, data from urinalysis adds little incremental benefit to the decision-making process.

   a. The presence of urobilinogen eliminates the possibility of complete biliary tract obstruction. That is, bile has entered the intestine, where it undergoes enterohepatic metabolism.
   b. The presence of bilirubinuria, on the other hand, suggests that conjugation is taking place.

6. **Coagulation studies** are useful in two areas.

   a. If an invasive intervention is considered, coagulation studies can be used to assess bleeding risk.
   b. If the prothrombin time is prolonged and other causes of coagulopathy are unlikely, chronic liver disease or hepatocellular etiologies become increasingly likely.

7. **Serum amylase** would be obtained in cases where extrahepatic obstruction is suspected on the basis of history and physical examination.

B. **Diagnostic imaging.** It is estimated that 25%–40% of common bile duct obstructions are missed by both ultrasound and CT scanning. However, when intrahepatic cholestasis or hepatocellular etiologies are suspected, then either of these noninvasive strategies is acceptable.

1. **Ultrasound:** This is the least invasive and lowest cost of the imaging procedures available to assess obstructive jaundice. Ultrasound determines the presence of obstructive jaundice by detecting dilated bile ducts.

   a. The sensitivity is 55%–93%, and the specificity is 71%–96%.
   b. False negatives are generally due to two factors:

      (1) Inability to visualize the biliary tree (often secondary to inter-posed bowel gas)
      (2) Absence of biliary dilatation in the presence of obstruction.

   c. Ultrasonography may be preferable, given its lower cost and radiation exposure.

2. **CT scanning** is slightly more sensitive (74%–96%) and specific (90%–94%) than ultrasound in detecting the presence of biliary obstruction.

   a. A CT scan is more likely to show the site and cause of obstruction when compared to ultrasound.
   b. CT also gives information in instances where staging a suspected neoplasm has clinical significance.

c. In patients where mass lesions (i.e., malignancy, abscess) are suspected or where technical limitations make ultrasound difficult to interpret, CT is preferred.

3. **Percutaneous transhepatic cholangiography (PTC):** The technical success rate of this procedure is approximately 90%–99%. Its use is limited by a major complication rate of 3%–5% and has been largely supplanted by endoscopic retrograde cholangiopancreatography (ERCP).

4. **ERCP** offers a lower complication rate than PTC and provides a greater number of therapeutic options (stone extraction, stent placement).

   a. This test could reasonably be used in patients with a high likelihood of extrahepatic obstruction (e.g., those who have had recent biliary surgery, symptoms of cholangitis, palpable gallbladder, pain or fever, pancreatitis).

   b. When palliation is the primary intent, ERCP is an appropriate initial procedure.

5. **Magnetic resonance cholangiopancreatography (MRCP)** is a radiologic technique that produces images of the pancreaticobiliary tree, which are similar in appearance to those obtained by invasive methods. It appears to have similar diagnostic accuracy to ERCP.

   a. MRCP is indicated for patients with allergies to iodinated contrast media, patients who have undergone unsuccessful ERCP (3%–10%), and patients with altered anatomy (i.e., secondary to surgical procedures or congenital abnormalities).

   b. ERCP has advantages over MRCP, which include the ability to perform therapeutic interventions, perform manometry or endoscopic ultrasound, directly visualize the ampulla, and biopsy lesions.

SUGGESTED READING

Scharschmid B, Goldberg H, Schmid R: Approach to the patient with cholestatic jaundice. *N Engl J Med* 308:1515–1518, 1983.
Siegel J, Yatto R: Approach to cholestasis. *Arch Intern Med* 142:1877–1879, 1982.

21

Ascites

Aftab Mohsin

I. **Definition.** Ascites is a **collection of free fluid in the peritoneal cavity.**
II. **Overview**

- A. **Chronic liver disease** (infectious hepatitis and alcoholism) causes 80% of cases of ascites.
- B. **Multiple causes,** including cirrhosis, peritoneal carcinomatosis, or tuberculous peritonitis, are responsible for 5% of cases.
- C. **Carcinomatosis** causes less than 10% of cases of ascites.
- D. **Heart failure** is responsible for less than 5% of cases, and **nephrotic syndrome** is a rare cause of ascites.
- E. **Cryptogenic cirrhosis** may account for as many as 10% of cases.

III. **Classification.** A list of causes of ascites is described in Figure 21–1. Ascites is currently classified as high gradient or low gradient, depending on the serum ascites albumin gradient (SAAG). Calculation of SAAG involves **the difference (not the ratio)** between serum values and ascitic fluid values.

- A. **High-gradient ascites** results from portal hypertension, whether cirrhotic or noncirrhotic. Nephrotic syndrome is an **exception** and will usually cause low-gradient ascites due to marked hypoalbuminemia.
- B. **Low-gradient ascites** usually occurs as the result of cardiac failure, malignant carcinomatosis of the peritoneum, infections (such as tuberculosis), perforation of the bowel, connective tissue diseases, and chemical inflammation as in pancreatitis.

IV. **Clinical Approach**

A. **History**

1. **Painless abdominal distention** is a common finding.
2. **Recent weight gain, increase in abdominal girth, and ankle edema** all increase the likelihood of finding ascites.
3. **Painful swelling** is associated with malignancy, tuberculosis, spontaneous bacterial peritonitis, pancreatitis, or other causes of acute abdomen (see Chapter 17).
4. **Dyspnea with orthopnea and dependent edema** in the setting of ascites favors congestive heart failure (CHF) as its etiology.
5. **History of alcohol intake, blood transfusions, high-risk sexual behavior, intravenous drug abuse, tattooing, ear piercing, and intake of any drug,** including alternative medicines, should be sought.

B. **Physical examination**

1. Note the presence of bulging flanks (81% sensitive; 59% specific), shifting dullness (77%/72%), and fluid wave (62%/90%).
2. Check for **lymphadenopathy.**

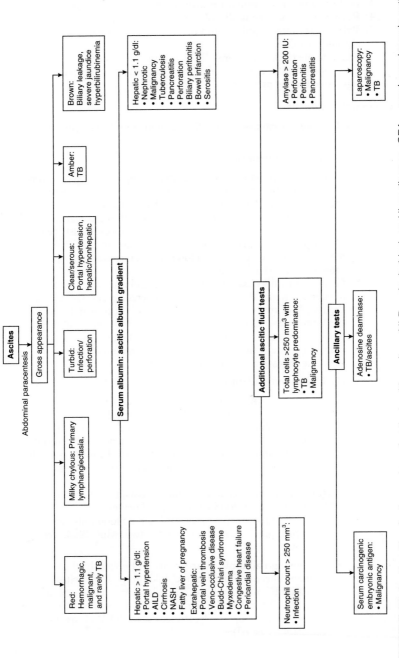

FIGURE 21–1. Algorithm for the workup of patients with ascites. *AILD* = alcohol-induced liver disease; *CEA* = carcinoembryonic antigen; *NASH* = nonalcoholic steatohepatitis; *TB* = tuberculosis; *TNC* = total neutrophil count.

3. Perform a **pelvic examination** with attention to the ovaries.

4. **Periumbilical and flank discoloration** suggests acute pancreatitis.

5. **Palmar erythema, spiders, and distended abdominal veins** favor chronic liver disease.

6. Examine the **neck veins** carefully. The presence of jugular venous distention (JVD) is crucial in identifying a cardiac etiology, denoting right-sided filling pressures.

V. Diagnostic Evaluation

A. Laboratory investigations. Ascitic fluid examination is the principle diagnostic tool.

1. Ascitic fluid examination

    a. Transparent to pale fluid is seen in cases of portal hypertension. Neutrophilia in excess of 1000/ml results in opalescence. Red blood cells in excess of 10,000/ml will give a faint pink tinge, and cell counts greater than 20,000/ml will color it red. A traumatic tap will be evident by a streak of blood rather than homogeneously red fluid and the tendency to clot. Hepatocellular carcinoma and, rarely, metastatic disease can cause a bloody tap. Tuberculosis is only a rare cause of hemorrhagic ascites.

    b. Chylous or milky ascites is rarely seen and is usually an indication of cirrhosis rather than lymphoma or tuberculosis as was previously thought. The triglycerides are > 1000 mg/dl in truly milky ascites. Dark-brown ascites may be seen in significant hyperbilirubinemia, biliary perforation (when ascitic bilirubin is higher than serum bilirubin), pancreatitis, and, rarely, in malignant melanoma.

    c. Baseline investigations in ascitic fluid

        (1) Cell count and differential

            (a) In **uncomplicated cirrhosis,** the total white blood cell count is less than 500 cells/ml with less than 250 neutrophils/ml. After diuresis, the total cell count may go up, but the neutrophil count remains below 250 cells/ml.

            (b) In **spontaneous bacterial peritonitis,** the total white blood cell count and neutrophil count are usually but not always raised.

            (c) In **tuberculosis and carcinomatosis,** the cell count rises but with a predominance of lymphocytes.

            (d) In **traumatic taps,** for every 250 red blood cells, one neutrophil is subtracted from the total white blood cell count.

        (2) Protein and albumin concentration: Previously, the total protein concentration of ascitic fluid categorized ascites into exudative (ascitic protein > 2.5 g/dl) or transudative (ascitic protein < 2.5 g/dl). The significance of this was never evaluated adequately and objectively. Presently, the SAAG is used for calculation (see III).

(3) **Culture of ascitic fluid:** Bedside inoculation of ascitic fluid in blood culture bottles has increased the positive bacterial yield to 80%, and it is now the recommended method. It must be interpreted in concert with the cell count.

(4) **Glucose:** The serum and ascitic fluid concentrations are nearly the same in uncomplicated portal hypertension. Large numbers of white blood cells, bacteria, or tumor cells consume glucose and may lead to diminished levels.

(5) **Amylase:** In pancreatitis and gut perforation, the amylase values may be about 3 to 5 times higher than the serum values.

(6) **Lactate dehydrogenase levels** rise because of release of lactate dehydrogenase from the neutrophils. The rise occurs in cases of secondary peritonitis, tuberculosis, and pancreatitis.

(7) **Gram staining** is of low yield. Even with **centrifugation**, it has 10% sensitivity in spontaneous bacterial peritonitis.

(8) **Acid-fast bacilli staining:** Culture and smear for tuberculosis have very low sensitivity. In an appropriate clinical setting of low-grade fever, malaise, and weight loss, a high cell count with lymphocytic predominance and low SAAG is suggestive of tuberculous ascites.

2. **Cytology** has limitations in the diagnosis of malignant ascites and has been replaced largely by laparoscopic examination of the peritoneum along with biopsy and culture.

B. **Ultrasonography** is useful for detecting the presence of ascites as well as for determining the etiology. It may reveal evidence of chronic liver disease, malignancy, hepatomegaly, and pancreatic disorder.

VI. Special Considerations

A. **Errors** may occur if serum albumin is very low or when serum and ascitic samples are not obtained within a short span of time from each other.

B. A high globulin level in serum may also give a **false result.**

SUGGESTED READING

Reynold, TB: Clinics in liver. *Disease* 4(1):151–168, 2000.

22

Hepatomegaly
Khoa Do

I. **Definition.** Hepatomegaly refers to **an enlarged liver with a vertical span greater than 12 cm as percussed in the midclavicular line.** Studies have suggested that by ultrasound, a midhepatic (sagittal) diameter greater than 15.5 cm indicates hepatomegaly in 75% of the cases. By radioisotope scanning, a span of greater than 15–17 cm in the midclavicular line indicates hepatomegaly.
II. **Overview.** Hepatomegaly may occur in the absence of pathology (i.e., normal variant), or as a result of a depressed right hemidiaphragm, Riedel's lobe, or subdiaphragmatic space occupying lesions.
III. **Differential Diagnosis.** The causes of hepatomegaly can be subdivided into processes involving (see Fig. 22–1):

A. Hypertrophy or hyperplasia of cells intrinsic to the normal liver parenchyma
B. Hepatomegaly secondary to infiltration of the liver by cells or organisms not normally present
C. Vascular causes resulting in congestion of the liver

IV. **Notes on the Differential Diagnosis** (Fig. 22–1)

A. **Common causes.** Fatty liver (NASH) is a common cause of hepatomegaly. The most common cause of fatty liver in the United States is chronic alcoholism. Other causes of fatty liver include diabetes, obesity, protein malnutrition, and prolonged total parenteral nutrition (TPN).
B. **Other causes.** In addition to infectious and drug-related causes, clinically important causes of hepatomegaly include hemochromatosis, α_1-antitrypsin deficiency, Wilson's disease, autoimmune hepatitis, systemic lupus erythematosus, and rheumatoid arthritis.
C. **Cholangiohepatitis** is a rare disorder in which intra- and extrahepatic bile ducts become obstructed with bile stones, leading to secondary inflammation of the liver.
D. **Congestion from heart failure** includes all causes of elevated right heart pressures (e.g., cor pulmonale, tricuspid regurgitation, constrictive pericarditis, ventricular dysfunction).
E. **Hepatocellular carcinoma** represents approximately 2.5% of all carcinomas in the United States and approximately 30%–50% of all carcinomas in Asians living in Asia, where chronic active hepatitis due to hepatitis B virus is common. Other risk factors include chronic hepatitis C or chronic liver disease of any type.
F. **Benign tumors** include adenomas, focal nodular hyperplasia, and hemangiomas. Adenomas are more commonly seen in women 30–40 years of age, mostly in the right lobe, and can be as large as 10 cm. There is often a history of oral contraceptive (estrogen) use. Focal nodular hyperplasia often presents as right-sided solid masses. Hemangiomas are most commonly benign, with hemorrhage and malignant transformation rarely occurring.

G. Budd-Chiari syndrome (hepatic vein thrombosis) usually presents with hepatomegaly, pain, and severe, intractable ascites. Risk factors include hypercoagulable states, polycythemia vera, myeloproliferative syndromes, paroxysmal nocturnal hemoglobinuria, and use of oral contraceptive pills (OCPs).

H. Metastatic tumors. After lymph nodes, the liver is the second most common metastatic site, probably due to its high vascularity from a dual arterial/venous blood supply. With the exception of primary brain tumors, any primary tumor can metastasize to the liver. The most common primary tumors derive from the gastrointestinal tract, lung, breast, and melanoma. The usual presentation is with nonspecific, systemic symptoms such as weight loss, fever, and loss of appetite.

I. **A tender liver mass** in a patient with an elevated white blood cell count and eosinophilia suggests a liver abscess and possibly parasitic infection.

V. Clinical Approach

A. History

1. Inquire about the patient's history of alcohol and drug use, sexual practices, toxic exposures at work, medications, neoplasms, travel, and military service.
2. **Family history:** Inquire about the family history of liver disease.
3. **Comorbidities:** Assess for comorbidities such as diabetes, obesity, and congestive heart failure (CHF).
4. **Assess associated symptoms**, including weight loss, jaundice, weight gain (fluid retention or ascites), fever, pruritus, and anorexia.

   a. Time course of symptoms may be abrupt or gradual.
   b. Light (acholic) stools and dark urine may precede scleral or skin icterus.
   c. Easy bruising (coagulopathy) or mental confusion (encephalopathy) suggests advanced chronic liver disease or acute fulminant disease.

B. Physical examination.
Overall, physical examination techniques have been shown to generally underestimate the liver size and have poor correlation to liver size as later demonstrated by imaging techniques such as ultrasound.

1. **Palpation:** During palpation, note the consistency (soft versus firm), tenderness, nodularity, presence of pulsations, and any irregularities in contour. Findings on palpation suggest the following:

   a. Very firm = possible metastatic infiltration
   b. Massively enlarged = myeloid metaplasia
   c. Nodularity = cirrhosis or tumor
   d. Tender = hepatitis

2. **Auscultation** may be used to assess for bruits or friction rubs. While uncommon, they are suggestive of tumor or infection. Auscultation is also used to assess the inferior hepatic border through the scratch test.

3. **Percussion** is generally thought to be more accurate as compared to palpation because in some situations such as overinflation of the lung, a "normal" sized liver can be pushed down, and the liver edge becomes palpable.

4. **Assess for other signs of liver disease,** such as ascites and jaundice, or **signs of chronic liver disease,** such as spider angiomas, palmar erythema, caput medusae, testicular atrophy, and gynecomastia. Look for parotid or lacrimal gland enlargement or Dupuytren's contractures as signs of alcohol abuse.

5. **Associated splenomegaly** suggests the presence of portal hypertension, which can be seen in cirrhosis or hepatitis.

6. **Skin examination** showing ecchymoses suggests prothrombin deficiency, whereas purpura suggests thrombocytopenia.

7. Assess for **lymphadenopathy.**

VI. Diagnostic Evaluation

A. **Laboratory evaluation** is dependent upon suspected etiologies. Refer to Figure 22–1 when considering further studies.

1. **Assessment of liver chemistry studies** [aspartate aminotransferase (AST), alanine aminotransferase (ALT), total bilirubin, alkaline phosphatase] can suggest hepatocellular damage, infiltrative disease, biliary obstruction, or cholestasis.

2. **Measurements of prothrombin time and albumin** can help assess hepatic synthetic function. Albumin is more reflective of chronic disease.

3. **Complete blood count** (CBC) with differential could suggest parasitic infection (eosinophilia), neoplastic disease (leukemia, lymphoma), or nonspecific infection (leukocytosis).

   a. Thrombocytopenia is suggestive of hypersplenism and disseminated intravascular coagulation.

   b. Polycythemia suggests the possibility of malignancy, hypercoagulability, or both.

4. **Alpha-fetoprotein** may be obtained if hepatocellular carcinoma is suspected. Because of recycling through the enterohepatic circulation, carcinoembryonic antigen may be falsely elevated in hepatobiliary disease.

5. **Hepatitis:** The evaluation of hepatitis is discussed in Chapter 24.

B. **Radiologic studies**

1. **Ultrasound** is considered the primary screening examination for hepatic disease. In general, ultrasound is better for focal lesions rather than parenchymal disease.

   a. The **advantages** include low cost, portability, and no ionizing radiation. Masses as small as 1 cm can be detected, and cystic masses or abscesses can be distinguished from solid masses. Doppler ultrasonography can assess the patency and direction of blood flow in the hepatic and portal veins (without contrast).

   b. The **disadvantages** include obscured images in the presence of bowel gas and obesity.

2. **Computed tomography (CT) scanning:** In general, anatomic definition is more complete than with ultrasound. CT scanning is also better than ultrasound for showing diffuse parenchymal liver disease (fat

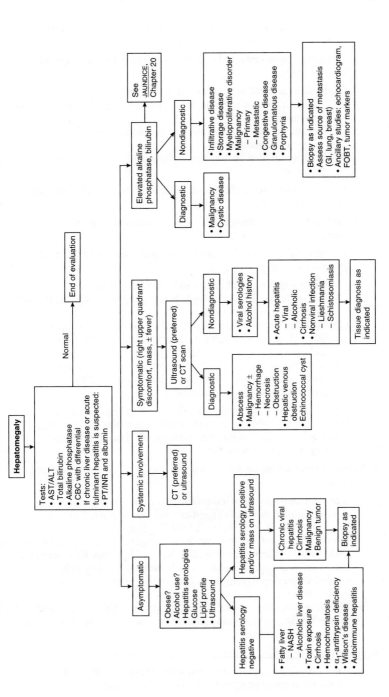

■ **FIGURE 22–1.** Algorithm for the workup of hepatomegaly, if the vertical span is > 12 cm by physical examination or imaging. *ALT* = alanine aminotransferase; *AST* = aspartate aminotransferase; *CBC* = complete blood count; *CT* = computed tomography; *FOBT* = fecal occult blood test; *GI* = gastrointestinal; *INR* = international normalized ratio; *NASH* = nonalcoholic steatohepatitis; *PT* = prothrombin time.

shows up as decreased density and hemochromatosis, or secondary iron overload shows up as increased density).

a. The **advantages** include the ability to image in the setting of obesity and bowel gas.

   (1) Lesions as small as 1 cm can be distinguished.
   (2) With intravenous contrast, abscesses can usually be distinguished from tumors.
   (3) Dynamic scanning with intravenous contrast may also show cavernous hemangiomas.
   (4) Mass lesions can be biopsied under either ultrasound or CT guidance.

b. The **disadvantages** include cost, radiation, and possible exposure to intravenous contrast.

3. Magnetic resonance imaging (MRI): Sensitivity is superior to CT scanning for mass lesions.

a. The **advantages** include lack of ionizing radiation and different planes of imaging.

   (1) It is the technique of choice to look for hemangiomas.
   (2) It is useful in distinguishing between a regenerating nodule and a tumor in the cirrhotic liver.
   (3) MRI can be used to monitor the liver for iron and copper deposition and with some modification can identify fatty liver and can produce an estimated quantification of fat content.
   (4) It can sometimes detect Budd-Chiari syndrome (hepatic vein thrombosis) without the need for intravenous iodinated contrast media (gadolinium is required).

b. The **disadvantages** include cost; slow time to acquire images, leading to more artifact; and limitations due to the use of a large magnet for patients with metal implants. MRI cannot distinguish a primary versus metastatic tumor.

4. Radioisotope scanning has been largely replaced by ultrasound and CT scanning.

a. Technetium-99m-labeled sulfur colloid scanning depends on uptake of phagocytic cells (Kupffer) and can help assess size and shape of the liver. Any disease where Kupffer cells are replaced by tumors, cysts, and abscesses produces a cold spot (adenomas); while with focal nodular hyperplasia, the liver will light up. Resolution for mass lesions is approximately 2 cm. Scintigraphy using radioactively labeled antibodies to tumor antigens is being developed as a diagnostic tool.

b. Gallium scanning uses gallium that is preferentially taken up in tissues synthesizing proteins (tumors or abscesses), and such areas show up as hot spots.

5. Imaging of the biliary tract

a. Endoscopic retrograde cholangiopancreatography (ERCP) allows for therapy (e.g., stone removal or stenting) as well as diagnosis.

   b. **Percutaneous transhepatic cholangiography** (PTC) allows for imaging of the proximal biliary ducts and some therapy (e.g., stent placement or percutaneous drainage) of the ducts.

   c. More recently, **magnetic resonance cholangiopancreatography** (MRCP) has demonstrated diagnostic accuracy similar to ERCP. The principle disadvantages include spatial resolution, which may not be as good as that achieved with ERCP; lack of therapeutic benefit; and decreased ability to visualize the ampulla.

SUGGESTED READING

Fauci, Anthony et al: *Harrison's Principles of Internal Medicine*, 14th ed. New York: McGraw-Hill, 1998, pp 579–581, 1660–1662, 1662–1663.

Zoli, Marco et al: Physical examination of the liver: Is it still worth it? *Am J Gastroenterol* 90(9):1428–1432, 1995.

23

Assessing Liver Chemistries
Fauzia Khan

I. **Introduction.** Liver chemistry tests may reflect liver cell damage, ability to excrete and metabolize, biosynthetic capacity, and cholestasis. According to one study, a single isolated liver test abnormality has an 84% chance of being false positive (see Table 23–1).

  A. **Bilirubin.** (See also Chapter 20, JAUNDICE.) Isolated hyperbilirubinemia distinguishes familial hyperbilirubinemia from the majority of other acquired cases of hyperbilirubinemia. Certain exceptions include conditions such as acquired hemolytic or megaloblastic anemias, transfusion of banked blood, massive hematomas, or aging infarcts.

  1. **Unconjugated hyperbilirubinemia** (indirect, water insoluble). Elevation of the unconjugated fraction results from increased bilirubin production (as in hemolysis), reduced hepatic uptake (as in Gilbert's syndrome), or reduced conjugation (as in jaundice). Hemolysis is the most common cause of unconjugated hyperbilirubinemia and acholic urine.

  2. **Conjugated hyperbilirubinemia** (direct, water soluble). The conjugated fraction of bilirubin is elevated when there is impaired secretion into the bile or an obstruction. The conjugated form is seen most commonly with hepatocellular disease (hepatitis, cirrhosis), malignancy, or cholestasis.

  a. The **distinction between intrahepatic and extrahepatic cholestasis** is made on clinical presentation with supplemental information from imaging and biopsy.

  (1) **Intrahepatic cholestasis** may be seen in sclerosing cholangitis, primary biliary cirrhosis, drugs, hormones, and in pregnancy.
  (2) **Extrahepatic cholestasis** may be caused by stones, neoplasms, strictures, cysts, and pseudocysts.

  b. **The highest bilirubin levels are found in cholestasis.** If hemolysis and renal failure are also present, these values are even higher.
  c. **Dipstick tests** may detect bilirubinuria even when there is a small increase in plasma conjugated bilirubin and may be positive before clinical jaundice.

  B. **Alkaline phosphatase.** There are high concentrations of alkaline phosphatase in bile duct epithelium, bone, intestinal mucosa, blood, and placenta (values rise in the third trimester). The most common causes for elevated levels include cholestatic liver disease, destructive bone disease, Paget's disease, childhood and adolescence, and incomplete and complete biliary obstruction.

TABLE 23–1. Patterns of Liver Chemistry Test Abnormalities

Pattern	Bilirubin	Alkaline Phosphatase	Amino-transferase	Albumin
Hemolysis	Usually elevated (mostly indirect)	Normal	Normal	Normal
Acute hepato-cellular disease (viral hepatitis, drugs, anoxia)	May or may not be elevated (both fractions)	Normal or < 3 times normal	Usually 400 u/L ALT > AST	Normal
Chronic hepato-cellular disease (alcoholic hepa-titis, cirrhosis)	May or may not be elevated (both fractions)	Normal or < 3 times normal	Usually < 300 u/L AST > ALT	May be decreased
Cholestasis	Usually elevated (both fractions)	> 4 times normal	Usually < 300 u/L	Usually normal
Infiltrative disorders	Usually normal	> 4 times normal	< 300 u/L	Usually normal

1. Alkaline phosphatase is **not helpful** in differentiating intrahepatic from extrahepatic obstruction.
2. An **isolated serum elevation** necessitates further chemical testing to determine its tissue of origin. An elevation of serum 5′nucleotidase or gamma-glutamyl transpeptidase (GGT) indicates a hepatic origin. Alkaline phosphatase isoenzymes may also be used to identify the tissue of origin (bone versus liver).

C. **Serum transaminases.** Aspartate aminotransferase (AST) and alanine aminotransferase (ALT) are intracellular enzymes. A high concentration is present in hepatocytes. AST derives from sources such as cardiac and skeletal muscle, kidney, brain, pancreas, leukocytes, and erythrocytes. ALT is therefore a more specific marker of liver disease.

1. **Liver injury:** Levels are increased in any form of liver injury. Though it may be necessary to measure both enzymes initially during patient evaluation, it is often possible to follow up with one enzyme. An AST/ALT ratio of 2 is seen in 70% of cases of **alcoholic hepatitis.**
2. **Viral hepatitis, ischemia, and toxins:** Levels are typically greater than 1000 IU.
3. **Systemic infection and decompensated congestive heart failure** (CHF) may also cause elevation of AST and ALT.
4. **Bile duct obstruction,** which interferes with enzyme secretion, may lead to mild elevations of AST and ALT.

D. GGT is found in the liver, kidney, pancreas, heart, and brain. This test is most commonly employed to determine whether alkaline phosphatase is of hepatic origin. It is also used as a marker of liver injury in alcohol-related liver disease.

   1. **Dramatic elevations** (> 500 μ/L) are associated with disorders of the liver and biliary tract, CHF, alcohol-related disease, and drug-induced liver dysfunction.
   2. **Abnormal enzyme activity** is 90% sensitive for liver disease but has lower specificity.
   3. **Hepatic enzyme-inducing drugs,** such as barbiturates, benzo-diazepines, phenytoin, and warfarin, cause plasma increases without evidence of liver disease. Serum levels fall with female sex hormones.

E. 5′Nucleotidase is found in the hepatocytes, heart, and pancreas. This test is most often employed to determine the source of elevated alkaline phospha-tase. It is as sensitive as alkaline phosphatase in detecting cholestatic conditions, hepatic infiltrative disorders, and hepatic mass lesions.

F. Albumin. Albumin levels can help differentiate between chronic and acute liver disease. Due to its half-life of 20 days, its levels are not affected significantly in acute states.

   1. **Child-Pugh score:** Albumin, bilirubin, and prothrombin times are laboratory tests included in the Child-Pugh score for assessment of liver disease. Low albumin is seen when the synthetic capacity of the liver is impaired.
   2. **Hypoalbuminemia** may also be caused by malnutrition, malabsorption, and malignancy. Increased loss due to proteinuria and enteropathy may result in low albumin. Increased catabolism, as in inflammation, results in low albumin.
   3. **Hemodilution,** as in overhydration, results in hypoalbuminemia.

G. Prothrombin time reflects hepatic synthetic function (see Chapter 43).

II. Clinical Application of Liver Chemistries

A. Approach. It is useful for the clinician to establish the pattern of abnor-mality when assessing abnormal liver chemistries. This is generally done with serial testing as dictated by the clinical picture. For example, mild elevation of the transaminases may be monitored over weeks, whereas moderate to severe elevations will require daily assessment.

B. Diagnosis. A particular pattern of liver injury may be identified by integrating the test results and the clinical picture (see Table 23–1).

SUGGESTED READING

Pratt DS, Kaplan MM: Primary care: Evaluation of liver enzyme. Results in asymptomatic pa-tients. *N Engl J Med* 342(17)1266–1271, 2000.

24

Diagnostic Approach to Additional Gastrointestinal, Hepatobiliary, and Pancreatic Disorders

Aftab Mohsin, Guenter L. Spanknebel,
Alicia M. DeTraglia, and Michael Mitchell

Acute and chronic viral hepatitis

Aftab Mohsin

I. Overview

A. Definitions. Acute hepatitis by definition is limited to a period of 6 months from the onset of symptoms.

B. Types of hepatitis

1. **Viral hepatitis** is the most common liver disorder and is caused by at least six known **hepatotropic viruses.** In addition, several other viruses can cause acute hepatitis, including Epstein-Barr virus, cytomegalovirus, HIV, and herpes virus.

2. **Nonviral hepatitis.** In clinical practice, before this diagnosis is reached, nonviral forms of hepatitis must be excluded.

C. Phases of infection. A large number of cases remain asymptomatic (70%–75%), but when symptoms develop there may be five distinct phases of viral infection:

1. Incubation phase or period
2. Prodromal phase
3. Icteric phase
4. Resolution phase
5. Chronicity phase (In certain instances, a phase of chronicity may follow an apparent resolution, or more commonly, an asymptomatic illness.)

D. Diagnosis and differentiation. Viral hepatitis may be diagnosed and differentiated on the grounds of **clinical, biochemical, serologic, and histologic findings.** These findings vary with the different viruses and will be discussed in reference to each individual virus.

II. Hepatitis B Virus

A. Definition. Hepatitis B virus (HBV) is a hepatotropic DNA virus (the only DNA genome among the A through G viruses) that is parenterally transmitted. It results in both acute and chronic hepatitis.

B. Overview

1. **Causes:** Parenteral transmission, sexual routes, and intravenous drug abuse are largely responsible for acquisition of new infections.
2. **Clinical course:** Most of the infections are either subclinical or anicteric; jaundice occurs in 25%–30% of patients. Aminotransferases are raised in almost all cases.
3. **Types of HBV infections**
   a. **Acute infection:** The incubation period ranges from 60–180 days.
   b. **Chronic infection.** Among those who become chronic carriers (5%), 50% will have evidence of **active viral replication.**
      (1) The risk of developing **cirrhosis** in patients with active viral replication is 15%–20% within 5 years.
      (2) The risk of **hepatocellular carcinoma** is increased as much as 300-fold in chronic carriers, particularly in those with active viral replication.

C. Clinical approach

1. The clinical presentation of **acute HBV infection** varies from asymptomatic infection to cholestatic hepatitis with jaundice and, rarely, to liver failure.
2. The clinical presentation of **chronic HBV infection** varies widely. Patients may be asymptomatic, have generalized symptoms of malaise and asthenia, or have one or more of the extrahepatic manifestations.
3. **Signs and symptoms** include:
   a. Extrahepatic manifestations
   b. Arthralgia and rashes (occur in 25% of patients)
   c. Polyarteritis nodosa with systemic vasculitis and membranoproliferative glomerulonephritis (as a result of deposition of immune complexes)

D. Diagnostic evaluation

1. **Biochemical diagnosis**
   a. The biochemical diagnosis of **acute hepatitis** consists of elevated serum bilirubin and aminotransferases. Biochemical findings coincide with the prodromal phase of the illness and may persist for 6 months.
   b. In **chronic infection,** alanine aminotransferase (ALT) levels may remain persistently abnormal (albeit moderately) but typically fluctuate, and a single normal reading may be misleading.
2. **Hepatitis B serology** (Figure 24–1)
3. **Liver biopsy** reflects disease severity, but the histologic appearance may be suggestive without being specific. It may range from being almost completely normal to showing various degrees of inflammation.

E. Complications

1. **Fulminant hepatic failure:** The most profound complication of HBV infection, albeit a rare one (< 1% of cases), is fulminant hepatic failure, defined as the onset of hepatic encephalopathy within 8 weeks of onset of symptoms.

    2. Cirrhosis: Patients with HBV infection are at risk of developing long-term complications that are related to the development of cirrhosis.

    3. Hepatocellular carcinoma: Patients with chronic liver disease, particularly those with established cirrhosis, are also at an increased risk of developing hepatocellular carcinoma.

III. Hepatitis A Virus

A. Description. Human hepatitis A virus (HAV), an RNA virus, has at least four distinct genotypes numbered in order of discovery; most human HAV belong to genotypes I and III. HAV has a single serotype.

B. Overview

  1. Incidence

    a. Worldwide distribution: Hepatitis A has a worldwide distribution. The prevalence of infection is related to the quality of the water supply, level of sanitation, and age.

    b. Seroprevalence: The seroprevalence in the United States is 38%, ranging from 11% in children younger than 5 years of age to 74% in adults 50 years of age or older.

  2. Transmission: The major mode of transmission is via the fecal-oral route.

  3. Incubation: The incubation period of the acute infection is 15–49 days. HAV titers are highest in acute-phase blood and fecal samples, and the period of host infectivity ranges from 14–21 days before the onset of jaundice, to 7–8 days after jaundice appears.

C. Risk factors. In 42% of cases, there is no known source of infection. The most common risk factors for HAV acquisition include:

  1. Personal contact with a person positive for anti-HAV (26% of patients)

  2. Day care association (15%)

  3. History of recent travel (5.5%)

D. Prognosis: The prognosis in acute HAV infection is excellent. The majority of patients recover completely within 2 months of the disease onset.

E. Diagnostic evaluation

  1. Serum bilirubin levels peak after the aminotransferase levels increase and are usually < 10 mg/dl. The bilirubin levels fall more slowly than the aminotransferase levels but will return to normal in 85% of patients by 3 months. Anicteric infections are 3.5 times more likely than icteric infections, with the vast majority of icteric infections occurring in children.

  2. Serum aminotransferase levels increase during the prodromal phase, and the peak is typically heralded by intense nausea, anorexia, and vomiting. Peak aminotransferase levels are commonly > 500 IU/L and decrease at the rate of 75% per week initially and then decline more slowly.

  3. Serology (see Figure 24–1)

    a. Detection of HAV immunoglobulin M (IgM) indicates acute HAV infection. Serum IgM usually persists for less than 6 months.

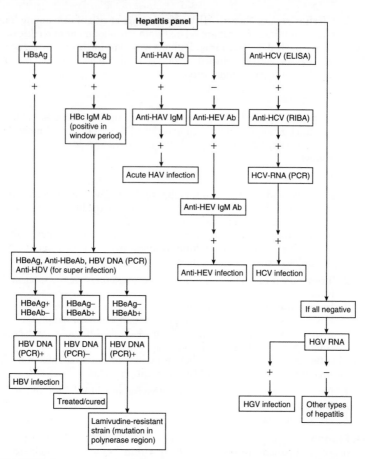

■ **FIGURE 24–1.** Algorithm for the workup of patients with hepatitis. *Ab* = antibody; *Ag* = antigen; *ELISA* = enzyme-linked immunosorbent assay; *HAV* = hepatitis A virus; *HBc* = hepatitis B core; *HBe* = hepatitis B early antigen; *HBs* = hepatitis B surface; *HBV* = hepatitis B virus; *HCV* = hepatitis C virus; *HDV* = hepatitis D virus; *HEV* = hepatitis E virus; *HGV* = hepatitis G virus; *IgM* = immunoglobulin M; *PCR* = polymerase chain reaction; *RIBA* = recombinant immunoblot assay.

    b. HAV immunoglobulin G (IgG) indicates previous exposure and/or immunity to HAV; however, a rising titer of HAV IgG is indicative of recent exposure. Anti-HAV IgG persists for decades.

IV. Hepatitis C virus

    A. Description. Hepatitis C virus (HCV) is a positive sense RNA virus. There are at least six different HCV genotypes based on major RNA sequence variation. Genotype group is indicated by number. Minor variation within different genotype groups result in identifiable subtypes, indicated by lower case letters after the genotype designation.

B. Incidence. HCV is a major cause of viral hepatitis and is estimated to cause 40% of chronic liver failure. In the United States, almost 4 million people have been infected by HCV and this infection accounts for approximately 25,000 deaths per year. The annual incidence of new infections has dropped dramatically because of public health interventions described below.

HCV infection is transmitted by direct percutaneous exposure to blood. The risk is directly related to the amount and frequency of blood exposure. Since 1994, the availability or techniques to screen for or inactivate HCV in transfusion products and organ donors has reduced the incidence of infection from transfusion and transplantation to very low levels. Currently, intravenous drug abuse is the major source of new infections. Exposure of hemodialysis patients contributes a small, but significant number of new infections. Acquisition of new infection is uncommon through tattooing, household, sexual, or perinatal exposure. Infection in Health Care Workers in not increased compared to the general population. A potential risk factor can be identified in at least 90% of patients with newly diagnosed HCV infection.

C. Clinical approach

1. HCV testing should be considered for patients with undiagnosed liver disease or high risk for infection, as in long-term hemodialysis or intravenous drug use. The incidence of HCV infection is increased in patients with documented HIV infection. Because asymptomatic chronic infection occurs, testing may be indicated for patients who received blood product transfusion or transplantation prior to the mid-1990s. Testing should be performed on infants born to mothers who are HCV RNA positive at the time of delivery. Testing may be indicated for the evaluation of Health Care Workers with a documented exposure to blood.

2. Approximately 70% of HCV infected patients develop chronic liver disease. Twenty to 25% of these patients will develop cirrhosis and approximately 3% of HCV infected patients will die as a result of cirrhosis, liver cancer, or other complication of infection.

3. There is considerable geographic variation in the distribution of HCV genotypes. Type 1 viruses cause most HCV infections in the United States. Infections caused by HCV type 1 viruses are more resistant to specific antiviral therapy and may require a longer duration of therapy to achieve durable remission.

D. Diagnostic evaluation

1. **Serology** (see Fig 24–1). Current HCV enzyme immunoassays will detect > 97% of HCV infected patients. Because of a small percentage of false positive results (e.g., in patients with rheumatoid factor), positive EIA results should be confirmed by an assay with high specificity, like a recombinant immunoblot (RIBA) or RNA quantification.

2. **Nucleic acid assays**

   a. HCV RNA is detectable as early as one week after acute infection, and may appear before ALT elevation, seropositivity, or other sign of infection. A positive HCV RNA assay may be used to confirm acute infection, while a negative RNA result may help identify patients with spontaneous resolution of active infection.

b. Techniques for HCV quantification include RT-PCR (nucleic acid amplification) and bDNA (signal amplification). These assays have lower levels of detection in the range of 200 to 550 genome copies/ml, respectively. The results of RT-PCR and bDNA assays are not strictly comparable, so the same assay should be used for serial testing. Following infected patients with serial nucleic acid testing, however, has not been definitively shown to improve clinical outcome. Newer qualitative assays are capable of detecting as few as 10 genome copies/ml.

c. Determination of HCV genotype may be determined by sequencing or use of an innovative line probe assay (LiPA). The HCV genotype may be critical for the determination of the optimal antiviral agents and duration of therapy.

3. Liver histology. Histologic examination of a liver biopsy is the most accurate mehtod for evaluating the extent of liver damage.

SUGGESTED READING

Laver GM, Walker BD: Hepatitis C virus infection. *N Engl J Med* 345:41–52, 2001.

Acute Pancreatitis

Aftab Mohsin

I. Definition. Acute pancreatitis is a **reversible inflammatory process of the pancreas,** usually associated with persistent severe upper abdominal pain and marked abdominal tenderness. If, however, inflammatory changes persist after the acute attack subsides, it may evolve to chronic pancreatitis.

II. Causes

A. Common causes of acute pancreatitis include **gallstones** (30%–70%), **alcohol consumption** (30%), and **hyperlipidemia** (4%). The cause is unknown in 30% of cases.

B. Uncommon causes of acute pancreatitis include hereditary pancreatitis, hyperparathyroidism, hypercalcemia, and medications such as azathioprine, 6-mercaptopurine, thiazide diuretics, furosemide, sulfonamides, estrogens (oral contraceptives), tetracycline, and valproic acid.

C. Other causes include infectious agents and toxins, vascular disease, postoperative pancreatitis, pancreatic trauma, endoscopic retrograde cholangiopancreatography (ERCP)-induced (< 5%), pregnancy, and cystic fibrosis.

D. Structural abnormalities that may cause acute pancreatitis include:

1. Congenital duodenal lesions and tumors
2. Choledochal cysts and sclerosing cholangitis
3. Stenosis or dyskinesia of the sphincter of Oddi

    4. Tumors, hook worms, and liver flukes in the main pancreatic duct

    5. Division of the accessory pancreatic duct

III. Clinical Approach

A. History

1. Almost all patients with acute pancreatitis experience diffuse **upper abdominal pain.** Pain may occasionally be localized to the epigastrium and left upper abdomen. In most cases, it reaches maximum intensity within 10–20 minutes.
2. Persistent **nausea, vomiting,** and **pain** are frequent complaints.

B. Signs and physical findings

1. Marked **abdominal tenderness with guarding and fever** is a typical presentation.
2. Patients may also be **disoriented, agitated,** and **hallucinating.**
3. **Dyspnea** may occur as a result of pleural effusions, atelectasis, or congestive heart failure (CHF).
4. If gallstones are present, they may lead to **jaundice.**
5. **Ecchymosis** in one or both flanks (Grey Turner's sign), **ecchymotic discoloration** of the periumbilical region (Cullen's sign), and brawny **erythema of the skin** in the flanks may be present.
6. On very rare occasions, **subcutaneous fat necrosis** may be seen. These tender nodules are 0.5–2.0 cm in size and located over the distal extremities.

IV. Diagnostic Evaluation

A. Laboratory diagnosis

1. **Amylase:** Serum amylase is increased by at least three times the normal level in 75% of cases of acute pancreatitis and remains elevated in most patients for 5–10 days.

    a. Normal serum amylase: A normal serum amylase is strong evidence against the diagnosis of acute pancreatitis. However, serum amylase levels may fail to rise significantly in cases of hyperlipidemia, in exacerbation of chronic pancreatitis, and if measured late in the course of the disease.

    b. Elevated serum amylase: Conditions other than pancreatitis associated with the elevation of serum amylase include salivary gland dysfunction, tumors such as carcinoma of lung and ovary, gynecologic conditions, cholecystitis, intestinal obstruction, and perforation and macroamylasemia in renal insufficiency.

    c. Measurement of isoenzymes increases specificity and helps to differentiate hyperamylasemia due to pancreatic causes from all other causes.

2. **Lipase** is invariably elevated on the first day and remains elevated longer than the serum amylase. It has sensitivity of 80% and specificity of 60%. With availability of the new turbidimetric assay, it is the single best test to perform. Other causes for increased lipase levels include cholelithiasis, nephrolithiasis, small bowel obstruction, and ruptured aortic aneurysm. However, the degree of elevation is less than in acute pancreatitis (three times versus five times). Amylase and lipase levels complement each other.

3. Miscellaneous tests

a. Pancreatitis-associated protein and **pancreatic-specific protein** are as accurate as serum amylase. There is evidence that serum pancreatitis-associated protein may help in establishing prognosis.

b. Trypsinogen assay, if available, is comparable to both lipase and amylase.

4. Additional blood tests

a. White blood cell count, serum glucose, serum aminotransferase, lactate dehydrogenase, alkaline phosphate, and triglyceride levels may all be elevated.

b. The serum calcium level may be depressed.

c. The serum hematocrit and renal chemistries should be obtained for consideration of prognostication using Ranson's criteria of severity (see V B).

B. Radiologic studies

1. On **abdominal flat plate,** gallstones, pancreatic stone, abnormalities of stomach, small or large bowel may be present.

2. Chest radiograph shows elevation of diaphragm, atelectasis, pleural effusion, and pulmonary exudates.

3. Barium studies, although not routinely obtained, may demonstrate anterior displacement of the stomach and the duodenum and widening of the duodenal loops.

4. Abdominal ultrasound is excellent for serial evaluation of pseudocysts, gallstones, dilation of the common bile duct, and ascites. Enlargement of the pancreas and change in echogenicity may be present.

5. ERCP is indicated when detection of gallstones in the common bile duct is necessary.

6. Contrast-enhanced computed tomography (CT) scan is the imaging procedure of choice. It may show inflammatory swelling of the pancreas. The presence of pancreatic parenchymal necrosis may be measured by comparing the pancreatic density after the contrast with that of the spleen. The density is reduced in the necrotizing type of pancreatitis.

7. Magnetic resonance imaging (MRI) can differentiate between fluid and solid inflammatory masses.

V. Complications. The severity of acute pancreatitis can be assessed by clinical evaluation or scoring systems.

A. Indicators of severity

1. Low hematocrit

2. Oliguria < 30 ml/hr

3. Systolic blood pressure < 90 mm Hg

4. Pulse > 120 beats per minute

5. O_2 saturation < 90%

B. Ranson's criteria of severity

1. Criteria: Age > 55 years, white blood cells > 16,000/mm³, glucose > 200 mg/dl, lactate dehydrogenase > 350 IU/L, aspirate transaminase > 250 IU/L

▲

2. **During initial 48 hours:** Hematocrit decreases > 10 mg/dl, blood urea nitrogen increases > 5 mg/dl (despite fluids), calcium < 8 mg/dl, PO_2 < 60 mm Hg, base deficit > 4 mEq/L, fluid sequestration > 6 L
3. **Prognosis:** Mortality ranges from 1% in mild cases (< 3 Ranson's criteria) to 50% in severe cases (> 4 Ranson's criteria).

VI. **Special Considerations.** It is not unusual to rely solely on amylase or lipase levels for diagnosis because both may be misleading. Amylase is rapidly cleared and may therefore be normal late in an attack. Serum amylase, lipase, and trypsinogen may all be elevated in renal disease.

SUGGESTED READING

Mergener K, Baillic J: Fortnightly review: Acute pancreatitis. *Br Med J.* 316:44–48, 1998.

Adult Upper Gastrointestinal Bleeding

Guenter L. Spanknebel

I. **Definition.** Upper gastrointestinal bleeding is defined as **coming from a source above the ligament of Treitz.**

A. **Onset.** The patient may present with stigmata of chronic blood loss (anemia and related symptoms) or acute blood loss (weakness or syncope).
B. **Incidence.** This is the **most common medical emergency** for gastro-enterologists.
C. **Mortality.** The mortality is approximately 8%, and it is not usually due to exsanguination but rather to the adverse effect on comorbid conditions.

II. **Differential Diagnosis** (Table 24–2)
III. **Notes on the Differential Diagnosis**

A. **Peptic ulcer disease** (PUD) is associated with risk factors including *Helicobacter pylori* infection, use of nonsteroidal anti-inflammatory drugs (NSAIDs), stress, and gastric acid. Risk factors for stress-related bleeding include respiratory failure and coagulopathy.
B. **Portal hypertension and varices** indicate the severity of a patient's underlying cirrhosis. These patients have an associated mortality of 50% even after control of the hemorrhage.
C. **Mallory-Weiss tears** occur in the distal esophagus, at the site of the gastro-esophageal junction, usually following a bout of retching. Most tears heal uneventfully within 24–48 hours. The diagnosis is made by endoscopic evaluation, at which time therapeutic interventions may be utilized as well as stratifying the risk of rebleeding.
D. **Neoplasm** accounts for less than 5% of all cases of severe bleeding. It is generally a late manifestation, and represents a negative prognostic feature. Uncommonly, tumors may metastasize to the gastric mucosa.

TABLE 24–2. Differential Diagnosis of Upper Gastrointestinal Bleeding

---

- **Peptic ulcer disease** (40%–50%; idiopathic, induced by drug, toxin, or stress, related to an infection, associated with Zollinger-Ellison syndrome)

- **Erosive esophagitis, gastritis, and duodenitis**

- **Portal hypertension and varices** (10%–15%; esophageal, gastric, duodenal, and portal hypertensive gastropathy)

- **Mallory-Weiss tear** (5%)

- **Rare causes**
  - Atriovenous malformations
  - Rendu-Osler-Weber syndrome
  - Watermelon stomach (gastric antral vascular ectasia)
  - Dieulafoy's lesion
  - Stomal ulcer
  - Neoplasm (benign, primary and metastatic malignancy)
  - Connective tissue disease (scleroderma, Ehlers-Danlos syndrome)
  - Aortic-enteric fistula
  - Hemobilia
  - Uremic gastritis
  - Foreign body

    E. Rendu-Osler-Weber syndrome is associated with telangiectasia of the lips, oral mucosa, and fingertips.

    F. Dieulafoy's lesion correlates with a dilated aberrant submucosal vessel, which erodes the overlying mucosa in the absence of an ulcer. This should be suspected in the patient with recurrent episodes of undiagnosed upper gastrointestinal bleeding.

IV. Clinical Approach. The clinician must discern true gastrointestinal bleeding from nongastrointestinal sources, such as epistaxis and hemoptysis.

    A. History

        1. Characteristics of bleeding: Upper GI bleeding presents as hematemesis (i.e., the vomiting of blood or coffee-ground-like material), melena (i.e., black or tarry stools), or hematochezia. Document the duration of bleeding and the number of episodes.

        2. Risk factor assessment: Note prior bleeding, prior surgery, use of aspirin, use of NSAIDs, alcohol or tobacco abuse, weight loss, early satiety, and dysphagia.

        3. Associated features include retching, lightheadedness, weakness, and use of antacids (both prescription and over-the-counter).

        4. Comorbid conditions include cirrhosis, coagulopathy, cardiac disease, aortic stenosis, aortic aneurysm, renal failure, and intensive-care-unit-related illness.

B. Physical examination

1. Check the skin for manifestations of coagulopathy, cirrhosis, jaundice, and telangiectasia.
2. Evaluate the patient for aortic stenosis murmur or CHF.
3. Check the abdomen for tenderness, hepatomegaly, a mass or bruit in the liver, splenomegaly, or aortic enlargement.
4. Evaluate the patient for encephalopathy and signs of alcohol withdrawal.

V. Diagnostic Evaluation

A. Initial assessment

1. **Assess magnitude of blood loss** [complete blood count (CBC), vital signs].
2. **Check coagulation studies** (prothrombin time, partial thromboplastin time, platelets).
3. **Type and crossmatch** number of units appropriate for severity of blood loss.

B. Following resuscitation and stabilization

1. **Esophagogastroduodenoscopy (EGD)** is the diagnostic procedure of choice for patients presenting with acute gastrointestinal bleeding. Advantages of early EGD include:

   a. Confirmation or modification of the working diagnosis, proposed by the history and physical examination
   b. Providing therapeutic measures, which lessen transfusion requirements and the need for surgery
   c. Potentially averting the need for hospitalization

2. **Upper gastrointestinal barium studies** are contraindicated in the setting of acute bleeding. The barium will interfere with subsequent studies (e.g., endoscopy).

SUGGESTED READING

Van Dam J, Brugge WR: Medical progress: Endoscopy of the upper gastrointestinal tract. *N Engl J Med* 341:1738–1748, 1999.

Small Intestinal Bleeding

Alicia M. DeTraglia

I. Overview. The small intestine is an uncommon site of hemorrhage accounting for only 3%–5% of gastrointestinal bleeding. Patients usually present with occult blood loss and may have evidence of melena or hematochezia.

II. Differential Diagnosis (Table 24–3)

TABLE 24–3. Differential Diagnosis of Small Intestinal Bleeding

- Angiodysplasia

- Small bowel tumors

- Less common causes:
  - Ulcerative diseases (most commonly Crohn's disease)
  - Meckel's diverticulum (the cause in two-thirds of men younger than 30 years of age)
  - Zollinger-Ellison syndrome (causes ulcerations)
  - Infections (e.g., tuberculosis, syphilis, typhoid, histoplasmosis)
  - Medications [e.g., potassium, nonsteroidal anti-inflammatory drugs (NSAIDs), 6-mercaptopurine]
  - Vasculitis
  - Radiation enteritis (injury can occur 6–24 months after exposure, secondary to the development of occlusive vasculitis)
  - Jejunal diverticula (< 5% actually bleed, but bleeding is usually massive, with mortality as high as 20%)
  - Vascular lesions (varices, venous ectasias, telangiectasias, hemangiomas, atrio-venous malformations)

III. Notes on the Differential Diagnosis

    A. Angiodysplasia accounts for the majority of small intestinal bleeding (70%–80%). Bleeding can be either brisk or occult. An isolated episode of bleeding does not mandate therapy, as the lesions do not usually rebleed (approximately 50%).

    B. Tumors account for 5%–10% of cases of small intestinal bleeding. Of these, one-third are benign (leiomyoma and adenomas most commonly) and two-thirds are malignant (45% adenocarcinoma, usually of the duodenum, 30% carcinoid, 14% lymphoma, and 11% leiomyosarcoma). The three most common malignancies are generally associated with chronic blood loss. Metastatic disease may also occur, most commonly from melanoma and breast cancer.

IV. Clinical Approach

    A. History

        1. Signs and symptoms of small intestinal bleeding include nausea, vomiting, hematemesis, melena, hematochezia, abdominal pain, bloating, anorexia, early satiety, weight loss, and change in bowel habits.

            a. Hematemesis almost always indicates a source above the ligament of Treitz, usually from a source proximal to the pylorus.

            b. Melena suggests a source below the pylorus, most commonly proximal to the jejunum. It can also indicate a colonic source if the bowel is obstructed distally. Melena is the presenting complaint in 25%–53% of patients with small intestinal bleeding.

            c. Hematochezia usually indicates a colonic source; blood from ascending colon produces black stool that is not as shiny or sticky as melena.

    d. Upper gastrointestinal bleeding usually leads to both hematemesis and melena, but either may occur alone. Small bowel lesions can give either melena or hematochezia.

  2. Past history should ascertain any occurrences of liver disease, intestinal polyps or cancer, ulcer disease, and other bleeding diatheses.

  3. Family history should be taken, with a focus on inheritable cancer syndromes.

  4. Medication and social history should include use of NSAIDs, alcohol, anticoagulants, and aspirin.

B. Physical examination. An assessment of hemodynamic stability should be the initial step.

  1. Assess the skin for cutaneous manifestations of underlying malignancy (e.g., acanthesis, nigricans, Kaposi's sarcoma), oral-pigmented lesions (e.g., Peutz-Jeghers syndrome), telangiectasia, or coagulopathy.

  2. Assess for stigmata of cirrhosis and hepatomegaly.

  3. Check for lymphadenopathy.

  4. Assess the abdomen for masses, splenomegaly, tenderness, and distention.

  5. Perform a rectal examination.

V. Diagnostic Evaluation

A. Plain abdominal films may show evidence of obstruction suggestive of stricture or tumor, but they are not likely to be diagnostic.

B. Contrast radiography

  1. Small bowel series have a low yield in identifying a bleeding source (i.e., a 5% detection rate). This may be increased to 10% with use of enteroclysis. If the bleeding source is a small intestinal malignancy, the yield is considerably better.

  2. Barium studies cannot diagnose angiodysplasias, but they may be useful in identifying mass lesions and mucosal defects.

  3. In spite of the low diagnostic yield, **contrast radiography** is the initial study in a patient where small intestinal bleeding is suspected (i.e., when the evaluation of upper and lower gastrointestinal tracts are non-diagnostic).

C. Endoscopic studies

  1. Routine EGD reaches the junction of the second and third portions of the duodenum.

  2. Conventional **push enteroscopy** (either a dedicated enteroscope or pediatric colonoscope) can reach the proximal jejunum. Yield with push enteroscopy varies from 24%–75% in detecting a bleeding source. Push enteroscopy also has therapeutic value.

  3. Sonde enteroscopy is a newer instrument that is being developed to visualize the entire jejunum and ileum. It is a flexible fiberoptic instrument carried through the bowel by peristalsis. It is not a routinely available procedure, and it is best reserved for those patients with comorbid conditions that may preclude intraoperative enteroscopy.

D. Angiography detects a bleeding rate of 0.5 ml/min. It can localize the site of bleeding in 50%–72% of cases if bleeding is massive, but in only

25%–50% of cases if bleeding has slowed. It has a low yield in diagnosing angiodysplasias and tumors.

E. Nuclear imaging

1. **Technetium-99 bleeding scan** may detect bleeding at a rate as slight as 0.1 ml/min. Like angiography, it is only of value in the setting of active bleeding. It can define a general area of bleeding, but it cannot identify the precise source.

2. **Technetium-99 Meckel's scan,** which is taken up by ectopic gastric mucosa in the diverticulum, is not useful if the diverticulum does not contain gastric mucosa.

F. Surgical evaluation

1. **Intraoperative enteroscopy** is a procedure whereby the bowel is manually advanced over an endoscope. It is the most common way to examine the entire small bowel. It is successful in identifying a bleeding source 83%–100% of the time.

2. **Exploratory surgery** is often considered in patients with recurrent gastrointestinal bleeding of unclear origin. Simple exploration has a low success rate, with a diagnostic yield of only 10% when unaccompanied by other evaluations (i.e., enteroscopy).

G. Stepwise approach to evaluation. In a study of 77 patients, the **interval from presentation to diagnosis** was > 20 months, owing to the relatively asymptomatic nature of the conditions and the difficulty in evaluating small bowel bleeding sources.

1. **Determine the source of bleeding**

   a. In those with a nondiagnostic evaluation of lower and upper gastro-intestinal tracts, **small bowel evaluation** will be necessary.

   b. Once the small bowel is assumed to be the bleeding source (i.e., standard examinations are nondiagnostic), proceed to **small bowel series.**

2. **If the source is not identified**

   a. Proceed to **push enteroscopy,** before considering repeat **EGD or colonoscopy.**

   b. **Sonde enteroscopy** may be considered as the next study if a bleeding source is not identified.

   c. Withhold **bleeding scans and angiography,** unless the patient is actively bleeding.

   d. **Exploratory surgery** can be done with intraoperative endoscopy if needed.

SUGGESTED READING

Lewis B: Small intestinal bleeding. *Gastroenterol Clin North Am* 23(1):67–91, 1994.

Adult Lower Gastrointestinal Bleeding, Acute

Guenter L. Spanknebel

I. Overview

A. Definition. Lower gastrointestinal bleeding is usually defined by **bleeding originating from below the ligament of Treitz.**

B. Lower versus upper gastrointestinal bleeding. If the initial assessment does not clearly distinguish between upper and lower sources of gastrointestinal bleeding, evaluation of the upper tract should be pursued, as this is the more common site of massive gastrointestinal bleeding.

II. Differential Diagnosis (Table 24–4)
III. Notes on the Differential Diagnosis

A. Angiodysplasia. In elderly patients, angiodysplasia is diagnosed with proportional greater frequency. Angiodysplasia are not visualized by barium enema. The bleeding tends to be self-limited, frequently arising from the right colon.

B. Benign anorectal pathology. In younger patients (< 35 years of age), benign anorectal pathology (e.g., hemorrhoidal bleeding) is the most common etiology.

C. Diverticulosis. Less than 15% of patients with diverticulosis develop significant bleeding. The bleeding is typically painless and occurs in the absence of diverticulitis. Although diverticuli are more commonly located on the left side of the colon, right-sided lesions account for a significant portion of diverticular bleeding.

D. Colon cancer accounts for 5%–10% of patients with lower gastrointestinal blood loss in patients older than 50 years of age.

E. Coagulopathy usually causes bleeding in patients with a comorbid gastrointestinal condition. Thus, a patient with coagulopathy always requires further evaluation.

F. Suspect upper gastrointestinal bleeding in patients presenting with **hematochezia.**

IV. Clinical Approach

A. History. The history should identify abdominal pain, cramping, persistent changes in bowel habits, bloating, perianal irritation, extraintestinal signs and symptoms of inflammatory bowel disease (IBD), laxative use, and long-distance running.

1. **Characteristics of bleeding.** Patients may have black, maroon, or bright red stools depending on the location of bleeding source, severity of bleeding, transit time, medications influencing intestinal motility, or bacterial flora.

2. **Past history.** Inquire about previous colorectal surgery, prior gastrointestinal investigations, previous diagnosis of neoplasia or IBD, unexplained anemia, and radiation therapy.

3. **Family history.** Ascertain any family history of neoplasia or IBD.

4. **Drug history.** Note use of acetylsalicylic acid (aspirin), NSAIDs, antibiotics, or anticoagulants.

TABLE 24–4. Differential Diagnosis of Lower Gastrointestinal Bleeding

- Diverticulosis (approximately 40%)

- Angiodysplasia (approximately 25%)

- Neoplasia (benign and malignant)

- Colitis (ulcerative, Crohn's, ischemic, pseudomembranous, infectious disease, radiation exposure)

- Hemorrhoid

- Less common causes:
  - Solitary ulcers
  - Nonsteroidal anti-inflammatory drugs (NSAIDs)
  - Venous lakes
  - Blue rubber nevus
  - Anastomotic ulcerations and suture lines
  - Mechanical trauma
  - Postbiopsy or polypectomy
  - Coagulopathy and anticoagulation therapy
  - Autoimmune disease (e.g., rheumatoid vasculitis, Henoch-Schönlein purpura)

B. Physical examination

1. Assess the skin for cutaneous manifestations of underlying malignancy (e.g., acanthosis nigricans, Kaposi's sarcoma), oral-pigmented lesions (e.g., Peutz-Jeghers syndrome), telangiectasia, coagulopathy, or IBD.
2. Check the abdomen for presence of masses, splenomegaly, tenderness, distention, stigmata of cirrhosis, hepatomegaly, and lymphadenopathy.
3. Perform a rectal examination.

V. Diagnostic Evaluation

A. Initial assessment

1. **Check coagulation studies** (prothrombin time, partial thromboplastin time, platelets, CBC).
2. **Type and crossmatch** number of units appropriate for severity of blood loss.

B. Endoscopic studies (assuming an upper gastrointestinal bleed is excluded by virtue of nonbloody bilious fluid obtained via nasogastric lavage)

1. **Anoscopy** may be performed to rule out bleeding hemorrhoids in appropriately selected patients.
2. **Colonoscopy** will identify a bleeding source in approximately 80% of patients. The procedure will help control bleeding in as many as 40% of patients. Other advantages include assisting in preoperative assessment

and specimen collection for histologic assessment. Colonoscopy should be considered the first procedure of choice given the superior diagnostic yield.

C. Radiographic studies

1. **Plain films** of the abdomen are useful for assessing free air (e.g., ruptured viscus) or the presence of ischemic changes (e.g., thumbprinting).
2. **Barium studies** will not identify angiodysplasia or evidence of acute colitis, and they may interfere with subsequent colonoscopic or surgical interventions.
3. **Radionuclide studies** may detect bleeding at a rate of 0.1–0.5 ml/min, provided the test is performed when the patient is actively bleeding. The principle advantage is the noninvasive nature of this test.
4. **Angiography** may detect bleeding at a rate of 1–1.5 ml/min. It is 100% specific but no more than 30%–50% sensitive.

   a. The **principle advantages** of angiography include the accurate anatomic localization and the lack of need for bowel preparation. It may also permit therapeutic interventions (e.g., vasopressin infusion and embolization).
   b. Unfortunately, **complications** are common with both angiography (renal failure) and the therapeutic interventions (rebleeding, intestinal infarction).

SUGGESTED READING

Chaudhry V, Hyser AM, Gracias VH, Gau FC: Colonoscopy: In the initial test for acute lower gastrointestinal bleeding. *Am Surg* 64:723–728, 1998.

Vernava AM III, Moore BA, Longo WE, Johnson FE: Lower gastrointestinal bleeding. *Dis Colon Rectum* 40:846–858, 1997.

General Medicine

25

Edema
Omar Ali

I. **Definition.** Edema is defined as **expansion of the interstitial volume,** which is clinically manifested by visible or palpable swelling.

II. **Overview.** An understanding of the relationship between hydrostatic and oncotic pressures on both sides of a semipermeable membrane serves as a foundation when approaching the patient with edema.

  A. **Starling's ultrafiltration equation** represents the forces that govern the flow of fluid out of the capillary space and the interstitium. An alteration in any one of the variables can result in a change in flow with the potential development of edema.

  $$\text{Flow} = K \, [\Delta \text{ Hydrostatic pressure} - \Delta \text{ Oncotic pressure}]$$

   1. The **Δ hydrostatic pressure** refers to the gradient between the hydrostatic pressure within the capillary and the hydrostatic pressure of the surrounding interstitial fluid.
   2. The **Δ oncotic pressure** refers to the gradient of pressure attributable to the difference in oncotic pressures created by osmotically active particles on either side of the membrane.
   3. The **sum total of the gradients** across the capillary membrane determines the direction and amount of fluid flux.
   4. **Factor (K)** represents capillary permeability.

  B. **Evaluation.** The evaluation of edema begins with the distinction of localized edema from generalized edema. While alterations in Starling's forces are present in both situations, the underlying disease states differ.

III. **Differential Diagnosis** (Table 25–1)

  A. **Venous insufficiency** (e.g., postphlebitic syndrome, valvular incompetency) is a common cause of localized edema in the lower extremities. The diagnosis is suspected on the basis of appropriate history and physical examination findings.

  B. **Idiopathic edema** is a common cause of generalized edema. In this condition, patients with no significant medical history present with chronic weight gain and fluid retention. These patients, usually middle-aged

TABLE 25–1. Differential Diagnosis of Edema

Localized edema

Increased hydrostatic pressure:
- Deep venous thrombosis (DVT)
- Tumor obstruction (e.g., superior vena cava obstruction)
- Rupture of popliteal cyst
- Thoracic outlet syndrome
- Lymphedema (as a result of a congenital defect, surgery, trauma, infection, radiation, compression by mass)
- Venous valve insufficiency
- Compartment syndrome

Decreased oncotic pressure:
- Reduced oncotic pressure typically does not result in local edema

Altered permeability:
- Cellulitis
- Bursitis
- Osteomyelitis
- Insect bite
- Burn
- Focal allergic reaction
- Reflex sympathetic dystrophy

Generalized edema

Increased hydrostatic pressure:
- Cardiac cause [e.g., congestive heart failure (CHF), restrictive and constrictive heart disease, cor pulmonale]
- Endocrine cause (and altered permeability)
  - Cushing's syndrome
  - Hyperaldosteronism
- Renal failure
- Beriberi
- Medications
- Large arteriovenous fistula
- Idiopathic edema
- Filariasis (and altered permeability)

Decreased oncotic pressure:
- Decreased albumin synthesis (malabsorption, cirrhosis, beriberi, kwashiorkor, food faddism, anorexia)
- Protein loss (proteinuria, protein-losing enteropathy)

Altered permeability:
- Histamine release
- Angioedema

continued

TABLE 25–1. Differential Diagnosis of Edema (*Continued*)

- Burns
- Anemia
- Vasculitis
- Thyroid disease
- Cushing's syndrome
- Acute respiratory distress syndrome or capillary leak syndrome

---

women, will retain fluid during the day, causing swelling of the hands, feet, breasts, and face. Usually, the fluid is mobilized with recumbency overnight, and nocturia results in fluid loss. Symptoms tend to worsen during the summer months. There exists a prominent postural component to the development of edema in these cases. The primary mechanism, however, is uncertain.

IV. **Clinical Approach** (see Table 25–1 and Figure 25–1). The initial approach is to distinguish between localized and generalized edema. The history and physical examination permit the distinction as well as guide the subsequent diagnostic approach. Bilateral lower-extremity edema may represent the clinical manifestation of either a local or a generalized process.

A. **History**

1. **Localized edema (acute)**

   a. **Assess for trauma, venous thrombosis risk** (see the THROMBOPHILIA section in Chapter 43), and **pain** (especially when related to significant physical activity, as in a ruptured gastrocnemius muscle or popliteal cyst).

   b. **Unilateral upper-extremity edema** without antecedent insult is cause for concern, because a malignant process may be secondarily compressing the vena cava or thoracic outlet.

2. **Localized edema (chronic)**

   a. Assess prior episodes of venous thrombosis, varicosities, and their chronicity. **Chronic incompetence of capacitance vessels** (venous or lymphatic) accounts for the majority of cases of chronic lower-extremity edema.

   b. Consider **lymphedema** as primary (congenital) or secondary (acquired). Acquired causes include trauma, surgery, infection, postradiation, or compression. In the absence of a clear explanation, malignant causes need to be considered.

3. **Generalized edema**

   a. **Comorbid conditions:** The evaluation of patients with generalized edema should focus on the identification of associated comorbid conditions, for which the edema is only one of the symptoms.

   b. **Underlying disorders:** Generalized edema commonly occurs in patients with a known underlying disorder. Common causes such as

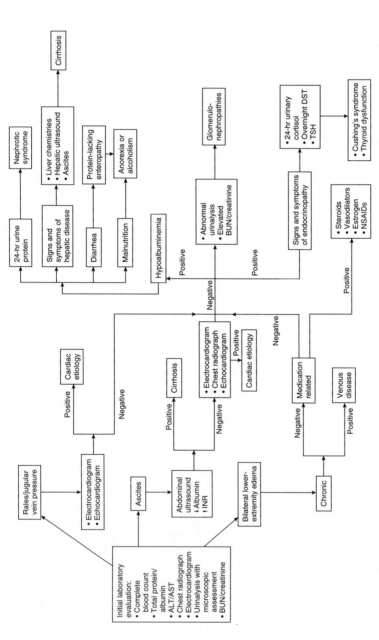

FIGURE 25–1. Algorithm for the diagnosis of generalized edema. A prudent approach to laboratory evaluation is encouraged. In the patient where the history and physical examination do not yield the diagnosis, these studies should be early considerations. *ALT/AST* = alkaline aminotransferase/aspartate aminotransferase; *BUN* = blood urea nitrogen; *DST* = dexamethasone suppression test; *INR* = international normalized ratio, NSAIDs = nonsteroidal anti-inflammatory drugs; *TSH* = thyroid-stimulating hormone.

congestive heart failure (CHF), cirrhosis, and renal disease can be determined by a thorough history.

c. **Pulmonary hypertension** occurs in a variety of diseases such as sleep apnea, chronic pulmonary emboli, intracardial shunts, chronic obstructive pulmonary disease, and primary pulmonary hypertension. Chronic pulmonary hypertension can result in isolated right heart failure and chronic lower-extremity edema. The history should focus accordingly on identifying features of dyspnea, fatigue, sleep disruption, venous thrombosis risk, tobacco use, and risk factors for occupational lung disease.

d. **Endocrine dysfunction:** The patient presenting with generalized edema in the absence of a prior history of cardiac, hepatic, or renal disease should raise suspicion for endocrine dysfunction. History should focus on symptoms of adrenal hyperfunction (e.g., Cushing's syndrome) or thyroid disease.

e. **Plasma protein production:** A reduction in plasma protein production can cause a reduced oncotic pressure and result in generalized edema. Thus, the history should focus on identifying those states identified in Table 25–1 associated with low oncotic pressure. Malabsorptive disorders may be associated with weight loss, diarrhea, and nutritional deficiencies and, when severe, are associated with an impaired ability to produce plasma proteins. Food faddists as well as alcoholics are also at risk for thiamine deficiency (beriberi).

f. **Medication history** should be elicited. Steroids, vasodilators, estrogen preparations, and nonsteroidal anti-inflammatory drugs (NSAIDs) are some of the more common offending agents that can cause generalized edema.

B. Physical examination

1. Local edema

a. **Unilateral lower-extremity edema:** The physical examination is of limited utility in the setting of unilateral lower-extremity edema. Physical evidence of injury or infection can be useful in situations of deep venous thrombosis (DVT), ruptured Baker's cyst, and compartment syndrome; however, the examination may be unremarkable. "Classic" DVT findings of calf tenderness, palpable cord, venous distention, and Homan's sign are frequently absent.

b. **Chronic lower-extremity edema:** In the setting of chronic lower-extremity edema, **venous insufficiency** may be differentiated from lymphedema by the presence of overlying hyperpigmentation or stasis dermatitis. Varicosities and peripheral stigmata further suggest venous disease.

c. **Underlying malignancy:** The examination should include a detailed assessment for underlying malignancy. Examine the lymph nodes. Perform a pelvic examination for gynecologic malignancy and a rectal examination for colon and prostate malignancy.

2. Generalized edema:

Once generalized edema is noted, the examination should focus on assessment for biventricular failure, stigmata of cirrhosis, and signs and symptoms of endocrinopathy (see DISORDERS OF THE ADRENAL GLAND and DISORDERS OF THE THYROID GLAND, Chapter 16).

V. Diagnostic Studies

A. **Local edema** is commonly caused by obstructive etiologies. **Thus, the workup is oriented toward regional conditions (e.g., venous disease, lymphatic obstruction).**

1. **Vascular duplex examination:** When DVT is suspected in a symptomatic patient, a vascular duplex examination is warranted and has excellent sensitivity and specificity (up to 86% and 98%, respectively). For those patients with multiple risk factors, a negative duplex examination may be insufficient to rule out the diagnosis. Greater than 30% of such patients will have thromboses and will require additional testing with serial examinations or a venogram.

2. **Magnetic resonance imaging** (MRI) **and ultrasound:** The diagnosis of a **ruptured gastrocnemius muscle** requires an MRI, whereas a **ruptured popliteal cyst** may be seen on MRI or ultrasound.

B. **Generalized edema** is predominantly caused by elevated hydrostatic gradients (cardiac disease) or oncotic pressure gradients (cirrhosis, nephrosis, enteropathy, nutritional deficiencies). In the absence of obvious etiologies, endocrinopathy should be considered.

1. **12-lead electrocardiogram (ECG), chest radiograph, and echocardiogram:** If suspicion of biventricular heart failure exists, these tests should be diagnostic.

2. **Liver chemistry tests** and **abdominal imaging** are obtained when the history and physical examination suggests cirrhosi. If cirrhosis is a likely consideration, an **abdominal ultrasound** is indicated, which might demonstrate a small nodular liver, splenomegaly, or ascites.

3. **Urinalysis** with microscopic examination of the urinary sediment, a **24-hour urinary protein collection, blood urea nitrogen,** and **creatinine determinations** are the initial steps when nephrotic and nephritic syndromes are possible.

4. **Serum total protein** and **albumin** are an integral part in evaluating patients with generalized edema.

5. **Hemoglobin** and **hematocrit** are used to identify anemia. Profound anemia may be associated with the edematous states.

SUGGESTED READING

Andreoli TE: Edematous states: An overview. *Kidney Int* Supplement 59:S2–S10, 1997.
Powell AA, Armstrong MA: Peripheral edema. *Am Fam Physician* 55:1721–1726, 1997.

26

Fatigue

Rebecca Spanagel

I. **Definition.** Fatigue is a **symptom in which patients describe a feeling of difficulty or exhaustion in pursuing or accomplishing activities.** This chapter will consider idiopathic fatigue that has been present for longer than 1 month. Chronic fatigue refers to fatigue that has been present longer than 6 months.

II. **Overview.** Fatigue should be considered a symptom, not a diagnosis.

   A. **Etiology**

   1. **Idiopathic fatigue.** Approximately 20% of cases have no identifiable cause.
   2. **Psychiatric disorders:** As many as 75% of patients with chronic fatigue have a psychiatric disorder. Depression is the most common of the psychogenic causes. Other causes include mood disorder, somatization disorder, and anxiety disorder.
   3. **Organic disease:** If fatigue develops in patients older than 40 years of age, the patient is twice as likely to have an organic disease as the cause.

   B. **Approach:** Patients with fatigue often receive either excessive or inadequate medical evaluations. Therefore, a judicious approach is necessary.

   1. The **primary purpose** of evaluating a patient with fatigue is to identify and treat any underlying or contributing factors.
   2. Exhaustive, unfocused evaluations are not likely to be revealing and in fact may be counterproductive, reinforcing that the patient has an insidious unidentified medical illness. This is particularly consequential in those with psychogenic components.
   3. When assessing the causes of fatigue using a relatively standardized diagnostic approach, it is rare to overlook important medical diagnoses. This is particularly true when patients are assessed serially.

III. **Differential diagnosis** (Table 26–1)

   A. **Physiologic fatigue** is found in situations that would cause most people to be fatigued. If a patient describes an overwhelming urge to sleep, even during the day, a sleep disorder should be suspected (see SLEEP DISORDERS, Chapter 53).
   B. **Muscular fatigue** can produce decreased performance in the setting of muscle overuse. It is relieved with rest and accentuated with physical activity. It may be localized to specific muscle groups or occur in a generalized distribution. Overdemand in the workplace, overuse of muscles, deconditioning, or true weakness from neurogenic or myopathic disease would be examples of muscular fatigue.
   C. **Medication-induced fatigue.** Fatigue is a common side effect of many medications, including prescription, over-the-counter, and drugs of abuse.

TABLE 26–1. Differential Diagnosis of Fatigue

Physiologic causes, including sleep disorders

Muscular disorders, including fibromyalgia, neuromuscular disorders

Systemic medical disorders
- Endocrine (hypothyroidism, diabetes, adrenal insufficiency, hypopituitarism)
- Cardiovascular (low output states)
- Respiratory (chronic obstructive pulmonary disorder, asthma, chronic hypoxia)
- Hematologic (anemia, myeloproliferative disorders)
- Infectious (HIV, hepatitis, tuberculosis, Epstein-Barr virus, cytomegalovirus disease, subacute bacterial endocarditis)
- Malignancy
- Neurologic (multiple sclerosis, Parkinson's disease, dementia)
- Rheumatologic (rheumatoid arthritis, vasculitis, systemic lupus erythematosus, Sjögren's syndrome)
- Renal insufficiency
- Electrolyte disturbance (especially hypercalcemia in the chronic setting)
- Hepatic insufficiency
- Obesity (body mass index > 45)
- Malnutrition or eating disorder
- Pregnancy

Pharmacologic causes
- Medication side effects, associated with over-the-counter medications, supplements, herbal medications, and prescription agents
- Substance abuse

Psychogenic disorder (most common)

Chronic fatigue syndrome

Undetermined etiology

A thorough medication history, including the temporal relation between the initiation of the medication and onset of fatigue is of paramount importance.

D. **Psychogenic fatigue.** Generally, the fatigue is present on awakening prior to getting out of bed. As the day progresses, or on weekends or holidays, it may improve. If this type of fatigue is found during the history, a thorough psychological assessment should be pursued.

E. **Fatigue related to a systemic illness.** This type of fatigue is generally absent upon waking but develops and progressively worsens during the day. Fatigue usually becomes worse unless the underlying disorder is diagnosed and treated. Relentlessly progressive fatigue may signal serious disease. Conditions in which fatigue may predominate are noted in Table 26–1.

F. **Idiopathic fatigue.** This type of fatigue is stable and does not change over time. If changes are noted, the patient should be reevaluated to identify intervening diagnoses. The approach to idiopathic fatigue is largely supportive, and patients may benefit from rescheduling activities and an exercise program.

IV. Clinical Evaluation

A. **History.** Eliciting important medical history or signs and symptoms of organic disease will permit a targeted evaluation, which will uncover the less common, yet potentially life-threatening medical causes of fatigue.

1. **Define fatigue.** It is very helpful to ask patients to define the fatigue they are experiencing. Fatigue has varying connotations such as weariness, weakness, fatigue with exertion, tiredness, boredom, lack of energy, and sleepiness. Asking why the patient feels fatigued can provide valuable insight into the meaning of fatigue for the patient.

2. **Onset of symptoms:** Explore medical and psychosocial circumstances present at the onset of symptoms. It is important to note that fatigue is rarely the only symptom present in medical conditions.

3. **Sleep history:** A detailed sleep history is mandatory, as sleep disorders are associated with excessive daytime somnolence. Questions that determine how many hours of sleep, quality of sleep, and daytime sleepiness can be revealing (see Chapter 53, SLEEP DISORDERS).

4. **Psychiatric history:** Obtain a relevant psychiatric history, including psychosocial stressors, major life changes, significant illness of family member or friend, current level of functioning, social supports, history of abuse (physical, mental, and substance), and coping skills.

5. **Review of symptoms:** A detailed review of symptoms, mandatory in all patients presenting with isolated fatigue symptoms, may be best obtained through the use of a standardized questionnaire.

B. **Physical examination.** Besides identifying important clues to underlying medical diagnoses, a complete physical examination also offers patients a message that their concern is being taken seriously. This is important not only diagnostically, but also as a tool when reviewing the syndrome with patients during the "therapeutic" interchange.

V. Diagnostic Evaluation (see Fig. 26–1)

A. **Laboratory evaluation.** If the history and physical examination do not identify a specific etiology or psychiatric diagnosis, a rudimentary laboratory evaluation is pursued, including a complete blood count (CBC) with differential, liver chemistries, electrolytes, creatinine, glucose, calcium, thyroid-stimulating hormone (TSH), and urinalysis.

B. **Supplemental studies.** The following should be considered in limited circumstances:

1. Where **rheumatic, inflammatory, or muscular conditions** are suspected, creatine phosphokinase (CPK), antinuclear antibodies, rheumatoid factor (RF), and erythrocyte sedimentation rate (ESR) should be considered (see also Chapter 79, MYALGIA). ESR is not recommended as a routine study since the diagnostic yield is low and will often generate other studies, which may be misleading.

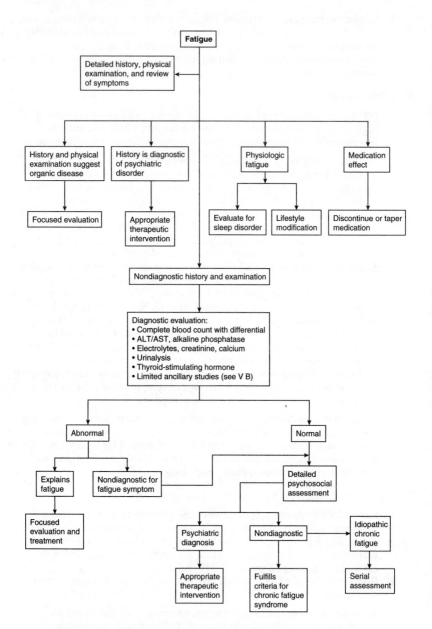

■ **FIGURE 26–1.** Algorithm for the diagnosis of fatigue. *ALT/AST* = alkaline aminotransferase/aspartate aminotransferase.

2. In **patients older than 50 years of age,** who are tobacco abusers, have known environmental exposures, and are at risk for occult pulmonary pathology (e.g., sarcoidosis, tuberculosis, neoplasm), a chest radiograph, intradermal tuberculosis test, and oximetry can be helpful.

3. **HIV testing** should be considered in any patient whose history or examination is suggestive of infection.

4. Patients should all be screened with age- and gender-specific **health maintenance recommendations.** Although identified pathology may not be causative of fatigue, the clinical presentation of fatigue affords the clinician an opportunity to pursue recommended screening procedures.

5. Where the clinical scenario is suggestive, an **overnight polysomnogram** should be considered (see SLEEP DISORDERS, Chapter 53).

SUGGESTED READING

Fukuda K, Straus S, Hickie I, et al: The chronic fatigue syndrome: A comprehensive approach to its definition and study. *Ann Intern Med* 121:953–959, 1994.

Komaroff AL, Buchwald DS: Chronic fatigue syndrome: An update. *Ann Rev Med.* 49:1–13, 1998.

27

Involuntary Weight Loss
Bruce Weinstein

I. **Definition.** No uniformly accepted definition exists. A reasonable working definition of significant involuntary weight loss (IWL) is **unintentional body weight loss of 5% or more within a 6-month period.**

II. **Overview**

   A. IWL is a **nonspecific sign or symptom** with numerous diagnostic possibilities that can be associated with a serious underlying disease or no discernable cause.

   B. **Etiology.** Clinical studies have shown that the prevalence of different causes of IWL depends in part on the clinical setting.

   1. **Physical causes** of IWL predominate in the inpatient setting.
   2. In the ambulatory setting, **nonphysical diagnoses,** including psychosocial and unknown causes, are more common.

III. **Differential Diagnosis**

   A. **Neoplastic disease,** rarely occult, is more common in the inpatient setting.

   B. **Gastrointestinal illnesses,** including malabsorption and "silent" peptic ulcer disease (PUD), are important causes of IWL.

   C. **Hyperthyroidism** is an uncommon cause of IWL, except in one study of ambulatory geriatric patients where it was not readily apparent by history and physical examination.

   D. **Medications** are an important cause of IWL, even with therapeutic doses, especially in the elderly. For example, anticholinergic effects of a drug may lead to dry mouth and attendant difficulty with eating and IWL in geriatric patients. In geriatric patients, alterations in taste, dentition, and swallowing all need to be considered.

   E. **Nonphysical diagnoses** include diagnoses like depression, bereavement, somatization disorders, and a number of social difficulties, such as financial difficulties, social isolation, and increased frailty. It is extremely important to obtain a thorough psychosocial history at the initial encounter when evaluating a patient with IWL.

   F. **Multifactorial causes** can contribute to IWL. This creates difficulty in assigning one unifying diagnosis. It is probably one of the reasons that many clinical studies have found no diagnosis for a number of patients with IWL.

IV. **Clinical Approach.** When evaluating the patient, it is important to note the clinical setting, perform a thorough history and examination, and order tests judiciously.

   A. **Initial approach.** The initial approach to evaluating a patient with IWL is to verify that weight loss has occurred, since a number of patients with complaints of IWL have not lost weight. This can be done directly by chart documentation, or indirectly by confirming weight loss with a reliable patient contact or by noting physical evidence of weight loss, such as a change in clothing size or the presence of cachexia.

B. **Determine cause.** Once weight loss is documented, the clinician needs to determine if the weight loss is from a physical or nonphysical cause.

1. When a **physical cause** of IWL is present, it is usually possible to make a diagnosis after a brief, directed evaluation.
2. When a **nonphysical cause** of IWL is suspected, watchful waiting and testing restraint are important considerations as part of the evaluation process.

C. **Perform a thorough history and physical examination**

1. **History**

a. **Changes in appetite:** Inquire about changes in appetite (increased appetite suggests endocrinopathies such as diabetes, hyperthyroidism, and pheochromocytoma) and food (caloric) intake; determine whether the weight loss is involuntary (patients with voluntary weight loss do not usually seek medical attention, unless in the setting of associated psychopathology); determine adult weight patterns.

b. **Medications:** Obtain a thorough medication and drug use history, including over-the-counter and recreational drugs.

c. **Known disease:** Establish whether the patient has a known disease associated with IWL (see III A–F).

d. **Psychiatric history:** Obtain a comprehensive psychiatric and social history.

e. **Review of systems:** Perform a symptom-specific system review. (A standardized questionnaire is useful.) As neoplasm and gastrointestinal illnesses predominate among the physical causes of IWL, a careful system review should be directed toward these categories of illness.

f. **Eating disorder:** Assess the possibility of an eating disorder (e.g., fear of weight gain, body image disturbance, amenorrhea, binge eating/purging).

2. **Physical examination**

a. The **initial physical examination** should be complete and thorough. Weight should be documented in the chart as part of the examination, and physical evidence of weight loss, such as cachexia, should be noted.

b. **Particular attention** should focus on thyroid findings, adenopathy, and indices of malnutrition. Breast, pelvic, and digital rectal examinations should be performed. The pulmonary and gastrointestinal organ systems should be assessed.

V. **Diagnostic Evaluation** (Figure 27–1). Order additional directed tests that target abnormalities revealed by the history and physical examination.

A. **Screening laboratory tests.** An initial panel of screening laboratory tests should include a complete blood count (CBC), glucose, liver chemistries, renal functions, thyroid-stimulating hormone (TSH), calcium, urinalysis, stool guaiac cards (for patients older than 50 years of age or suspected of having a gastrointestinal cause of IWL), chest radiograph, and age- and

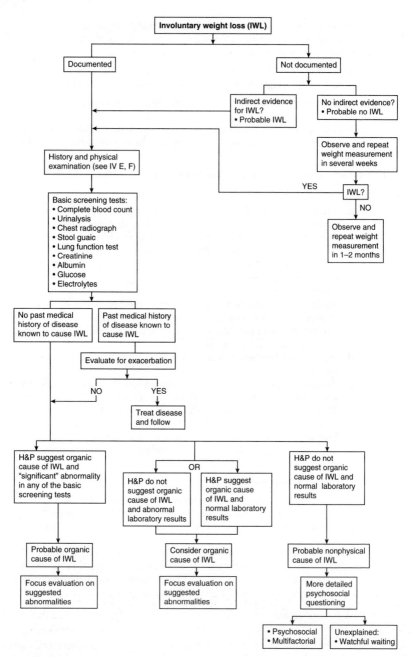

FIGURE 27–1. Algorithm for the diagnosis of involuntary weight loss (*IWL*). *H&P* = history and physical examination. (Adapted with permission from Weinstein B: Involuntary weight loss. In Greene HL, Johnson WP, Maricic MJ (eds): *Decision Making in Medicine.* Philadelphia: B.C. Decker (Mosby-Year Book, Inc), 1993.)

gender-appropriate health screens. With extremes of weight loss, albumin and total protein levels should be noted.

B. HIV testing should be considered in the patient with risk factors.

C. Nondirected testing. Additional, nondirected testing cannot be recommended unless the history or examination points toward a particular abnormality. More extensive blood work or other imaging studies, including nondirected computed tomography (CT), magnetic resonance imaging (MRI), or endoscopic studies, are not recommended as part of the evaluation.

SUGGESTED READING

Thompson MP, Morris LK: Unexplained weight loss in the ambulatory elderly. *J Am Geriatrics Soc* 39:497–500, 1991.

Weinstein B: Involuntary weight loss. In Greene HL, Johnson WP, Maricic MJ (eds): *Decision Making in Medicine.* Philadelphia: B.C. Decker (Mosby-Year Book, Inc), 1993.

28

Obesity
Christian Potter

I. Definition

A. The National Institutes of Health (NIH) currently recommends **body mass index (BMI)** as the most useful means of diagnosing and following overweight and obese individuals. Other recommended strategies include estimations of total body fat, waist circumference, and waist-to-hip ratio.

$$BMI = weight\ (kg)\ /\ height\ (m)^2$$

or

$$BMI = weight\ (lb)\ /\ height\ (in)^2 \times 704.5$$

1. Obesity is defined as a **BMI greater than 30 kg/m²**. Overweight is defined as a **BMI of 25 to 29.9 kg/m²**. This general classification is based on risk stratification, but the relationship between BMI and disease varies among individuals. Muscular individuals or those under 5 feet may have elevated BMI with no increase in total body fat or increased risk of disease.

2. **Waist-to-hip circumference is an indirect measurement of abdominal obesity**, which is an independent predictor of morbidity and mortality. High-risk individuals are defined as those with a waist circumference greater than 102 cm (40 inches) in men or greater than 88 cm (35 inches) in women. This is especially important in individuals with a BMI between 25 and 35 kg/m² because increased waist circumference confers additional risk beyond that of an elevated BMI alone. For those individuals with a BMI greater than 35 kg/m², there is little additional risk at high waist circumferences.

B. Obesity most commonly derives from an **imbalance between caloric consumption and energy expenditure.**

II. Clinical Approach.
In evaluating an individual who is overweight or obese, the emphasis is twofold:

A. Screen for **secondary causes of obesity,** which account for less than 1% of all cases, but often present as the patient's primary concern.

B. Screen for **comorbid conditions,** which have been shown to increase morbidity and mortality in those patients with primary obesity.

III. Differential Diagnosis (Table 28–1 and Figure 28–1)
IV. Notes on the Differential Diagnosis

A. Sedentary lifestyle and excess caloric consumption. The vast majority of patients with obesity have no identifiable etiology other than sedentary lifestyle and excess caloric consumption.

TABLE 28–1. Differential Diagnosis of Obesity

Lifestyle factors (sedentary lifestyle, excess caloric intake, tobacco cessation)
Insulinoma
Hypothyroidism
Cushing's syndrome
Polycystic ovary syndrome
Medications
Hypothalamic disorders
Congenital disorders

B. **Adenoma or carcinoma.** An insulin-secreting adenoma or carcinoma may be associated with weight gain. However, exogenous insulin and sulfonylurea-associated hyperinsulinemia are also associated with weight gain.

C. **Medications.** Certain medications have been associated with weight gain, such as tricyclic antidepressants, phenothiazines, estrogens, serotonin antagonists, and glucocorticoids. Other medications may cause weight gain, but the extent and causation are not well documented.

D. **Congenital disorders** (e.g., Froehlich syndrome, Prader-Willi syndrome, and Laurence-Moon-Biedl syndrome) are usually seen in childhood and are associated with mental retardation, hypogonadism, and other endocrinologic disorders.

E. **Hypothalamic disorder.** Rarely, an acquired hypothalamic disorder can be associated with obesity. These include tumors (e.g., craniopharyngioma), inflammatory disorders (e.g., tuberculosis, sarcoid), and trauma.

V. **Clinical Evaluation.** Most patients with secondary causes of obesity can be identified by a thorough history and physical examination, with diagnostic tests done for confirmation.

A. **History**

1. **Baseline weight:** Obtain a baseline weight (the "ideal body weight"), the duration of obesity, previous weight loss experience, and dietary history (e.g., meal patterns, caloric consumption).

2. **Family history:** Inquire about a family history of thyroid disease or symptoms of endocrinopathy such as fatigue, lethargy, constipation, cold intolerance, muscle cramping, menorrhagia, weight gain (hypothyroidism), muscle weakness, pathologic bone fractures, and mental status changes.

3. **Fasting hypoglycemia:** Assess for symptoms of fasting hypoglycemia. In the setting of hyperinsulinemia (insulinoma), symptoms may be either related to adrenergic hyperreactivity (tachycardia, palpitations, anxiousness, diaphoresis, tremulousness) or the neuroglycopenic effects (mental impairment, headache, slurred speech, psychological alterations, visual disturbances, confusion, coma). Symptoms are generally relieved after glucose correction.

4. **Hyperandrogenism:** Assess for signs of hyperandrogenism, such as oligomenorrhea, infertility, and acne.

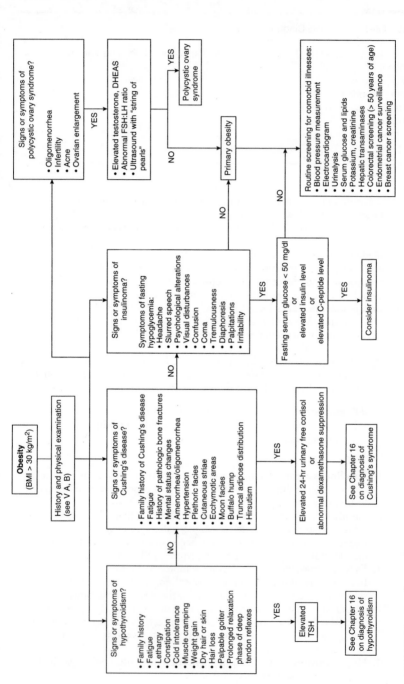

■ **FIGURE 28–1.** Algorithm for the workup of obesity. *BMI* = body mass index; *DHEAS* = dehydroepiandrosterone sulfate; *FSH:LH* = follicle-stimulating hormone:luteinizing hormone; *TSH* = thyroid-stimulating hormone.

TABLE 28–2. Comorbid Conditions Associated with Obesity

Hypertension
Type II diabetes mellitus
Coronary artery disease
Congestive heart failure
Cerebrovascular disease
Hepatic steatosis
Cholelithiasis
Osteoarthritis
Obstructive sleep apnea
Colon cancer
Endometrial cancer
Cholangiocarcinoma
Breast cancer
Depression

   5. Medication history: Obtain a medication history (see IV C).

B. Physical examination

   1. Obtain height, weight, BMI, waist circumference, waist-to-height ratio, and blood pressure.

   2. Assess for dry hair or skin, evidence of ongoing hair loss, palpable goiter, and a prolonged relaxation phase of deep tendon reflexes.

   3. Assess for hypertension, plethoric facies, cutaneous striae, ecchymoses, moon facies, buffalo hump, truncal adipose distribution, and hirsutism.

   4. Assess for acne, acanthosis nigricans, and ovarian enlargement.

VI. Diagnostic Evaluation. Diagnostic evaluation should be focused on the secondary etiologies and complications of obesity.

   A. Pursuit of secondary causes should only be undertaken as indicated by the history and physical examination. Thus, studies may include thyroid-stimulating hormone (TSH), dexamethasone suppression testing [or 24-hour urinary free cortisol (UFC)], fasting glucose, serum androgens [testosterone, dehydroepiandrosterone sulfate (DHEAS)], or pelvic ultrasound (to assess polycystic ovary syndrome in women).

   B. Comorbid conditions associated with obesity are noted in Table 28–2. Although there are no specific recommendations regarding screening for these conditions in the obese, the pretest probability of detecting pathology is higher than that of the general population. The clinician should be aware of these associations.

SUGGESTED READING

National Institutes of Health: Clinical guidelines on the identification, evaluation and treatment of overweight and obesity in adults—the evidence report. *Obes Res* 6:51s, 1998.

29

Tumor Markers

Fauzia Khan, Aftab Mohsin, Armando Fraire,
and Howard Sachs

I. Introduction

A. Tumor markers are **usually proteins that can be detected in peripheral blood, body fluids, solid tumors, and bone marrow.**

B. Tumor markers may be **used for diagnosis, staging, screening, and serial evaluation of tumors** (see also Chapter 37, Ovarian Cancer Screening).

1. Serum tumor markers, with the exception of prostate-specific antigen (PSA), are used for follow-up of disease progression and response to therapy rather than for tumor diagnosis.

2. In general, serum tumor markers rise too late in the course of disease to be of clinical benefit for screening.

II. Carcinoembryonic Antigen

A. **Description.** Carcinoembryonic antigen (CEA) is a glycoprotein normally found only in the gastrointestinal epithelium of the fetus.

1. Conditions associated with elevated CEA levels include gastric carcinomas (86%), pancreatic carcinoma (85%–100%), and breast cancer (45%–60%). Approximately 97% of patients with colon carcinoma are positive for CEA. Small and localized tumors are less likely to be positive.

2. Benign conditions associated with elevated CEA levels include alcoholic cirrhosis, common bile duct obstruction, and active ulcerative colitis. About 20% of normal smokers also have elevated CEA levels.

3. CEA titers greater than four times the upper reference limit (> 10 ng/ml) are usually associated with advanced colorectal carcinomas and imply a poor prognosis.

B. **Indication.** CEA is used for serial monitoring of patients with an established diagnosis of colon cancer. Given the low value early in the course, it is not recommended for screening.

C. **Measurement protocol.** CEA titers are measured at baseline, preoperative, and every 2 months (time varies in different protocols) to detect recurrence after treatment. Levels may rise before a recurrence is clinically evident.

D. **Performance characteristics**

1. **Interassay test precision** is about 10%; therefore, it is recommended to use the same assay consistently.

2. **Colon cancer:** Twenty percent of patients with progressive colon cancer do not have rising CEA levels.

3. **Fluctuating levels:** Technical reasons including inflammation, acute infection, and smoking may result in significant fluctuations of CEA levels.

III. Alpha-Fetoprotein

A. Description. Alpha-fetoprotein (AFP) is an α_1-globulin normally present in high concentration in serum only during the fetal life. Synthesis of the globulin appears to be age related; younger patients are more likely to have elevated serum values.

1. **Elevated serum levels of AFP** (> 500 ng/ml) are a strong indicator of hepatocellular carcinoma (HCC) and hepatoblastoma.
2. AFP is also expressed in testicular and ovarian carcinoma.
3. AFP is elevated in some benign conditions, such as chronic active hepatitis (up to 30%), cirrhosis, Crohn's disease, and benign gynecologic disease (approximately 20%).

B. Performance characteristics

1. About 20%–30% of patients with HCC do not produce AFP. These tumors do not differ biologically. Attempts to correlate the degree of differentiation of HCC with production of AFP have not resulted in a clear answer.
2. Elevated serum levels do not correlate with either clinical or biochemical features of the disease, the size and stage of the tumor, long-term survival, or sex of the patient.

C. Indications

1. **High-risk populations:** AFP and ultrasonography are used for screening in high-risk populations such as the Japanese, who have a high incidence of HCC. Its value as a screening tool in the United States is still debated.
2. **Screening for testicular cancer:** AFP has no value in screening testicular cancer because only 20% of early-stage tumors produce this marker. AFP eventually is positive in as many as 90% of patients with testicular cancer. It may be used for serial monitoring of patients.
3. **Triple screen:** AFP is offered to pregnant women between 16 and 18 weeks' gestation as a part of the "triple screen." The other two markers are human chorionic gonadotropin (HCG) and unconjugated estriol. The triple screen can positively predict 90% of neural tube defects and 60% of Down's syndrome and trisomy 18 cases.

D. Modifications

1. **Fucosylated AFP:** Fucosylated AFP is a subtype of alpha protein. It is useful in differentiating HCC from other tumors, especially when AFP is below the diagnostic level of 500 ng/L.
2. **Des-gamma-carboxy prothrombin:** Serum concentrations of des-gamma-carboxy prothrombin, also called **prothrombin induced by vitamin K absence or antagonism II** (PIVKA II), are elevated in the majority of patients with HCC. In populations where incidence of this tumor is low, the abnormal prothrombin may prove to be more reliable than AFP.

IV. Prostate-Specific Antigen

A. Description. PSA is a neutral serine protease expressed by epithelial cells of normal and neoplastic prostate tissue.

1. Conditions associated with elevated PSA values include:

   a. Benign prostatic hyperplasia (50% of men with PSA 4–10 ng/ml have benign disease)

   b. Prostate cancer (the level may be normal in 25%–40% of men with localized disease)

   c. Prostatitis

   d. Prostate trauma (urinary retention, infarction, recent instrumentation)

2. The PSA level is decreased in men treated with finasteride.

B. Performance characteristics

1. **Assays:** A number of assays are available to measure serum PSA.

2. **Abnormal values:** A serum concentration of 4 ng/ml or higher is generally considered abnormal.

3. **Adaptations:** In an attempt to increase the specificity of the test, a number of adaptations have been developed with varying degrees of clinical utility. These include the age-adjusted value, the PSA density (i.e., PSA corrected for prostate gland volume), the PSA velocity (i.e., the annual rate of rise for PSA), and the percentage of free PSA (i.e., the relative amount of unbound circulating PSA).

   a. **PSA density** refers to the numerical ratio determined by dividing the PSA concentration by the volume of the prostate gland. An elevated density (> 0.15) is suggestive of prostate cancer, because prostate cancer elaborates more PSA per gram of tissue than noncancerous tissue. Unfortunately, the sensitivity of PSA screening is diminished when relying on this measure alone. Also, determination of prostate volume requires the use of transrectal ultrasound, which limits the application of this method.

   b. **PSA velocity** refers to the rate of change in PSA over time. A change of 0.75 ng/ml per year is suggestive of prostate cancer. In clinical practice, an elevated PSA level will generally be evaluated upon initial identification. The velocity becomes clinically useful in patients evidencing acceleration within the normal range and for those patients whose initial evaluation failed to identify prostate cancer.

   c. **Free PSA:** PSA circulates in the serum bound primarily to protease inhibitors. For reasons that are uncertain, a lower percentage of unbound (free) PSA is observed in those patients with prostate cancer. That is, the percent of free PSA is lower. Values < 5% to 10% should be viewed with heightened suspicion. Conversely, values of free PSA > 25% are more commonly seen in benign disease. Free PSA is most appropriately reserved for following those patients with total PSA values in the 4- to 10-ng/ml range after initial evaluation reveals no evidence of cancer. Serum concentrations > 10 ng/ml need aggressive evaluation regardless of the free PSA percentage.

C. **Indications.** PSA is used for screening prostate cancer, assessing tumor burden, and serial monitoring patients following diagnosis and treatment.

V. CA19–9

A. **Description.** Although originally derived from a colorectal cell line, CA19–9 is most specific for pancreatic carcinoma and is positive in 70%–90% of all cases of pancreatic carcinoma. It is also positive in colon, breast, and ovarian mucinous adenocarcinomas. The positive predictive value in patients who do not have jaundice, but have a confirming computed tomography (CT) scan is considerable at levels above 200 ng/ml.

B. Indications. A combination of CEA and CA19–9 may be used for screening pancreatic cancer in high-risk populations. It may also be used for serial follow-up in patients with an established diagnosis.

SUGGESTED READING

Lindblom A, Lilijegren A: Tumor markers in malignancies. *Br Med J* 320:424–427, 2000.

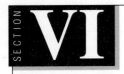

Gynecology

30

Abnormal Uterine Bleeding

Gertrude Manchester

I. Definition

A. **Normal uterine bleeding** is considered to be flow of 2–6 days, blood loss of 20–60 ml, and cycle length of 21–35 days.

B. **Abnormal uterine bleeding (AUB)** can be defined in absolute terms as any menstrual bleeding that falls outside of these defined norms or in relative terms as any significant departure from the patient's previously established pattern of menses.

II. Overview

A. Menstrual abnormalities associated with **ovulatory cycles** include menorrhagia (i.e., excessive flow or days of bleeding) and metrorrhagia (i.e., irregular bleeding between cycles). Ovulatory cycles are usually associated with an organic cause.

B. Menstrual abnormalities associated with **anovulatory cycles** include menometrorrhagia (i.e., irregular heavy menses) or polymenorrhea (i.e., frequent bleeding and spotting). Anovulatory cycles are frequently idiopathic.

III. Differential Diagnosis (Table 30–1)

A. **Dysfunctional uterine bleeding (DUB)** is defined as excessive, prolonged, unpatterned bleeding from the endometrium that is unrelated to structural or systemic disease. It is thus a diagnosis of exclusion. DUB results in an anovulatory pattern of bleeding 85% of the time. The hallmark of DUB is the relative deficiency of progesterone (either in absolute terms or relative to estrogen levels).

B. The **patient's age** is an important consideration in developing a patient-specific differential diagnosis.

1. **Adolescence**

   a. An **anovulatory cycle** related to an immature hypothalamic-pituitary-ovarian axis is the most common cause for AUB in adolescence (accounts for 95% of cases).

TABLE 30–1. Abnormal Uterine Bleeding

The broad differential diagnosis falls into four major categories:

1. **Reproductive tract disease**
   a. **Complications of pregnancy**
      - Threatened, incomplete, or missed abortion
      - Ectopic pregnancy
      - Trophoblastic disease
      - Placental polyp
      - Subinvolution of the placental site
   b. **Malignancy**
      - Endometrial
      - Cervical
      - Vaginal
      - Vulvar
      - Ovarian
   c. **Infection**
      - Endometritis
      - Salpingitis
      - Severe vaginitis
   d. **Other benign pelvic disorders**
      - Traumatic lesions
      - Foreign bodies
      - Cervical or endometrial polyps
      - Cervical erosion
      - Cervicitis
      - Submucosal uterine leiomyomas
      - Adenomyosis
      - Endometriosis
      - Intrauterine device

2. **Systemic causes**
   a. Hypothyroidism
   b. Cirrhosis
   c. Coagulopathy (von Willebrand's disease most frequently)

3. **Pharmacologic causes**
   a. Sex steroids (oral contraceptives)
   b. Psychotropic agents
   c. Autonomic drugs
   d. Digitalis
   e. Phenytoin
   f. Anticoagulants
   g. Nonsteroidal anti-inflammatory drugs (NSAIDs)
   h. Corticosteroids
   i. Ginseng (has estrogen-like effect on endometrium)

continued

TABLE 30–1. Abnormal Uterine Bleeding (*Continued*)

4. Dysfunctional uterine bleeding (DUB)
  a. Hypothalamic-pituitary-ovary axis immaturity in adolescence
  b. Anovulatory cycles in perimenopausal women
  c. Obesity
  d. Polycystic ovary syndrome (PCOS)

    b. Coagulation defects such as von Willebrand's disease are the most common organic cause of AUB in this age group.
    c. Pregnancy and genitourinary infection are also important considerations for those patients who are sexually active. AUB in a **woman of reproductive age** must be considered a complication of pregnancy until proven otherwise.

  2. Young adults (15–35 years of age)

    a. Pregnancy, endometritis, and oral contraceptive pills (OCPs) are the most common organic causes.
    b. Trophoblastic disease is an uncommon but important cause to rule out, as good prognosis depends on early diagnosis.

  3. Middle-aged women (35–45 years of age). The causes are similar to those for young adults, with the important additions of **uterine fibroids** (prevalence increases with age) and **endometrial carcinoma**.

  4. Peri- and postmenopausal women

    a. Endometrial carcinoma is the most important and common organic cause of AUB. In patients with AUB, 5% of perimenopausal women and as many as 20% of postmenopausal women are ultimately diagnosed with endometrial carcinoma.
    b. AUB should be considered the result of **malignancy** until proven otherwise.

IV. Clinical Evaluation

  A. History

    1. Gynecologic considerations: The onset, frequency, duration, severity, and pattern of bleeding (cyclic versus irregular), as well as any change from a previously established pattern of bleeding are all essential components of the history. Age, parity, marital status, sexual history, previous gynecologic disease, contraceptive history, medications, and dates of past pregnancies may contribute important clues.
    2. Medication: Note temporal relationships between onset of AUB and initiation of a new medication, including over-the-counter drugs and herbal preparations.
    3. Bleeding: Unusual bleeding from other sites, family history of blood dyscrasia, easy bruisability, or a history of excessive bleeding suggests the possibility of coagulopathy.

    4. Endocrinopathies

        a. Weight gain, fatigue, cold intolerance, constipation, and goiter all suggest **hypothyroidism.**

        b. Onset of voice change, hirsutism, and acne suggest **hyperandrogenism.**

B. Physical examination

    1. Pay particular attention to vital signs, the presence or absence of orthostasis, and abdominal or pelvic tenderness when **ectopic pregnancy** is being considered.

    2. Assess the **thyroid gland** for size and nodularity.

    3. Assess for **stigmata of liver disease** (e.g., palmar erythema, spider angiomata, ascites).

    4. Perform a **pelvic examination and Pap smear,** and assess for signs of infection, cervical abnormalities, or structural abnormalities (e.g., enlargement of the uterus, the presence of an adnexal mass).

V. Diagnostic Evaluation (Figure 30–1)

    A. Initial evaluation should include a complete blood count (CBC), thyroid-stimulating hormone (TSH), Pap smear, coagulation profile (include bleeding time if von Willebrand's disease is suspected),

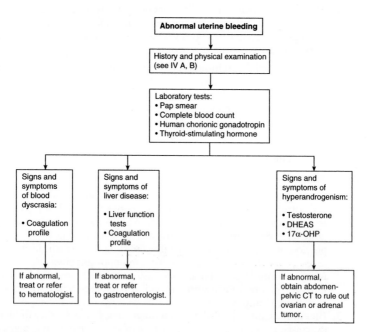

■ **FIGURE 30–1.** Algorithm for the evaluation of abnormal uterine bleeding. *17α-OHP* = 17α-hydroxyprogesterone; *CT* = computed tomography; *DHEAS* = dehydroepiandrosterone sulfate.

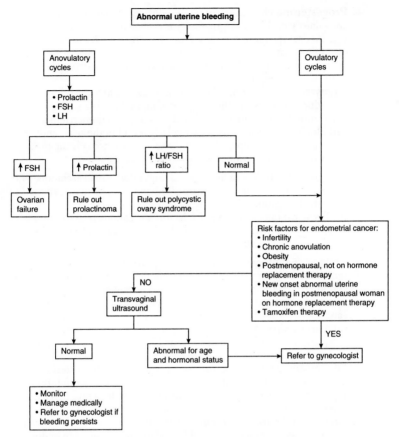

■ **FIGURE 30–1.** (*Continued*) Algorithm for the evaluation of abnormal uterine bleeding. *FSH* = follicle-stimulating hormone; *LH* = luteinizing hormone.

and human chorionic gonadotropin (HCG) in women of reproductive age.

B. Additional studies (as suggested by the history and physical examination) include:

1. **Serum quantification:** If ectopic pregnancy is a consideration, a urinary HCG may be insufficient. If suspicious and the urinary test is negative, a serum quantification should be pursued.

2. **Dehydroepiandrosterone sulfate** (DHEAS), **testosterone,** and **17α-hydroxyprogesterone** (17α-OHP) should be obtained if signs and symptoms of hyperandrogenism are present.

3. **Prolactin, follicle-stimulating hormone** (FSH), and **luteinizing hormone** (LH) should be tested for anovulatory cycles. The FSH is best obtained on the third day of the menstrual cycle.

4. **Progesterone challenge** should be considered in all patients with anovulatory cycles, after pregnancy is excluded. The clinician usually uses medroxyprogesterone at a dose of 10 mg daily for 7–10 days. If bleeding occurs 2–7 days following the medication, anovulatory cycles are confirmed. If no bleeding occurs, consider hypoestrogenic states or outflow obstruction.

5. **Transvaginal ultrasound** is the least invasive and lowest-cost procedure for assessing the endometrium, as there is a strong correlation between increasing thickness of the endometrium and pathologic involvement. It is particularly useful in the peri- and postmenopausal groups, where endometrial carcinoma is the most worrisome consideration.

   a. A patient with low or average risk for endometrial carcinoma who has a normal endometrial stripe (< 5 mm) can be managed medically with close monitoring.

   b. Those patients who have risk factors for endometrial carcinoma or an abnormal ultrasound require further evaluation (sensitivity 88%–97%, specificity 89%).

6. **Endometrial biopsy** is a simple office procedure that has 90%–98% sensitivity (when an adequate tissue sample is obtained) for detecting endometrial carcinoma in both peri- and postmenopausal patients. Although this procedure carries high sensitivity for endometrial carcinoma, localized pathology such as endometrial polyps and submucous myomas may be missed, and it may not be possible to obtain adequate tissue samples in as many as 15% of patients with atrophic endometrium.

7. **Sonohysterography** is performed by instilling 10 ml of sterile saline into the endometrial cavity prior to obtaining an ultrasound. It is superior to standard transvaginal ultrasound in detecting polyps, submucous fibroids, and focal areas of endometrial thickening.

8. **Dilation and curettage** is done under anesthesia, is highly sensitive, and was once considered the gold standard for diagnosis of endometrial pathology. The office endometrial biopsy procedure carries equally high sensitivity, with less cost, risk, and inconvenience for the patient.

9. **Hysteroscopy** is a direct visualization technique employed to assist with a directed biopsy or excision of a localized abnormality within the uterus. Hysteroscopy combined with directed biopsy is superior to dilation and curettage or office endometrial biopsy alone.

SUGGESTED READING

Long, CA: Evaluation of patients with abnormal uterine bleeding. *Am J Obstet Gynecol* 175(3): 784–786, 1996.

31

The Palpable Breast Mass
Michael Wertheimer

I. **Definition.** A palpable breast mass is defined as a **new, unexplained, three-dimensional finding that has describable features of size, margins, texture, and location.**

II. **Overview**

   A. **Breast cancer** is newly diagnosed in 180,000 women per year in the United States.

   B. Given the public's heightened awareness of breast cancer, an increasing number of women can be expected to seek consultation for the evaluation of a palpable breast mass.

III. **Clincial Evaluation.** When a careful and thorough **physical examination,** an accurate **mammographic evaluation,** and a **fine-needle aspirate cytology** are performed on a suspicious breast mass, the correct diagnosis can be obtained in 99% of patients.

   A. **History**

   1. **A complete medical and family history is essential.** In addition to obtaining basic health and demographic information, the history should include age of menarche, age of menopause, number of pregnancies and deliveries, and any exogenous hormone therapy.

   2. **Family history** in the evaluation of breast disease is very important and includes any breast or genital malignancies in first- and second-degree relatives.

   3. The **history of all previous breast surgeries** with their histopathology as well as prior mammographic patterns and abnormalities should be included in the history.

   4. Inquire about the practice of **breast self-examination** and any findings or symptoms of current or recent breast disease.

   B. **Physical examination**

   1. A thorough and complete **physical examination of the breast and all regional node basins** (axilla, cervical, supraclavicular) is a critical component in the evaluation.

   2. The examination is always performed with the patient disrobed and in an examination gown, opened in the front. The examination is always **performed in at least two positions—supine and upright.**

   3. Note any **skin changes or nipple abnormalities. Palpate the breast parenchyma** by pressing the tissue against the chest wall using finger-tips. The breast should be examined either in circumferential "time zones" or by quadrant.

   4. **All lumps must be evaluated and characterized to a logical conclusion without delay.** A basic principle for breast lump diagnosis is

that **virtually all lumps can be characterized nonoperatively or preoperatively.** It has become increasingly uncommon to perform open, surgical diagnostic biopsies of the breast. Cysts may be eliminated by fine-needle aspiration (FNA). Benign solid tumors too may be characterized and cancers may be routinely diagnosed by FNA.

IV. Diagnostic Evaluation

A. **FNA biopsy.** Figure 31–1 illustrates the most efficient diagnostic approach in the evaluation of a solitary mass.

1. **Technique.** FNA biopsy is performed with the examiner standing on the side opposite the breast lump and trapping the lump between the fingers. The mass is compressed against the chest wall, and a 5-cc syringe with a 22-gauge needle is inserted into the lump (usually without the need for local anesthesia).

2. **Cyst versus solid mass:** The examiner can usually determine whether the lump is a cyst or a solid mass.

a. **Cystic lumps** are aspirated dry.

(1) If the physical finding completely disappears, and if the fluid is clear, the patient can be reassured. The fluid may be discarded as cytologic evaluation of clear cyst fluid yields 0.1% results. The patient should be examined and aspirated again in a month to determine reoccurrence.

(2) A residual mass or thickening after aspiration or a nontraumatic bloody tap mandates referral and excisional biopsy.

b. **Solid structure:** If a solid structure is encountered on entry of the needle, a repetitive, piston-like motion in and out of multiple regions of the mass will yield a reliable cytologic preparation that can differentiate benign from malignant cells in most cases.

B. **Diagnostic imaging in the evaluation of breast lumps**

1. **Breast imaging** now includes standard diagnosis by mammography, digital mammography, and breast ultrasound. Also used are adaptations

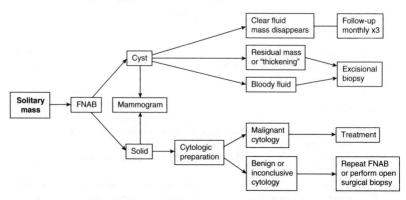

■ **FIGURE 31–1.** Diagnostic algorithm for fine-needle aspiration biopsy (FNAB).

of existing technologies for minimally invasive stereotaxic (mammography-based) or ultrasound-guided FNA cytology. Similarly, core histopathologic biopsy of occult, mammographically detected tumors including solid masses and microcalcifications can be evaluated in this manner.

2. **Biopsies formerly performed by surgeons** are now handled by breast imagers, traditional radiologists, and mammographers who perform as many as 50%–60% of all breast biopsies in large centers.

C. **Breast ultrasound**

1. **Ultrasound** will differentiate between a benign simple cyst, a complex cyst, or a suspicious solid density.

   a. Benign simple cysts might be safely ignored or aspirated.
   b. Complex cysts and solid tumors discovered mammographically and confirmed ultrasonographically may be biopsied with needle core technique under ultrasound guidance with the same reliable result that FNA biopsy, stereotactic fine-needle biopsy, or core biopsy can achieve.

2. **Diagnostic ultrasound** has developed an increasing role in breast diagnosis. It is primarily indicated for the **further evaluation of nonpalpable, occult, mammographic densities seen on mammography.**

D. The **careful integration** of imaging technology with the clinical evaluation and the judicious use of fine-needle or core-biopsy techniques can lead to the accurate diagnosis in the vast majority of breast lumps.

SUGGESTED READING

Donegan W: Evaluation of a palpable breast mass. *N Engl J Med* 327:937–942, 1992.

32

Amenorrhea
Marjorie Safran

I. **Definition.** Amenorrhea is the **absence of menarche at puberty (primary amenorrhea) or the absence of menses for three cycles in a woman who was previously menstruating (secondary amenorrhea).**

II. **Differential Diagnosis** (Table 32–1). It is useful to classify cases into primary or secondary causes. The primary causes are not commonly seen in the adult population.

III. **Notes on the Differential Diagnosis** (see Table 32–1)

   A. **Ovarian and hypothalamic causes** account for nearly 75% of secondary amenorrhea.

   B. **Hypothalamic disorders** are characterized by loss of gonadotropic-releasing hormone pulsatility, with associated loss of luteinizing hormone surge.

   C. **Pituitary causes.** The most common pituitary cause is hyperprolactinemia. It is associated with galactorrhea in 50%–80% of the cases.

   D. **Ovarian causes.** The ovarian causes are dominated by premature ovarian failure and hyperandrogenic states.

   1. **Premature ovarian failure** is a relatively common cause of amenorrhea and is suggested by an elevated level of follicle-stimulating hormone (FSH). Causes include genetic disorders (e.g., galactosemia, X-chromosome abnormalities), and immune, chemical (alkylating agents), and radiation insults.

   2. **Hyperandrogenic states** are dominated by polycystic ovary syndrome (PCOS), although androgen-producing neoplasms or exogenous androgen use are additional considerations. PCOS is a chronic anovulation syndrome, which is associated with hyperandrogenism, oligomenorrhea or amenorrhea, infertility, elevated levels of circulating androgens, obesity, and insulin resistance. Cutaneous manifestations include acanthosis nigricans, acne, and hirsutism. Most women will have morphologically abnormal ovaries, although this is not a diagnostic requirement.

IV. **Clinical Approach**

   A. **History** should make the distinction between primary and secondary amenorrhea.

   1. Assess for weight changes, stressors, exercise, galactorrhea, signs or symptoms of thyroid dysfunction, and medication use.

   2. Assess previous uterine procedures or injury, fertility history, and signs of hyperandrogenism (e.g., acne, hair growth, unusual menstrual pattern).

   B. **Physical examination**

   1. Observe the body habitus.

TABLE 32–1. Causes of Amenorrhea

1. Outflow tract or uterine abnormality
- Asherman's syndrome (intrauterine adhesions)
- Mullerian agenesis or anomalies*
- Testicular feminization* (XY with congenital androgen insensitivity)

2. Ovarian causes
- Turner's syndrome* (gonadal dysgenesis, XO)
- Gonadal agenesis*
- Premature ovarian failure, menopause

3. Pituitary causes
- Hyperprolactinemia (prolactinoma, drugs)
- Nonsecreting pituitary tumor

4. Hypothalamic dysfunction
- Craniopharyngioma
- Chronic illness (Crohn's disease, cystic fibrosis, anorexia)
- Anovulation (extreme weight loss or gain, stress, exercise)
- Delayed puberty*
- Infiltrative disorders (hemochromatosis, sarcoidosis, lymphoma)

5. Inappropriate feedback
- Neoplasms producing androgens or estrogens
- Neoplasms producing human chorionic gonadotropin (HCG)
- Liver and renal disease
- Obesity
- Congential adrenal hyperplasia
- Polycystic ovary syndrome (PCOS)

6. Miscellaneous
- Hyper- or hypothyroidism
- Cushing's syndrome
- Acromegaly
- Exogenous androgen use

*This finding indicates primary amenorrhea.

2. Check for breast discharge.
3. Perform a pelvic examination with focus on the vagina, cervix, and uterus.
4. Check for ovarian or thyroid gland abnormalities, and signs of hyperandrogenism (e.g., acne, acanthosis nigricans).

V. Diagnostic Evaluation (Figure 32–1)

A. Pregnancy. The first step in evaluating all patients with secondary amenorrhea is to rule out pregnancy. Human chorionic gonadotropin (HCG) should be obtained in all patients.

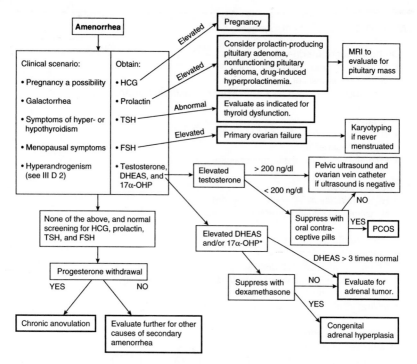

■ **FIGURE 32–1.** Algorithm for the workup of amenorrhea. *17α-OHP* = 17α-hydroxyprogesterone; *DHEAS* = dehydroepiandrosterone sulfate; *FSH* = follicle-stimulating hormone; *HCG* = human chorionic gonadotropin; *MRI* = magnetic resonance imaging; *PCOS* = polycystic ovary syndrome; *TSH* = thyroid-stimulating hormone.

*17α-OHP should be drawn at 8 AM during the follicular phase.

    B. **Metabolic, psychosocial, and uterine factors.** The clinician next distinguishes among the metabolic factors (e.g., liver, renal disease), psychosocial factors (e.g., stressors, exercise, weight loss), and uterine factors (e.g., Asherman's syndrome).

    C. **Hypothalamic-pituitary-ovarian axis abnormalities.** Once accomplished, the challenge lies in assessing any hypothalamic-pituitary-ovarian axis abnormalities.

        1. **Hormonal evaluation:** The hormonal evaluation includes prolactin, thyroid-stimulating hormone (TSH), and FSH.

        2. **Hyperandrogenism:** If signs or symptoms suggest hyperandrogenism, dehydroepiandrosterone sulfate (DHEAS) and testosterone should be obtained.

    D. **Further evaluation.** Abnormalities on any of these studies require appropriate further evaluation. It should be noted that most women undergoing a hormonal assessment will have a nondiagnostic evaluation. An uncertain percentage of these women may in fact have PCOS, while others have functional hypothalamic amenorrhea.

E. Karyotype studies are recommended for patients with premature ovarian failure manifesting before 30 years of age.

SUGGESTED READING

American College of Obstetrician and Gynecologists: ACOG Technical bulletin #202. Hyperandrogenic chronic anovulation. *Int J Gynaecol Obstet* 49:201–208, 1995.

Watson RE, Bouknight R, Alguire PC: Hirsutism: Evaluation and management. *J Gen Intern Med* 10:2832–2892, 1995.

Goudas VT, Dumesic DA: Polycystic ovary syndrome. *Endocrinol Metab Clin North Am* 26: 893–912, 1997.

33

Infertility
Elaine R. Evans-Metcalf

I. **Definition.** Infertility is defined as **failure of a couple to establish pregnancy after 1 year of unprotected intercourse.**

    A. **Primary infertility** is infertility occurring with no previous pregnancy.

    B. **Secondary infertility** is that associated with a history of prior pregnancy.

II. **Overview**

    A. **Conception rate.** The definition is based on an expected monthly conception rate among healthy couples of 20%–25%.

    B. **Etiology.** A cause can be identified in **85%** of couples; in the remaining 15%, standard investigations yield normal results and infertility is thus "unexplained."

        1. **Male factor infertility** (35%–40%). The most common correctable cause of male factor infertility is a **varicocele.**

        2. Ovulatory defects (20%–25%)

        3. Tubal and peritoneal factors (25%–30%)

        4. Cervical or uterine factors (10%)

    C. **Pregnancy without treatment.** After 1 year of infertility, as many as 50% of couples will ultimately achieve pregnancy without treatment. Each month, approximately 3% of couples with unexplained infertility conceive on their own.

    D. **Influencing factors.** Factors that influence the likelihood of pregnancy include the duration of infertility, the age of the woman, and the cause of infertility. Bilateral tubal obstruction, azoospermia, and prolonged amenorrhea decrease the likelihood of unassisted conception.

    E. **Time frame for fertilization.** It is estimated that the human egg is fertilizable for 12–24 hours after ovulation and that sperm are able to fertilize for 24–48 hours. This information is used to **maximize coital efficiency** while attempting to conceive.

III. **Clinical Evaluation.** Evaluation is generally initiated after a 12-month trial, but it should be pursued sooner (after 6 months) in high-risk groups, such as women older than 35 years, women who are anovulatory, or if either partner has had a prior sterilization procedure.

    A. The **initial assessment** should include both partners.

        1. **General approach.** The approach to evaluation varies, but generally the initial assessment includes a history, physical examination, semen analysis, documentation of ovulation [using basal body temperature (BBT) or urinary luteinizing hormone (LH)], and documentation of tubal patency.

        2. **Hormonal evaluation.** Because of the low incidence of endocrinologic

disorders in the infertile population, many clinicians limit hormonal evaluation to patients with irregular menses and for the assessment of "ovarian reserve" [see IV B 1 c (6)].

B. History

1. **Reproductive history:** Note the prior reproductive history of both partners, duration of attempt at conception, and frequency and timing of coitus.

2. **Gynecologic history** should include menstrual regularity, dysmenorrhea, pelvic pain, use of intrauterine device, sexually transmitted disease, pelvic inflammatory disease, endometriosis, surgical procedures involving the cervix, and pelvic surgery.

3. **Endocrinology assessment:** Assess for dysfunction of the thyroid, adrenal (hyperandrogenism), and pituitary glands, including any history of galactorrhea, acne, and hirsutism. Inquire about symptoms of weight change, menopause, and medication use.

4. **Male partner:** The male partner should be assessed for prior surgery, history of drug use, toxin exposure, sexual and pubertal development, testicular abnormalities, ejaculatory disturbance, and erectile dysfunction.

C. Physical examination

1. **Female partner:** Assess the body habitus, hair distribution, and thyroid. Also check for any signs of acanthosis nigricans and galactorrhea. A careful pelvic examination is important, including Pap smear, and where indicated, cervical cultures for gonorrhea and chlamydia.

2. **Male partner:** Note surgical scars, penile anomalies, and testicular size and consistency. Palpate the vas deferens for varicocele.

IV. Diagnostic Evaluation

A. Male factors

1. **Semen analysis**

   a. **Technique.** The patient should be abstinent for 2–3 days. A semen specimen is collected through masturbation and is delivered to the lab within 1 hour, kept at body temperature.

   (1) "**Normal**" **parameters** (World Health Organization) include a volume > 2 ml, a sperm concentration ≥ 20 million/ml, motility ≥ 50% progressively motile, and morphology > 30% normal forms. Some laboratories also include leukocytes < 1 million/ml.

   (2) **Abnormal analysis:** If the semen analysis is abnormal, repeat specimen and refer the patient to a urologist if there is persistent abnormality.

   b. **Limitations** of semen analysis include:

   (1) A lack of sperm function evaluation (e.g., capacity for fertilization)

   (2) Sperm counts can fluctuate

   (3) The overlap between fertile and subfertile

2. **Hormonal evaluation** (which is rarely indicated except when hypo-gonadism is suspected) includes follicle-stimulating hormone (FSH), testosterone, and prolactin. Hyperprolactinemia is unlikely to be found as an etiology in the absence of erectile dysfunction.

B. Female factors

1. Ovulatory factors

a. **Anovulation** is likely if there is amenorrhea, or cycle length > 42 days. However, anovulation can still be present with regular menstrual cycles.

b. **Guiding coital activity:** Documentation is necessary as part of the infertility workup, but it can also be used to guide coital activity (coitus every 36–48 hours 3–4 days prior to and 2 days after expected ovulation maximizes the chance of conception).

c. **Documentation:** Techniques for documentation include:

(1) **BBT:** Temperature is taken daily for 1–2 months immediately upon awakening in the morning and charted along with coital activity.

(a) Ovulatory cycles have a biphasic curve due to a 0.5- to 1°F-temperature rise in the luteal phase from progesterone secretion.

(b) The rise should be sustained for 11–16 days.

(c) Ovulation typically occurs on the day **prior** to first temperature elevation and, thus, can only be identified retrospectively.

(d) Monophasic cycles (i.e., cycles without the temperature spike) do not exclude ovulation.

(2) **LH monitoring** (urinary LH) is used to document the LH surge that precedes ovulation by approximately 24–48 hours.

(3) Midluteal serum progesterone: Serum progesterone > 3 ng/ml (10 nmol/L) 5–7 days prior to anticipated menses (days 21–23 of ideal 28-day cycle) confirms ovulation. Low levels are not diagnostic of anovulation. This is not a first-line test for ovulation detection.

(4) **Endometrial biopsy** is performed in the office 2–3 days before expected menses. A secretory endometrium confirms ovulation. This test is generally reserved for women with long-standing anovulation to rule out hyperplasia, and to exclude luteal phase defects, rather than ovulation documentation alone.

(5) **Hormonal assessment**

(a) If anovulation is suspected, evaluation should include thyroid-stimulating hormone (TSH) and prolactin.

(b) If hirsutism is present, dehydroepiandrosterone sulfate (DHEAS), testosterone, and 17α-hydroxyprogesterone (17α-OHP) should be included.

(c) If Cushing's syndrome is suspected, a 24-hour urinary cortisol secretion or an overnight dexamethasone suppression test is warranted.

(6) Assessing ovarian reserve: To test "ovarian reserve" (i.e., ovarian age), FSH performed on day 3 of the cycle may be useful. This test is generally reserved for women 35 years and older or those with unexplained infertility.

   (a) An FSH $\geq$ 15 IU/l is associated a poor likelihood of in vitro fertilization.
   (b) A level $\geq$ 25 IU/l suggests a low likelihood of achieving pregnancy by any means.
   (c) FSH levels > 40 IU/l are consistent with complete cessation of ovarian function.

2. **Tubal and peritoneal factors**
   a. **Tubal patency** must be assessed. This is most commonly done by hysterosalpingography, which also serves to evaluate uterine contour. The false–positive rate is approximately 15% due to proximal tubal spasm; false negatives are rare.
   b. **Laparoscopy** with simultaneous injection of blue dye through the cervical os and observation for spill from the tubes is informative and permits visualization of the peritoneal cavity. If adhesions or early-stage endometriosis is present, surgical treatment can be concomitantly undertaken. Given the associated costs and risks, laparoscopy is not considered part of the initial assessment.

3. **Cervical factors** include structural abnormalities and abnormal mucus production. A **postcoital test** was historically used to evaluate for cervical factors; however, this test has lost much favor due to its poor reproducibility and predictive value. Because test results do not affect treatment decisions, there is no clear consensus as to its role in infertility evaluation.

4. **Uterine factors** may include infection, fibroids, intrauterine scarring, congenital malformations, and foreign bodies. Typically, hysterosalpingography is performed with other tests (e.g., hysteroscopy, saline infusion ultrasound, endometrial biopsy) as indicated.

SUGGESTED READING

Speroff L, Glass RH, Kase NG: *Clinical Gynecologic Endocrinology and Infertility*, 5th ed. Baltimore: Williams & Wilkins, 1994.

34

Vaginitis
Kathleen Goonan

I. Definition. Vaginitis is an **inflammation of the vagina that may be characterized by one or more of the following symptoms: increased volume of discharge, abnormal color or odor of discharge, itching, irritation, burning, and dyspareunia.**

II. Overview

    A. Normal vaginal secretions are clear with gram-positive bacilli present, and are either odorless or smell like "sour milk."

        1. During the menstrual cycle, vaginal secretions may vary with an increase in clear discharge around the time of ovulation.

        2. Normal secretions also increase with pregnancy and sexual excitement.

    B. Symptoms of vaginitis. The symptoms of vaginitis are nonspecific, and therefore, identifying the causal diagnosis can be challenging. Diagnostic tests can be misleading if not interpreted in the appropriate clinical setting.

III. Differential Diagnosis (Table 34–1)

    A. Normal secretions are formed by a combination of factors that include mucoid endocervical secretions, sloughed epithelial lining cells, and the normal vaginal flora. The normal pH ranges from 3.8–4.2.

    B. Bacterial vaginosis (BV)

        1. Signs. The hallmark of BV is a reduction in the concentration of lactobacilli, which are present in the normal vaginal flora. The resultant increase in bacteria (mostly anaerobic organisms) is thought to contribute to the characteristic clinical symptoms. BV typically causes either no discomfort or mild burning and itching. Patients lack a significant inflammatory response. The patient may report a "fishy" odor. The discharge can vary from gray to yellow-green and tends to be thin. Recurrences are common.

        2. Diagnosis. The diagnosis of BV is made in a patient presenting with a typical discharge, vaginal pH > 4.5, a positive whiff test (see V B 2), and the presence of "clue cells" on wet mount. Gram stain is more reliable than wet mount for the diagnosis of BV, although not routinely performed.

            a. Clue cells are characterized by the presence of short, motile rods yielding round, moth-eaten cell borders or stippled epithelial cells. Clue cells are thought to be clinically relevant when they comprise > 20% of the epithelial cells assessed.

            b. Other important findings include **the lack of normal flora** (i.e., lactobacilli), white blood cells (noninflammatory condition), and other pathologic conditions (e.g., candidiasis, trichomoniasis).

    C. Candida is increasingly common due to the widespread and injudicious use of antibiotics. Other predisposing factors include the use of corticosteroids

TABLE 34–1. Causes of Vaginitis

Normal secretions

Peri-ovulatory
Pregnancy
Sexual arousal

Infectious causes

Bacterial vaginosis (BV)
Vulvovaginal candidiasis
Trichomoniasis

Noninfectious causes

Allergic or contact dermatitis
Chronic activity-induced trauma
Atrophic vaginitis
Idiopathic

or the presence of diabetes mellitus (DM). The range of disease includes asymptomatic colonization, episodic or recurrent episodes, and candidiasis-complicating dermatitis.

1. **Symptoms.** The predominant symptom is pruritus. Other symptoms include irritation, soreness, and dyspareunia. The discharge (often, there is none) is typically described as white and clumpy ("cottage cheese").
2. A **potassium hydroxide (KOH) wet prep** has a 50% specificity; cultures may be negative; and 20%–30% of asymptomatic women have positive yeast cultures. *Candida albicans* accounts for 90% of cases, although other Candidal species (namely, glabrata) may account for infection.

D. **Trichomonas vaginalis.** This condition has a clear pattern of sexual transmission.

1. **Symptoms** include discharge, pruritus, dyspareunia, dysuria, urinary frequency, and abdominal pain. It may be asymptomatic. Vaginal erythema and edema are seen on examination. Symptoms range from a scant discharge to profuse, foul-smelling frothy discharge with burning introitus. The discharge may occur without inflammation in chronic infection.
2. Trichomonas infection may be difficult to see on **saline smear** (especially on a dry slide or if insufficient fields are assessed). Swishing the swab in a sterile tube with saline and transporting for immediate review will maximize the yield of a wet prep.

IV. **Clinical Approach** (Figure 34–1 and Table 34–2). A thorough history and physical examination are essential in order to make the correct diagnosis. Because women are often self-conscious about vulvovaginal complaints, be attentive to their need for privacy and reluctance to offer a full history. Be alert to signs or suggestions of physical abuse.

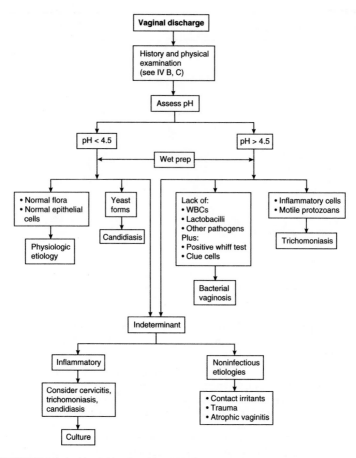

■ **FIGURE 34–1.** Vaginitis algorithm *WBCs* = white blood cells.

A. History

1. **Discharge:** Describe the discharge (e.g., amount, color, consistency, odor, duration, timing).
2. **Associated symptoms:** Determine associated symptoms, including itching, burning, discomfort, and dyspareunia. Inquire about the presence of any pain (abdominal, pelvic, back) and urinary symptoms.
3. **Sexual history:** Obtain a sexual history (e.g., number of partners, new partners, symptoms in partner) and gynecological history.
4. **Symptom provocation and relief:** Elicit activities that provoke the symptom as well as interventions that have led to symptom relief. Note other medication use [e.g., steroids, antibiotics, oral contraceptive pills (OCPs)].
5. **Personal habits:** Assess personal hygiene habits (including the type of underclothing) and lifestyle (including participation in sports).

TABLE 34–2. Clinical Aspects of Common Vaginal Infections

Characteristic	Normal Condition	Bacterial Vaginosis	Candidiasis	Trichomoniasis
Symptoms				
Itching	−	−	+++	+/−
Burning	−	+	++	+
Dysuria	−	+	++	+/−
Discharge				
Amount	Slight	Moderate	Variable	Moderate
Color	Yellow-white	Gray-white	White	Yellow-green
Odor	−	+++	−	+
Character	Thin	Thin, homo-geneous	Thick, curdy	Frothy
Adherence	Minimal	Moderate	Strong	Minimal
pH	3.4–4.5	5–5.5	4–5	6–7
Findings				
Gross	Normal	Minimal erythema	Erythema, excoriation	Petechiae
Microscopic	Few WBCs	"Clue cells"	Hyphae on KOH	Trichomonads
"Whiff test"	−	++++	−	+

Adapted with permission from Smith RP: *Gynecology in Primary Care.* Baltimore: Williams & Wilkins, 1996, p 617.

KOH = potassium hydroxide; WBCs = white blood cells.

    6. Self-treatment: Note that women frequently self-treat with over-the-counter preparations for Candida before seeing a physician.

B. Physical examination

    1. Inspect the vulvar area for abnormalities (e.g., erythema, ulcers, rash, fissure).

    2. Check vaginal pH on a sample from the lateral vaginal wall or the anterior fornix (see V A 1, 2).

    3. Inspect vaginal secretions, and obtain specimens for microscopic examination and cultures (where appropriate). **The appearance of the secretions should not be used in isolation to make a clinical diagnosis.** A wet prep review should be performed to confirm the clinical hypotheses.

4. **Obtain a Pap smear,** unless the patient has had a normal test within 12 months.

5. **Perform a bimanual examination** to assess the adnexa and uterus for mass or tenderness.

6. **Perform a rectal examination** to test for mass or tenderness.

V. **Diagnostic Evaluation** (see also IV)

A. **Vaginal pH assessment.** This is a vital step in assessing vaginitis and is often overlooked.

1. **The normal pH ranges from 3.8–4.2:** pH above this range is abnormal. When assessing pH, it is necessary to use detection methods that distinguish pH over a narrow range (4.0–4.9).

a. **If the pH is normal,** infectious vaginitis other than candidiasis is ruled out.

b. **If the pH is elevated** (> 4.5), consider bleeding, menopausal atrophic vaginitis, recent intercourse, contamination from cervical secretions, or an infectious cause of vaginitis (e.g., BV, trichomonas).

2. The pH should be sampled on a **specimen from the lateral vaginal wall or the anterior fornix.** A specimen obtained from the posterior fornix may give erroneous readings if exposed to intravaginal preparations or semen (which has an alkaline pH).

B. **Microscopic assessment of vaginal discharge** (i.e., wet prep). This component of the evaluation is often diagnostic when taken in the context of the medical history and physical examination. Slide preparation should include the following:

1. **Slide #1 (saline prep):** Place 1 drop of vaginal fluid on the slide; add 1 drop of warm **saline** and a coverslip. An alternative method uses a small sterile tube that is filled with 2–3 drops of saline. A swab containing the vaginal specimen is added to the saline and swished vigorously. The fluid is then poured onto a microscope slide and visualized after application of the coverslip. Examine under high power, looking for normal epithelial cells, gram-positive bacilli (normal), and clue cells. Absence of bacilli suggests infection (BV), especially in the absence of an inflammatory response. Motile protozoan of Trichomonas vaginalis may be seen and is diagnostic of trichomoniasis.

2. **Slide #2 (KOH prep):** Place 1 drop of vaginal fluid on slide; add 1 drop of 10% KOH and a coverslip. KOH dissolves most cellular material.

a. **Perform the whiff test:** This corresponds to the aromatic release of amines ("fishy odor") when KOH is added to a preparation in a patient infected with BV.

b. **Examine under low power,** looking for branching pseudohyphae and oval yeast forms, of which *C. albicans* is most common.

C. Other findings on microscopic assessment

1. **Atrophic vaginitis:** Parabasal cells commonly indicate a low estrogenic state ("fried egg"–appearing epithelial cells); the pH may also be elevated (> 4.5).
2. **"Inflammatory" smear:** In a high-risk patient with high numbers of polymorphonuclear leukocytes and no identified source, cervicitis should be considered. Appropriate testing should be pursued to assess for both *Neisseria gonorrhoeae* and *Chlamydia trachomatis*.

D. Cultures

1. **The majority of patients presenting with vaginal discharge do not require a culture.** If other conditions are suspected (e.g., cervicitis, endometritis, urinary tract infection), then appropriate cultures should be obtained.
2. **In patients with refractory symptoms or uncertain diagnosis,** culture should be considered. Trichomonads are cultured on Diamond's medium, with a high sensitivity. Such testing should be considered in a high-risk patient who failed treatment and has evidence of an elevated pH in the setting of an inflammatory discharge. It is important, in such cases, to treat the sexual partner.
3. The presence of ***Gardnerella vaginalis*** on a culture does not confirm BV. BV is diagnosed when at least three of the four criteria are fulfilled (see III B 2).

   a. *G. vaginalis* on culture result is not part of the diagnostic criterion.
   b. Although present in the majority of women with BV, *G. vaginalis* is also present in 50%–60% of healthy, asymptomatic women.

E. Pap smear

1. On occasion, a Pap smear may return with information **suggestive of infection.** Interpretation of this information is dependent on the entire clinical picture.

   a. **If Trichomonads are noted,** the patient requires further evaluation to eliminate the possibility of a false positive.
   b. **If Candida and BV are present,** treatment should be predicated upon clinical symptoms. **If the patient is devoid of symptoms,** then treatment may be reasonably withheld.

2. It is worth noting that a Pap report identifying **clue cells** is 90% sensitive and 95% specific for the presence of BV. On the other hand, a report that identifies the presence of ***Gardnerella*** is only 25% sensitive and 58% specific for the presence of BV.

SUGGESTED READING

Smith RP: *Gynecology in Primary Care*. Baltimore: Williams & Wilkins, 1996.

35

Sexually Transmitted Diseases
Michael Mitchell and Jennifer Daly

I. **Definition.** A sexually transmitted disease (STD) is a **disease that is transmitted through sexual contact.**

II. **Syphilis.** This disease is caused by the spirochete *Treponema pallidum*. There has been a marked increase in syphilis cases coincident with the HIV epidemic.

A. **Clinical features**

1. **Primary syphilis** occurs about 3 weeks after infection (range: 3–90 days). A painless papule appears at the site of contact. The papule erodes into an ulcerated, wet chancre. Moist chancres are teeming with spirochetes, rendering the patient highly infectious. Regional adenopathy may occur.

2. **Secondary syphilis:** Signs and symptoms of secondary syphilis occur 2–8 weeks after the chancre disappears. During this stage, spirochetes disseminate to all organs of the body. Systemic symptoms include a macular rash, generalized lymphadenopathy, fever, and malaise.

3. **Latent stage of syphilis:** During the latent phase of syphilis, patients are asymptomatic, but seropositive. The latent stage may last for years.

4. **Tertiary syphilis:** The chronic symptoms of tertiary syphilis may occur months to years after primary infection.

B. **Laboratory diagnosis**

1. **Culture of *T. pallidum* in vitro is not available.** Therefore, diagnosis is made by demonstrating *T. pallidum* directly in infected tissue or by serology.

2. **Direct examination:** Spirochetes may be demonstrated by specific or nonspecific staining. Darkfield examination of fluid exuded from infected lesions may be diagnostic, if the typical *T. pallidum* morphology and motility are noted.

3. **Serologic testing:** Antibody response can usually be demonstrated between 3–10 weeks after infection. Two types of assays are used.

   a. **"Nontreponemal" assays** measure antibodies formed in response to *T. pallidum*-induced tissue damage; these antibodies are cross-reactive with cardiolipin.

      (1) The rapid plasma reagin (RPR) assay is the most commonly used nontreponemal assay, whereas the Venereal Disease Research Laboratory (VDRL) assay is the only assay standardized for testing cerebrospinal fluid.

      (2) Because biological false positives occur in nontreponemal assays, all positive results must be followed up with a treponemal assay (see II B 3 b). The titer of nontreponemal assays may fall (or disappear) in late tertiary syphilis and must be interpreted with caution in late chronic disease.

b. **Treponemal assays** are based on specific *T. pallidum* antigens. They are most useful in confirming positive nontreponemal assay results and may be the most accurate tests in tertiary syphilis. False–positive reactions are rare.

   (1) The microhemagglutination-*T. pallidum* (MHA-TP) assay measures agglutination of erythrocytes sensitized with *T. pallidum* antigen. The assay has been miniaturized in a microtiter plate format.

   (2) In the fluorescent treponemal antibody, absorbed (FTA-ABS) assay, antibodies in test serum react with *T. pallidum* organisms that have been fixed to a slide. Specific antibodies in the serum reactive with surface antigens on the organisms are detected using labeled antihuman antibodies.

   (3) False–negative reactions may occur in primary syphilis, but sensitivity increases with longer duration of disease.

III. **Gonorrhea.** Gonorrhea is caused by the Gram-negative diplococcus, *Neisseria gonorrhoeae*.

A. Clinical features

   1. Symptoms usually occur within 7 days after exposure.

      a. **Men** who are infected usually have urethritis, epididymitis, or prostatitis.

      b. **Women** who are infected typically have cervicitis, urethritis, salpingitis, pelvic inflammatory disease (PID), or perihepatitis (i.e., Fitz-Hugh Curtis syndrome). PID may occur in 10% of women with cervical infection. Infertility is a major complication.

   2. Disseminated gonococcal infection develops in 1%–2% of patients. Certain complement deficiency states increase the risk for disseminated gonococcal infection. Myalgia, arthralgia, polyarthritis, tenosynovitis, and peripheral dermatitis characterize this bacteremic illness.

B. Laboratory diagnosis

   1. Direct examination

      a. In men, a Gram stain of urethral discharge showing bunches of intracellular Gram-negative diplococci is diagnostic.

      b. Genital secretions in women should not be stained because of nonpathogenic Gram-negative diplococci in normal vaginal flora.

   2. Cultures of local lesions are frequently negative. Clinical diagnosis and culture of the primary site of infection is critical.

      a. **Handling of specimen.** Isolates are fastidious and lose viability quickly. Therefore, special handling of specimens is critical. The use of charcoal-containing transport media for swabs may ensure viability for 12–24 hours.

         (1) The requisition for throat swabs submitted to rule out gonorrhea pharyngitis must specifically indicate that *N. gonorrhoeae* is suspected.

  (2) The anticoagulant sodium polyanethol sulfonate (SPS), present in most commercial blood culture media, may inhibit isolates of *N. gonorrhoeae.*

  b. Sensitivity of culture. Cultures of secretions show high sensitivity for detecting gonorrhea in men. Sensitivity of culture is somewhat lower in women (80%–90%), due in part to problems associated with appropriate specimen collection.

  c. Proctitis. If proctitis is suspected, obtain sample secretions from the anal crypts. Discard swabs stained with stool.

3. Molecular genetic testing: Direct probe or molecular amplification techniques are available for the detection of *N. gonorrhoeae* infection.

  a. Cervical and urethral specimens may be submitted for molecular diagnosis.

  b. Because molecular genetic testing offers increased sensitivity, urine may be tested by molecular amplification tests.

  c. Use of molecular tests may eliminate the transport problems associated with cultures of *N. gonorrhoeae.*

  d. Susceptibility testing is unavailable for infections documented by molecular genetic testing.

IV. Chlamydia. Chlamydia is caused by the intracellular pathogen *Chlamydia trachomatis,* which is the most common cause of bacterial STD.

  A. Clinical features. The spectrum and clinical features of *C. trachomatis* infection may be indistinguishable from gonorrhea.

  1. Intrapartum infection may result in inclusion conjunctivitis, mucosal infection, and pneumonitis in newborns.

  2. Lymphogranuloma venereum (LGV) is an uncommon presentation of *C. trachomatis* infection caused by serotypes L1–3.

    a. In the primary stage of LGV, a painless ulcer forms at the site of inoculation.

    b. Subsequently, during the second phase, painful regional (typically inguinal) adenopathy develops.

    c. During the tertiary phase of LGV, systemic symptoms, local cutaneous changes, draining sinuses, and lymphatic obstruction may develop.

  B. Laboratory diagnosis

  1. Direct detection

    a. Inclusion conjunctivitis caused by *C. trachomatis* may be accurately detected (~90%) by the direct staining of corneal specimens using a tagged monoclonal antibody.

    b. The sensitivity for cervical or urethral specimens is only about 75% sensitive compared with culture.

    c. Similar sensitivity has been reported for *C. trachomatis* detection by enzyme immunoassay (EIA). The specificity of EIA testing may limit its usefulness for screening low prevalence populations unless confirmatory testing is performed.

d. Detection of *C. trachomatis* using direct hybridization of nucleic acid probes may be comparable to detection by culture.

2. Culture: It is critical to sample infected **epithelial cells** for the diagnosis of *C. trachomatis* infection. Purulent discharge should be removed before vigorously sampling the epithelial surface of infected tissue.

    a. Specimens for *C. trachomatis* culture should be placed in transport media and sent to the laboratory on wet ice.

    b. Specimens acceptable for *C. trachomatis* culture include cervical os, urethra, corneal scraping, fallopian tube biopsy, lymph node aspirate, and anal swab.

    c. Subculture of initially negative cultures increases the sensitivity of detection. Properly performed, around 80% of patients with *C. trachomatis* infection can be identified by culture.

3. Amplified nucleic acid tests

    a. Polymerase chain reaction (PCR), ligase chain reaction (LCR), transcription-mediated amplification (TMA), and other assays have been developed to amplify specific *C. trachomatis* sequences in clinical material before detection with specific probes.

    b. Amplification techniques can identify 90%–95% of infected patients. A small number of infected patients may not be detected because of substances in the specimen that inhibit the amplification reaction.

    c. Use of urine specimens in amplified nucleic acid tests yield detection comparable with *C. trachomatis* culture and may be a suitable noninvasive specimen type.

V. Genital Herpes. Herpes simplex virus (HSV) causes genital herpes infection. **HSV type 2** causes most cases, although a significant number of cases (10%–40%) are caused by HSV type 1.

A. Clinical features

1. Most genital HSV infections are asymptomatic, which may contribute to the spread of the disease.

2. Symptomatic disease tends to be more severe in women, especially in those patients with primary infection. Typical infection consists of a localized vesicular rash that may be preceded by pain or tenderness.

    a. Symptoms usually occur **within 7 days after infection.** New vesicles form for a week or more. As vesicles rupture, local spread to the urethra, anus, and adjacent mucosal and cutaneous sites is common. Virus shedding may continue for weeks after symptom onset.

    b. Herpetic lesions may be **exquisitely sensitive** with intense local inflammation including lymphadenopathy.

    c. Urethritis and dysuria are common symptoms in women.

    d. Systemic symptoms of fever, headache, and malaise also occur more commonly in women.

    e. Infection in men is frequently localized and associated with lower incidence of symptoms.

3. Infection at nongenital sites may occur by primary sexual or genital contact (pharyngitis, proctitis, neonatal infection), viremic spread (disseminated rash), or neural spread (meningitis in patients with lumbosacral symptoms).

4. Recurrent HSV infections occur in most patients due to reactivation of latent virus.

B. Laboratory diagnosis. Virus shedding is greatest in vesicular and wet ulcerative lesions compared with crusted lesions.

1. Direct detection: Cells scraped from the base of unroofed vesicles or wet ulcers may be stained for rapid identification.

a. Multinucleated giant cells demonstrated by a Tzanck stain are consistent with HSV infection, but cannot distinguish lesions from *Varicella zoster* virus.

b. The use of tagged monoclonal antibodies gives HSV results that are 80%–90% sensitive compared with culture.

2. Culture detection: Mucocutaneous lesions may be sampled by Dacron swab early in infection. Calcium alginate swabs may be inhibitory and should not be used. Swabs should be placed in viral transport media and sent to the laboratory on wet ice. Specimens are often positive within 2 days.

3. Serological testing may identify prior infection, but is of limited value in the diagnosis of acute HSV infection.

SUGGESTED READING

Gorbach, SL, JG Bartlett, NR Blacklow (eds): *Infectious Diseases*, 2nd ed. Philadelphia: WB Saunders Co., 1998.

Murray, PR, EJ Baron, MA Pfaller, et al: *Manual of Clinical Microbiology*, 7th ed. Washington, DC: ASM Press, 1999.

36

Interpretation of the Abnormal Pap Smear
Elaine R. Evans-Metcalf

I. Overview

A. Cervical anatomy

1. The **cervix** is composed of columnar epithelium lining the endocervical canal and squamous epithelium covering the exocervix; they meet at the squamocolumnar junction.

2. **Squamous metaplasia:** The squamocolumnar junction moves over the lifetime from its original location on the exocervix toward the endocervix in response to various hormonal influences. Squamous metaplasia results from transforming columnar cells into squamous cells; the **transformation zone** is thus created.

3. **Cervical intraepithelial neoplasia (CIN):** In most cases, CIN (also known as dysplasia) originates in the transformation zone, and thus Pap smears must sample this area.

B. Pap smear as a screening tool

1. **Purpose:** The purpose of the Pap smear is **to detect preinvasive disease** so that appropriate evaluation and treatment can be initiated.

2. **False-negative rate:** The exact false-negative rate is unknown, but it may be as high as 10%; therefore, a normal Pap smear does not rule out an underlying abnormality. If there is a gross abnormality present, further investigation, including a biopsy of the lesion, is mandatory.

3. **Frequency of Pap smears:** The American College of Obstetricians and Gynecologists recommends that annual Pap smear screening begin when women become sexually active or reach 18 years of age.

   a. If three or more consecutive annual examinations have been normal, they may be performed less frequently (e.g., every 2–3 years), depending on risk factors and the discretion of the physician and patient.

   b. A Pap smear should be performed no less than annually if risk factors are present [e.g., early age at first intercourse, multiple sexual partners, smoking, infection with human papilloma virus (HPV) or HIV, and immunosuppression such as from whole-organ transplantation or Hodgkin's disease].

4. **Recent developments in Pap smear screening**

   a. **Thin-layer technology** (ThinPrep®; AutoCyte(R) PREP®) was initially approved by the Food and Drug Administration in 1996 as an alternative to conventional Pap smear screening. Several studies have demonstrated that this technique increases detection of cervical disease and improves specimen adequacy.

   b. **Automated cytological testing** has been approved for primary screening (AutoPap 300®) and for rescreening negative conventional smears with the aim of reducing the false-negative rate.

II. Clinical Approach—General Evaluation of the Abnormal Pap

A. History should include interval since last Pap smear; frequency of Pap smears; prior history of abnormal smears or treatments to the cervix; history of sexually transmitted diseases (STDs), including HPV infection; menstrual history; postcoital bleeding; and family history of gynecologic malignancies.

B. Physical examination

1. If there is **suspicion of malignancy,** assess sites of spread (e.g., lymph nodes, parametria adjacent to cervix).
2. If the **cervix appears abnormal,** consider performing a biopsy despite a normal Pap smear.

III. Interpretation of the Pap Smear

A. The **Bethesda system** was created in 1988 and revised in 1991 and 2001 in an effort to provide uniform guidelines for reviewing and reporting Pap smears.

1. This system was designed to be **clinically relevant** and reflect **current understanding** of the biology of cervical disease.
2. All samples should include an **assessment of the specimen adequacy and categorization,** and they may also include a descriptive diagnosis of abnormal findings.

B. Adequacy of the specimen: The aim is to reduce the false-negative rate. The Bethesda 2001 system categorizes specimens as follows:

1. **Satisfactory:** Quality limitations (e.g., absence of endocervical component or partially obscuring blood/inflammation) have not been associated with an increased rate of CIN in retrospective studies. An early repeat Pap smear is not necessary; however, attention to regular screening is suggested.
2. **Unsatisfactory:** Specimen is unreliable for the detection of epithelial lesions and must be repeated. For those patients with unsatisfactory Pap smears, more intraepithelial lesions appear during follow-up. Information about the Pap smear aids further patient management:

   a. Specimen rejected or not processed (specify reason)
   b. Specimen processed or examined, but unsatisfactory for evaluation of epithelial abnormality (specify reason)

C. Interpretation of results. The Bethesda 2001 system eliminated the category of "benign cellular change," and modified atypical squamous cell (ASC) results. Smears are now designated as "negative for intraepithelial lesion or malignancy" (with descriptive terms as applicable), "epithelial cell abnormality," or "endometrial cells present."

1. **Negative for intraepithelial lesion or malignancy**

   a. Organisms: If the description includes *Trichomonas, Candida, Actinomyces, Herpes,* or a shift in flora suggestive of bacterial vaginosis, repeat the Pap test as routinely indicated. Treatment of infection depends on symptomatology of the patient (see Chapter 34 V E).

b. Other nonneoplastic findings

   (1) Reactive changes associated with inflammation, radiation, and an intrauterine device

   (2) Glandular cells status posthysterectomy. Possible origins include fallopian tube prolapse, vaginal endometriosis, fistula, vaginal adenosis without diethylstilbestrol (DES) exposure, and prior radiation or chemotherapy. This finding is considered benign, even in patients with a history of malignancy.

   (3) Atrophy

2. Epithelial cell abnormality

   a. Squamous

   (1) ASC: Cytologic changes suggestive of a squamous intraepithelial lesion that are quantitatively or qualitatively insufficient for a definitive interpretation.

   (a) ASC reports should not exceed 5% of total diagnoses; the rate varies among centers.

   (b) ASC is associated with many causes, including HPV (30%–60% prevalence), vaginal infection, CIN (5%–15% prevalence of high grade), and cancer.

   (c) The Bethesda 2001 system includes two subcategories of ASC:

   (i) ASC-US: ASC of undetermined significance

   (ii) ASC-H: Cytologic changes that are suggestive of high-grade squamous intraepithelial lesion (HSIL), but lack criteria for definitive interpretation

   (d) Management of ASC (Tables 36–1 and 36–2)

   (2) Low-grade squamous intraepithelial lesion (LSIL): Cellular changes associated with HPV (e.g., koilocytosis) and CIN I.

   (a) Background

   (i) Approximately 75% of LSIL Pap smears are associated with CIN (with at least 15%–18% of cases associated with high-grade CIN).

   (ii) Approximately 50% of cases of CIN I will regress within 1–2 years, while about 15% will progress to high-grade CIN.

   (b) Management strategies for LSIL include initial colposcopy with follow-up Pap smears, or Pap smears repeated at 4- to 6-month intervals.

   (i) Initial colposcopy is recommended if risk factors are present (Table 36–3).

   (ii) Once three consecutive Pap smears are normal (either as initial management or following colposcopy), annual surveillance can be resumed. If a subsequent Pap smear is abnormal, management options include:

   ■ Colposcopy for **any** abnormal Pap test (most sensitive for detection of CIN)

TABLE 36–1. Management Options for ASC*

ASC-US

1. Perform HPV DNA testing using a sensitive molecular test.† [Sensitivity for high-grade CIN is equal to colposcopy (80%–100%). Negative predictive value is greater than 95%.]
   - If the results are positive for high-risk HPV, perform a colposcopy. If colposcopy is negative, repeat Pap smear in 1 year.
   - If the results are negative for high-risk HPV, repeat Pap smear in 1 year.

2. Immediately perform a colposcopy.
   - If colposcopy is negative, repeat Pap smear in 1 year.

3. Repeat Pap smears at 3- to 4-month intervals until two consecutive smears are negative, then return to routine screening. This approach is acceptable, but not optimal.
   - If another Pap smear is abnormal, perform colposcopy.

ASC-H

1. HPV testing is less useful because ASC-H is associated with a higher prevalence of high-grade CIN (24%–94%) and HPV DNA (at least 70%).

2. Colposcopy is appropriate.

---

*The management approach may be influenced by the patient's history, compliance, preference, and cost.

†If the initial ASC Pap smear used liquid-based technology, "reflex" HPV testing can be performed without a return patient visit, making this the preferable approach in this situation.

ASC = atypical squamous cells; CIN = cervical intraepithelial neoplasia; HPV = human papilloma virus.

> ■ Colposcopy only for Pap tests with severe results (e.g., HSIL or worse)
> ■ Colposcopy if less severe Pap results (e.g., LSIL, ASC-US) persist for 24 months
>
> **(c) Special situations**
>
>   **(i)** If LSIL is accompanied by an identifiable infection, treat the patient initially with the appropriate antibiotics and then manage as described in III C 2 a (2) (b).
>
>   **(ii)** If LSIL is suggestive of atrophy (in a postmenopausal patient), initiate a 3-week course of intravaginal estrogen, repeat Pap smear 1 week after completion of estrogen, and then manage as described in III C 2 a (2) (b).
>
> **(d) HPV DNA testing** has not been found to be universally useful in triage.

TABLE 36–2. Special Circumstances in the Management of ASC

Patient Circumstance	Acceptable Approach
Postmenopausal women	Repeat Pap smear 1 week after a 3-week course of vaginal estrogen cream (1 gram QHS) and 3–4 months later. Return to routine screening if both Pap smears are normal. HPV testing may be used.
Patients with inflammation or vaginal infections	Treat the specific infection,* followed by a repeat Pap smear 4–6 weeks later. If the repeat Pap smear is negative, return to regular screening. Approaches in Table 36–1 may also be used.
Immunosuppressed patients	Because the risk of high-grade CIN is increased, immediately perform colposcopy.
Pregnant women	Manage the patient as though she were not pregnant.

*Empiric treatment of inflammation is not indicated.

ASC = atypical squamous cells; CIN = cervical intraepithelial neoplasia; HPV = human papilloma virus.

    (3) HSIL: This report indicates cellular changes associated with moderate and severe dysplasia (e.g., CIN II, CIN III, and carcinoma in situ). These patients must have colposcopy with directed biopsy.

    (4) Squamous cell carcinoma: This report implies the probable presence of invasive tumor.

  b. Glandular

    (1) Atypical glandular results should comprise less than 1% of smears.

      (a) Studies indicate a 5%–54% likelihood of high-grade CIN on follow-up of atypical glandular cells of undetermined significance (AGUS) [Bethesda 1991 category].

      (b) Other associated findings include endocervical polyps, endometrial hyperplasia or adenocarcinoma, and extrauterine cancer.

    (2) Categorization. The Bethesda 2001 system eliminates AGUS. Categories now include:

      (a) Atypical endocervical, endometrial, or glandular cells (unqualified)

      (b) Atypical endocervical or glandular "favor neoplastic"

TABLE 36–3. Risk Factors Influencing Management of LSIL

History of CIN, vulvar intraepithelial neoplasm, vaginal intraepithelial neoplasm, or cancer

Poor patient compliance

Tobacco use

Immunosuppression

Relevant family history

A Pap smear suggesting more severe lesions or lack of atrophic change in the post-menopausal woman

CIN = cervical intraepithelial neoplasia; LSIL = low-grade squamous intraepithelial lesion.

        (c) Endocervical adenocarcinoma in situ (AIS)
        (d) Adenocarcinoma (endocervical, endometrial, extrauterine, or not otherwise specified)

    (3) Management

        (a) All glandular abnormalities: Perform colposcopy with endocervical sampling.

            (i) If the test is negative, repeat Pap smears every 4–6 months until three tests are normal, then return to routine surveillance.
            (ii) If repeat Pap tests are abnormal, perform another colposcopy.
            (iii) Perform a cone biopsy if repeat Pap results indicate HSIL or atypical glandular cells (AGCs).

        (b) If initial or subsequent Pap results indicate **favor neoplasia, probably AIS, or AIS:** Cone biopsy must follow initial colposcopy unless invasive cancer is identified.
        (c) If **cone biopsy fails to identify the source:** Perform endometrial sampling.
        (d) If **colposcopy, cone biopsy, or endometrial biopsy fails to identify the source:** Perform a pelvic ultrasound, and if negative, follow with abdominal or pelvic computed tomographic imaging. Hysteroscopy should be considered for women older than 35 years.
        (e) If a **woman is older than 35 years,** or has **unexplained vaginal bleeding or atypical endometrial cells:** Perform endometrial sampling as part of the initial workup. Some clinicians recommend endometrial sampling for all patients with unexplained AGCs regardless of their age.
        (f) Individualize management if the patient has a history of DES exposure, previous treatment for neoplasia, or immune deficiency.

3. Other: Endometrial cells

a. **Causes.** In women 40 years of age or older, this finding may be due to menstrual bleeding, inadvertent sampling of the lower uterine segment, or endometrial polyps, hyperplasia, or cancer.

b. **Investigation** (e.g., endometrial biopsy) is generally recommended, particularly in those postmenopausal women who are not taking hormone replacement therapy.

SUGGESTED READING

Bernstein SJ, Sanchez-Ramos L, Ndubisi B. Liquid-based cervical cytologic smear study and conventional Papanicolaou smears: a metaanalysis of prospective studies comparing cytologic diagnosis and sample adequacy. *Am J Obstet Gynecol* 185(2):308–317, 2001.

Kurman RJ, Henson DE, Herbst AL, et al: Interim guidelines for management of abnormal cervical cytology. The 1992 National Cancer Institute Workshop. *JAMA* 271(23):1866–1869, 1994.

NCI Bethesda System 2001. Retrieved December 27, 2001 from the World Wide Web: http://www.bethesda2001.cancer.gov/

Solomon D, Schiffman M, Tarone R: Comparison of three management strategies for patients with atypical squamous cells of undetermined significance; baseline results from a randomized trial. *J Natl Cancer Inst* 93:293–299, 2001.

Spitzer M: Cervical screening adjuncts: Recent advances. *Am J Obstet Gynecol* 179(2):544–556, 1998.

37

Ovarian Cancer Screening
Howard Sachs

I. Overview

A. Incidence. Each year there are approximately **25,000 new cases of ovarian cancer,** resulting in 14,000 deaths.

B. Risk factors include nulliparity, more than two pregnancies, breast cancer, talc and asbestos exposure, genetic factors (e.g., family history of ovarian cancer or the familial ovarian cancer syndrome), and increasing age (for epithelial tumors). Use of infertility drugs has been suggested to increase the risk (odds ratio of 2.8), whereas oral contraceptive use appears to reduce the risk.

C. Familial ovarian cancer syndrome. The familial ovarian cancer syndrome (< 1% of cases) is characterized by cancers in multiple members of 2 to 4 generations and a younger age at diagnosis. These patients may benefit from a strategy of heightened surveillance, although the best approach is not defined at this time and treatment options remain controversial.

D. Pathology

1. Tumors can arise from **all histologic components of the ovary,** including epithelial, stromal, and germ cells.

   a. **Epithelial cell tumors** account for approximately 90% of all tumors in the adult.

   b. **Stromal cell tumors** account for the majority of hormone-secreting tumors. Most of these are granulosa cell tumors. Given the effects of the hormones (feminizing/masculinizing symptoms) and their more indolent nature, these tumors tend to be found at an earlier disease stage.

   c. **Germ cell tumors** tend to be unilateral, often with hematogenous spread to the lungs. Peritoneal implantation and ascites are rare. They may be associated with tumor marker production [alpha-fetoprotein, beta-human chorionic gonadotropin (HCG)].

2. **Metastases**

   a. The **pattern of spread** for epithelial tumors begins locally (ovary and pelvis), followed by diffuse peritoneal implantation of serosal surfaces and metastases to regional lymphatics.

   b. **Metastatic tumors** to the ovary comprise approximately 10% of all ovarian masses.

E. Survival in patients with ovarian cancer is related to the stage of disease at the time of detection.

II. Differential diagnoses of the adnexal mass include functional cyst, ovarian cancer (primary or metastatic), endometrioma, uterine fibroid, tubo-ovarian abscess, diverticular or appendiceal abscess, teratoma, and pregnancy.

III. Clinical Approach. Given the lack of specific symptoms, ovarian cancer is frequently detected (approximately 75% of cases) at an advanced stage. Current screening methods lack sensitivity and specificity, leading to unnecessary invasive interventions, which have significant associated morbidity.

    A. History. The symptoms of ovarian cancer are nonspecific. They may include abdominal discomfort or pain, nausea, bloating or increasing abdominal girth, anorexia, and menstrual irregularities.

    B. Physical examination

        1. Perform a **pelvic examination**. It is estimated that one tumor is detected for every 10,000 routine pelvic examinations. However, early-stage tumors are rarely found.

        2. If the ovaries are abnormal, check for palpable fullness or a frank mass. Note the size (normal ovary is $3.5 \times 2 \times 1.5$ cm before menopause), contour (smooth versus irregular), texture (soft versus firm), and mobility of the mass.

        3. Assess for **hepatic lesions** (e.g., mass or enlargement, bruit, rub, tenderness), **ascites,** and **lymphadenopathy.**

IV. Diagnostic Evaluation

    A. CA-125 antigen

        1. Technique. Serum measurement of this glycoprotein is the most widely studied of the biochemical screening methods for ovarian cancer. It is measured using a monoclonal antibody (OC-125) directed against the CA-125 antigen. CA-125 antigen is not detected in normal ovary tissue.

            a. Elevated in epithelial tumors: Although consistently elevated in epithelial tumors, it is not an adequately sensitive or specific screening test.

            b. Elevated in stage III and IV ovarian cancer: CA-125 is elevated in more than 80% of patients with stage III and IV ovarian cancer, although less frequently in women with earlier-stage disease.

            c. Approximately 29% of patients with nongynecologic malignancies (of the pancreas, stomach, colon, and breast), 6%–40% of patients with benign disease (fibroids, endometriosis), and 1% of healthy women have elevated levels of CA-125 (> 35 U/ml).

        2. Sensitivity: The average reported sensitivity is 29%–75% for stage I cancer and 67%–100% for stage II cancer. The specificity is reported as high as 97%–99%.

        3. Mortality: There are no randomized trials that demonstrate reduced mortality with this screening strategy. It is uncertain whether tumor markers become elevated early enough in the natural history to provide adequate sensitivity for effective screening, relative to the risks.

        4. Disease regression or progression: CA-125 does provide evidence of disease regression or progression, and it can reflect overall tumor burden.

    B. Ultrasound

        1. Role of ultrasound: Data assessing the role of ultrasound in the setting of ovarian cancer are derived from two general approaches.

a. **Known diagnosis:** The first method reflects women with a known diagnosis of ovarian cancer. Ultrasound is used in an effort to determine the performance characteristics. In these studies, ultrasound has a reported sensitivity of 80%–100%.

b. **Screening studies:** The second method of assessing efficacy is derived from screening studies. That is, ultrasound is performed on healthy women, and the diagnostic efficiency is determined. Limitations in interpreting these studies include the low prevalence of the disease (need a very specific test), the short-term nature of the trials (short trials may overestimate sensitivity), and the lack of data on tumor stage at the time of diagnosis (i.e., the net benefit).

2. **Sensitivity:** The reported sensitivity is 50%–100%, and the specificity is 76%–97%. The positive predictive value is reported to be as low as 2.6%.

3. **Drawbacks:** It has been estimated that ultrasound screening of 100,000 patients older than 45 years of age would detect 40 cases of ovarian cancer, but at a cost of 5,398 false positives and more than 160 complications from diagnostic laparoscopy.

SUGGESTED READING

Jacobs I: Screening for early ovarian cancer. *Lancet* 2:171–172, 1988.

US Preventive Services Task Force: Screening for Ovarian Cancer. In: *Guide to Clinical Preventive Services,* 2nd ed. Baltimore: Williams & Wilkins, 1996, pp. 159–166.

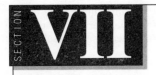
38

Lymphadenopathy

Mike Zavarin

I. **Definition.** Lymphadenopathy refers to **any disease process affecting the lymph nodes.** This condition usually results in lymphadenitis (i.e., inflammation of the lymphatic lymph node) or lymphadenectasis (i.e., distention of the lymph node).

II. **Incidence**

A. In **referral centers,** 16% of cases have a malignancy as their cause (e.g., lymphoma or metastatic cancer) and 84% are benign (of which 63% are idiopathic and 37% are infectious).

B. In **primary care settings,** 0.4% of patients less than 40 years of age have malignancies, and 4% of those patients older than 40 years of age have malignancies.

III. **Differential Diagnosis**

A. **Idiopathic causes.** The vast majority of patients with lymphadenopathy in the primary care setting will have a benign, idiopathic cause. Before proceeding with further evaluation, a 2- to 4-week watchful waiting period may be appropriate for patients younger than 40 years of age who have no suspicion of serious illness.

B. **Medications.** Phenytoin, hydralazine, allopurinol, gold, atenolol, captopril, cephalosporins, penicillins, and sulfonamides can cause lymphadenopathy.

C. **Infectious causes**

1. **Viral infections** [e.g., infectious mononucleosis with Epstein-Barr virus (EBV), cytomegalovirus (CMV), HIV, rubella, varicella-zoster virus, herpes simplex virus (HSV), infectious hepatitis, adenovirus, measles, mumps]

2. **Bacterial infections** [e.g., staphylococci, streptococci, *Brucella, Francisella tularensis, Listeria monocytogenes, Pasteurella pestis, Haemophilus ducreyi, Bartonella henselae* (cat-scratch disease), chlamydia, mycobacterium (tuberculosis, leprosy, scrofula), spirochete]

3. **Parasitic infections** (e.g., toxoplasmosis, leishmaniasis, trypanosomiasis, filariasis)

4. **Fungal infections** (e.g., histoplasmosis, coccidioidomycosis, paracoccidioidomycosis)

D. Immunologic diseases. Rheumatoid arthritis, systemic lupus erythematosus, dermatomyositis, eczema, Sjögren's syndrome, serum sickness, angioimmunoblastic lymphadenopathy, and drug reactions may result in lymphadenopathy.

E. Malignancies

1. **Hematologic malignancies** (e.g., Hodgkin's disease, non-Hodgkin's lymphoma, acute or chronic leukemia)
2. **Metastatic solid tumors** (e.g., head and neck, breast, lung, thyroid, melanoma)

F. Endocrine diseases. Hyperthyroidism, hypothyroidism, and adrenal insufficiency may occasionally result in lymphadenopathy.

G. Lipid storage diseases. Gaucher's disease, Niemann-Pick disease, and Fabry's disease are congenital lipidoses, which may be associated with infiltrative lymphadenopathy.

IV. Notes on the Differential Diagnosis

A. Supraclavicular lymphadenopathy has a high likelihood of a malignant cause and should be biopsied.

1. When **supraclavicular nodes** are affected, consider primary tumors of the breast, lung, and esophagus.
2. When **nodes on the left side** are affected, consider intrathoracic or intra-abdominal malignancy (including stomach, pancreatic, renal, testicular, and ovarian cancers).
3. **Virchow's node** is a left supraclavicular node that is associated with metastatic cancer from the gastrointestinal tract.
4. **Sister Mary Joseph's node** is a paraumbilical node suggestive of abdominal or pelvic neoplasm.

B. Bacterial pneumonias generally do not cause mediastinal lymphadenopathy.

C. Infections or **malignancies** in the internal pelvic organs and testes drain via the iliac nodes to the internal abdominal nodes, and thus do not cause inguinal lymphadenopathy.

D. Hematologic malignancies

1. **Hodgkin's disease** (see also Chapter 43). Peak incidence is in the 3rd and 6th decades. Patients present with a painless, prominent lymph node associated with fever, night sweats, and weight loss. Fevers are often cyclical, with 1- to 2-week febrile periods alternating with afebrile periods. Two-thirds of patients will have accompanying mediastinal lymphadenopathy, and some cases will involve pelvic and retroperitoneal nodes, usually sparing the mesenteric nodes. Some patients will complain of increased pain in lymph nodes after ingestion of alcoholic beverages.
2. **Non-Hodgkin's lymphoma** (see also Chapter 43). Patients often present with fever, night sweats, and weight loss associated with widespread lymphadenopathy. Depending on the type of lymphoma, the lymphocytic infiltration often involves the cerebrospinal fluid, liver, bone marrow, and gastrointestinal tract. Mediastinal involvement is less common.

E. The **site and pattern of adenopathy** lends insight to the underlying etiology.

1. **Causes of generalized lymphadenopathy** (two or more noncontiguous areas involved)

a. **Medications:** Phenytoin, hydralazine, allopurinol

b. **Systemic infections:** EBV, CMV, toxoplasmosis, HIV, tuberculosis, fungal infection (e.g., histoplasmosis, coccidioidomycosis), viral hepatitis, syphilis

c. **Malignancy**

d. **Immunologic causes:** Rheumatoid arthritis, systemic lupus erythematosus, sarcoidosis

e. **Other:** Angioimmunoblastic lymphadenopathy, angiofollicular lymph node hyperplasia (i.e., Castleman's disease)

2. **Causes of localized lymphadenopathy** (only one area involved)

a. **Infections and granulomatosis** are noted in the following regions:

(1) Occipital (conjunctivitis, scalp inflammation)
(2) Submandibular (pharyngitis, mononucleosis)
(3) Cervical (assess face, teeth, ears, and pharynx)
(4) Axillary and epitrochlear (assess skin)
(5) Mediastinal (tuberculosis, sarcoidosis, fungal infection)
(6) Inguinal [assess skin, or for a sexually transmitted disease (STD) such as syphilis, chancroid, genital herpes, lymphogranuloma venereum]

b. **Certain malignancies** are noted in the following regions:

(1) Submandibular (thyroid, nasopharyngeal)
(2) Cervical (lymphoma, thyroid, nasopharynx or larynx)
(3) Supraclavicular (breast, lung, esophagus)
(4) Axillary (melanoma, lymphoma, lung, breast)
(5) Epitrochlear (melanoma)
(6) Mediastinal (lung, lymphoma)
(7) Inguinal (melanoma, lymphoma)

V. **Diagnostic Approach** (Figures 38–1 and 38–2)

A. **Objectives.** The objectives in evaluating a patient with lymphadenopathy include:

1. Minimizing the biopsy rate for benign disease
2. Maximizing the biopsy rate for pathologic processes (e.g., malignant disorders, granulomatous disease)
3. Efficient use of ancillary testing

B. **History.** A focused history is a necessary first step in the evaluation of lymphadenopathy.

1. **Associated symptoms:** Attempt to determine if the lymphadenopathy is in response to a localized or generalized disease process.
2. **Age** is important because the incidence of malignancy increases with age, especially after 40 years. Furthermore, infectious mononucleosis is exceedingly rare after 30 years of age.

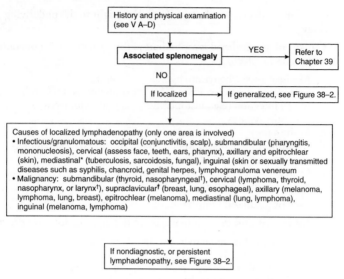

■ **FIGURE 38–1.** Algorithm for the workup of localized lymphadenopathy.

*Mediastinal adenopathy will require computed tomography (CT) scan for confirmation.

†If the patient is older than 40 years of age, consider endoscopy to rule out nasopharyngeal malignancy, especially if the patient abuses alcohol or tobacco.

‡Supraclavicular nodes should be aggressively assessed. Maintain a low threshold for biopsy.

3. **Past medical history:** Inquire about previous blood transfusions (risk for HIV and CMV), previous treated malignancies, rheumatologic illnesses, and STDs.

4. **Medications:** Specifically inquire about phenytoin, hydralazine, and allopurinol, which are the most common drugs to cause lymphadenopathy. These agents can usually be substituted or deleted in the initial workup of lymphadenopathy.

5. **Allergies:** Check for atopic dermatitis (eczema), which is a common cause of localized lymphadenopathy.

6. **Social history:** Inquire about sexual promiscuity (risk for HIV, syphilis, HSV, viral hepatitis, or CMV), intravenous drug abuse (risk for HIV or viral hepatitis), occupation, pets (risk of cat-scratch disease, toxoplasmosis), smoking (lung cancer), alcohol use (throat cancer), travel (southwestern United States: coccidioidomycosis; Ohio central valley: histoplasmosis), outdoor activities, and tick bites (Lyme disease and tularemia).

7. **Family history of cancer** (especially breast and ovarian) or **autoimmune disorders**

C. **Physical examination**

1. **Palpable lymph nodes** may signify a normal anatomical state, a transient benign process, a serious treatable illness, or a terminal

▲

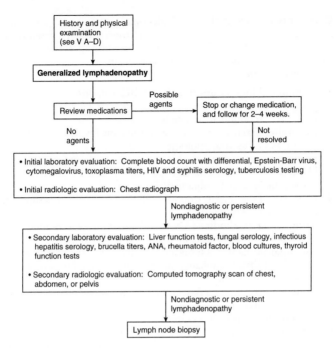

■ **FIGURE 38–2.** Workup for generalized lymphadenopathy. *ANA* = antinuclear antibodies.

disease. Especially in thin individuals, palpable lymph nodes can often be found in the submandibular, axillary, or femoral region. **Any lymph node in excess of 1 centimeter should be considered pathologic,** except if in the supraclavicular area, where they are always abnormal.

2. **Normal lymph node texture** is soft, nontender, and mobile.

  a. Infections cause warm, soft, or erythematous lymph nodes.
  b. Metastatic, solid malignancies cause fixed, firm lymph nodes.
  c. Lymphoma may cause rubbery, mobile lymph nodes.

3. **Tenderness** is not very helpful, although rapid enlargement suggests infections or leukemia. Lymphadenopathy in Hodgkin's lymphoma is nontender, but it may become tender after alcohol ingestion.

4. Note the **extent** of lymphadenopathy, especially in the occipital, submandibular, cervical, supraclavicular, axillary, epitrochlear, umbilical, inguinal, and popliteal regions.

5. Examine for **splenomegaly.** If present, proceed with a splenomegaly workup as described in Chapter 39.

6. Thoroughly assess, as indicated by symptoms and lymph node regions affected, the **skin** (for infection, cancers, or inflammation), the **thyroid** (for nodules), the **liver** (for a mass or tenderness), the **genitalia and pelvic organs,** the **oropharynx,** the **head and neck,** and the **breasts.**

D. Laboratory assessment. Lymphadenopathy often has an obvious etiology and does not require extensive testing. However, when a diagnosis is suspected, it may be confirmed by laboratory testing. If there is no obvious cause, laboratory studies may be needed to eliminate some of the more common etiologies.

1. **Complete blood count** (CBC): A CBC with differential may be suggestive of possible malignancy (e.g., leukemia, lymphoma), or infections (e.g., HIV, mononucleosis, endocarditis).
2. **Liver chemistries** are used to assess hepatic involvement of visceral disease as well as viral etiologies.
3. **Serology:** Studies for fungal infections (histoplasmosis, coccidioidomycosis), viral infections (hepatitis, HIV, EBV, CMV), syphilis, and toxoplasmosis may be obtained.
4. **Cultures** of the throat, wound, or blood are obtained as supported by the clinical presentation.
5. **Antinuclear antibodies (ANA)** and **anti-double-stranded DNA** are useful in diagnosing systemic lupus erythematosus.
6. **Rheumatoid factor:** This is an ancillary test in the diagnosis of rheumatoid arthritis. Lymphadenopathy may be seen, but it is not usually a presenting symptom.
7. **Bone marrow biopsy:** Assess for hematologic malignancy, metastases, and infectious etiologies.
8. **Tuberculosis testing** is employed to assess for mycobacterial infection.
9. **Thyroid studies:** Use thyroid-stimulating hormone (TSH) to assess for hyper- or hypothyroidism and fine-needle aspirate biopsy to assess for nodular disease.

E. Imaging

1. **Chest radiography** is used to assess for mediastinal or hilar adenopathy (suggestive of sarcoidosis or lymphoma), interstitial disease (suggestive of infectious etiologies), and neoplasm (primary or metastatic).
2. **Computed tomography (CT)** of the chest, abdomen, or pelvis is useful in assessing other sites of visceral involvement and extent of disease.
3. **Mammography** is used to assess for breast cancer when appropriate.
4. **Testicular ultrasound** is useful in the assessment of testicular cancer when suspicious of an occult primary source.

F. Biopsy. If a diagnosis is not achieved through noninvasive means, or if the lymphadenopathy persists despite adequate treatment or time, a biopsy is often required.

1. **Avoid biopsy of inguinal, femoral, or upper cervical nodes** that may demonstrate abnormal architecture from chronic reactions to common infections.
2. **Needle biopsy of a lymph node is not useful** since preservation of the architecture by excisional biopsy is required for accurate pathologic diagnosis.
3. **If biopsy is nondiagnostic,** continue to follow the patient for any new signs of lymphadenopathy that may point to another area for biopsy.

SUGGESTED READING

Haynes, BF: Lymphadenopathy. In Fauci, AS, et al (eds): *Harrison's Principles of Internal Medicine*, 14th edition. New York: McGraw-Hill, 1997.

39

Splenomegaly
Howard Sachs

I. Definition. Splenomegaly is **enlargement of the spleen** that is palpable on physical examination or seen on imaging techniques as greater than 13 cm in length by plain film or 250 cm³ by computed tomography (CT), ultrasound, or radioisotope scintiscan.

II. Overview

    A. Splenic enlargement should always be evaluated. It is rarely a normal variant (range 0.3%–3%). The spleen functions as the site of blood formation in utero. This activity resumes in adults only in pathologic conditions, when it results in enlargement.

    B. It is important to note that the spleen is rarely the site of primary disease. Rather, as a lymphoid organ it is usually involved in systemic inflammatory, metabolic, and generalized hematopoietic disorders. Processes that stimulate any of these functions may contribute to splenic enlargement. Examples include:

        1. Immune system activation (e.g., infection, inflammation)

        2. Enhanced phagocytic activity (e.g., autoimmune disease, physical or immunologic abnormalities of the red blood cell)

        3. Infiltrative disease (e.g., hematologic malignancies)

        4. Vascular congestion [e.g., portal hypertension, congestive heart failure (CHF)]

        5. Extramedullary hematopoiesis (e.g., myeloid metaplasia, myelofibrosis)

III. Differential Diagnosis. See Table 39–1 for a list of conditions associated with splenic enlargement.

IV. Notes on the Differential Diagnosis

    A. When splenomegaly is discovered through imaging (as opposed to clinical examination), infectious causes and other rare conditions (see Table 39–1) occur at a higher frequency. This is especially true in the HIV-infected population.

    B. Congestive heart failure as an etiology is usually seen only in severe heart disease, and in particular when there is complicating rheumatic valvular disease and endocarditis.

    C. Hematologic disorders, storage disease, and some infections (e.g., malaria, leishmaniasis) generally account for massive splenomegaly.

    D. Immune thrombocytopenic purpura (ITP) is not associated with splenomegaly; splenomegaly in the setting of ITP should alert the clinician to seek alternative diagnoses.

V. Clinical Approach (Figure 39–1)

    A. History. The history should be considered in the context of spleen-related functions (see II B). The clinician should also focus on consequences of

TABLE 39–1. Differential Diagnosis of Splenomegaly

Congestive splenomegaly

Portal hypertension (cirrhosis, portal/splenic vein thrombosis, Budd-Chiari syndrome), severe congestive heart failure (CHF)

Nonmalignant hematologic disorders

Hemolytic/megaloblastic anemias, hereditary spherocytosis/elliptocytosis, hemoglobinopathies, thalassemia major

Hematologic malignancies

Lymphomas, leukemias, myeloma, myeloproliferative disorders, primary splenic tumors, myeloid disorders

Infectious causes

Viral infections [Epstein-Barr virus (EBV), cytomegalovirus (CMV), HIV], bacterial infections (typhoid fever, brucellosis, subacute bacterial endocarditis, abscess), mycobacterial disease, fungal infections (disseminated histoplasmosis), spirochete (congenital syphilis), parasitic infections (toxoplasmosis, malaria, leishmaniasis, schistosomiasis, echinococcus)

Inflammatory/immunologic diseases

Drug (phenytoin), granulomatous disease (sarcoidosis), systemic lupus erythematosus, rheumatoid arthritis (Felty's syndrome), thyrotoxicosis

Infiltrative processes

Amyloidosis and storage disease (especially Gaucher's disease)

Other

Cyst, aneurysm, arteriovenous malformation, infarction, hematoma

---

splenomegaly (i.e., symptoms related to size and hypersplenism). The history should document the presence or absence of:

1. Fever, night sweats, anorexia, pharyngeal symptoms, fatigue, travel history (including previous residences)
2. Bruising, anemia, or history of thrombocytopenia, especially as a manifestation of **hypersplenism** (i.e., cytopenias resulting from trapping of red cells, white cells, or platelets by macrophages of an enlarged spleen)
3. Dyspnea, orthopnea, leg swelling, abdominal distention, alcohol and intravenous drug abuse, hepatitis
4. Joint swelling, bone pain, morning stiffness, skin rash, history of a

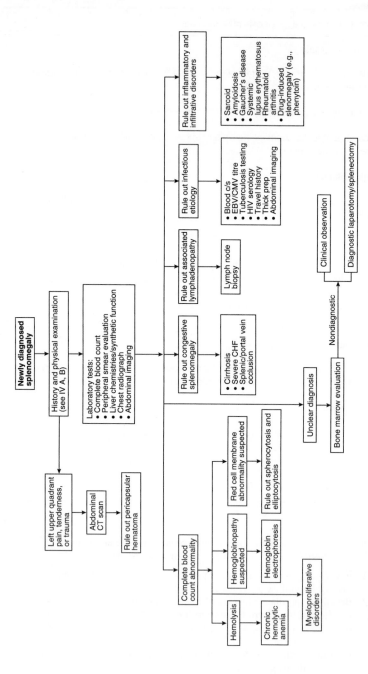

FIGURE 39–1. Differential diagnosis of splenomegaly. *CT* = computed tomography; *CHF* = congestive heart failure; *CMV* = cytomegalovirus; *EBV* = Epstein-Barr virus.

sexually transmitted disease (STD), aphthous ulcers, symptoms of serositis, renal disease, paresthesia or numbness
5. Early satiety, abdominal pressure

B. **Physical examination.** Note the presence of the following:
1. Fever
2. Petechiae, ecchymoses, or skin rash
3. Hepatomegaly or lymphadenopathy
4. Jugular venous distention (JVD), right-sided CHF, ascites, palmar erythema, spider angiomata, pedal edema, or joint deformity

VI. Diagnostic Evaluation

A. **Complete blood count (CBC).** A CBC is useful in the initial assessment of splenomegaly. It lends insight into the myriad of etiologies in addition to assessing the presence and degree of hypersplenism, which tends to be more pronounced when caused by congestive disorders rather than infiltrative ones. Platelets are especially likely to be sequestered in an enlarged spleen.

B. **Peripheral smear.** Examination of the peripheral smear may identify red cell abnormalities, parasites, immature white cell forms, or atypical lymphocytes.

C. **Hepatic function.** Given the high frequency of portal hypertension as a cause of splenomegaly, hepatic function should be assessed.

D. **Infectious etiologies.** A selective approach is recommended when evaluating for infectious etiologies. Thus, testing will be dictated by associated clinical findings. Examples include testing for Epstein-Barr virus (EBV) in the patient with posterior cervical adenopathy and blood cultures in patients at high risk for subacute bacterial endocarditis. In these instances, splenomegaly is an associated finding of systemic disorders.

E. **Lymph node biopsy** may be helpful diagnostically if lymphadenopathy is identified (see Chapter 38).

F. **Bone marrow examination** is indicated when the etiology of splenomegaly could not be made through the aforementioned evaluation or in further assessment of identified disease entities (e.g., hematologic malignancies). Bone marrow studies are useful in identifying myeloproliferative disorders, chronic infections, and infiltrative disorders, and they should be performed prior to splenectomy.

G. **Imaging studies**
1. **Chest radiography** is recommended, as it may identify associated pathology in addition to identifying a potential site for obtaining a diagnostic tissue specimen.
2. **Abdominal imaging** by ultrasound or CT scan is useful in confirming the presence of splenomegaly, assessing the presence of associated pathology, identifying anatomic or vascular abnormalities, and following up with patients for clinical observance or treatment.

H. **Diagnostic splenectomy.** In some patients with isolated splenomegaly, the workup may not reveal a cause. In these instances, the clinician must decide whether to proceed with a diagnostic splenectomy. (Splenic biopsy is not recommended because of its high morbidity).

1. In young, asymptomatic patients with only mild splenomegaly, a course of watchful waiting may be advocated. Close follow-up of these patients is advised. This approach is predicated on studies identifying palpable spleens in 3% of healthy college students.
2. In a series of patients with splenomegaly of unknown etiology who underwent laparotomy, abnormal findings were common. This series reported lymphoma in one-third of the patients, congestive splenomegaly in one-fourth, and inflammatory causes in one-fifth.

SUGGESTED READING

Haynes BF: Splenomegaly. In Fauci AS, et al (eds): *Harrison's Principles of Internal Medicine*, 14th edition. New York: McGraw-Hill, 1997.

O'Reilly RA: Splenomegaly in 2505 patients at a large university medical center from 1913–1995 (1963–1995: 449 patients). *West J Med* 169:88–97, 1998.

40

Bruising
Ahmad-Samer Al-Homsi

I. **Definition.** Bruising is a **confluent purplish discoloration of the skin** due to extravasation of blood from cutaneous and subcutaneous blood vessels.

II. **Overview**

   A. **"Easy bruisability"** in isolation is an infrequent presentation for disorders of hemostasis.

   B. **Evaluation.** The evaluation of patients complaining of excessive bruising requires adroit **history taking.** In fact, 55% of normal women and 22% of healthy men consider themselves "easy-bruisers." On the other hand, many patients with dramatic bleeding disorders do not volunteer any related complaints.

III. **Differential Diagnosis** (See Table 40–1)

IV. **Clinical Approach**

   A. **History**

      1. Question patients about persistent **bleeding from shaving wounds and menstrual flow.** Menstrual flow may be quantified using a pictorial chart.

      2. More objective information is also valuable, such as **history of bleeding requiring medical attention, iron-deficiency anemia,** or **blood transfusions.**

      3. Patients must be insistently asked about **medication intake,** including over-the-counter drugs and herbal remedies.

      4. Many bleeding disorders are inherited; therefore, a thorough **family history** is mandatory.

      5. A number of bleeding disorders are characterized by normal hemostatic and coagulation profile and should be considered when suggested by a **bleeding history.** These include dysfibrinogenemic conditions and factor XIII deficiency.

      6. **Monoclonal gammopathies** and **increased fibrinogen degradation products (FDP)** must be considered in patients with "easy bruisability."

   B. **Physical examination**

      1. Evaluate for signs of **cutaneous hemorrhages and joint deformities,** the latter being the hallmark of hemophilia A and B.

      2. Distinguish between **petechiae** (punctate hemorrhages) seen with thrombocytopenias and **ecchymoses** (large bruises) seen with more severe bleeding abnormalities.

V. **Diagnostic Evaluation** (Chapter 43 V C)

   A. **Template bleeding time test** reflects the **hemostatic vascular efficiency,** the **platelet count and function,** and certain **coagulation factors,** such as

TABLE 40–1. Differential Diagnosis of Bruising

Diagnosis	Manifestations
Structural malformation of vessels	
Hereditary hemorrhagic telangiectasia	Mucocutaneous telangiectasia appearing in the third decade
Ehlers-Danlos syndrome	Skin hyperextensibility and joint hyper-mobility
Osteogenesis imperfecta	Retinal angioid streaks and yellow cuta-neous plaques in flexural sites
Pseudoxanthoma elasticum	Retinal angioid streaks and yellow cuta-neous plaques in flexural sites
Vitamin C deficiency or scurvy	Perifollicular bleed
Multiple myeloma and amyloid disease	Periorbital and pinch purpura
Hyper- and cryoglobulinemic purpura	
Steroid-excess purpura	Purpura associated with red-brown skin pigmentations
Small vessel vasculitis	Purpura associated with red-brown skin pigmentations
Skin diseases	
Quantitative and qualitative platelet disorders	
von Willebrand's disease and other coagulation defects	
Traumatic purpura	
Senile purpura	
Love bites or "hickeys"	
Others	
Purpura simplex	
Psychogenic purpura	Bruising associated with the menstrual cycle

von Willebrand's factor and fibrinogen. It may also be abnormal in patients with monoclonal paraproteins and increased FDP. However, it must be kept in mind that the bleeding time depends on the technologist's skill.

B. **Automated platelet count** must always be confirmed by **blood smear review.**

   1. **Mean platelet volume** is increased in a wide variety of disorders, including some inherited platelet dysfunction disorders, such as Bernard-Soulier syndrome.
   2. **Platelet morphology** is sometimes diagnostic, such as in the gray platelet syndrome.
   3. **Platelet aggregation studies** help assess the functional status of platelets (i.e., the ability of platelets to aggregate in the presence of different agonists). Platelet aggregation is affected by the intake of several drugs and foods, including aspirin, nonsteroidal anti-inflammatory drugs (NSAIDs), ticlopidine, beta-lactam antibiotics, garlic and onion extracts, and cumin. On the other hand, these studies may occasionally be normal in patients with platelet dysfunction disorders such as storage pool diseases.

C. **Von Willebrand's disease** is the most common inherited bleeding disorder, yet no single sensitive screening test is available for diagnosis. Furthermore, von Willebrand's factor levels vary over time physiologically and in response to stress and estrogens. Therefore, diagnosis must rely on repeated testing (see Chapter 43). In addition, interpretation of results must take into account that normal values vary according to blood groups.

D. **PT, PTT.** See Chapter 43 V C.

SUGGESTED READING

Kitchens CA: Approach to the bleeding patient. *Hematol Oncol Clin North Am* 6:983–989, 1992.

41

Complete Blood Counts and Diagnostic Approach to Anemias

Fauzia Khan and Liberto Pechet

Complete Blood Counts

Fauzia Khan

I. **Overview.** A complete blood count (CBC) is performed in most laboratories using automated hematology analyzers. It may include red cell indices, mean platelet number and volume, and a white cell differential.

II. **Indications for Ordering a Complete Blood Count**

A. Order a CBC in the following cases:

1. **Suspicion of anemia, infection,** or **a low platelet count**
2. **Assessment and serial evaluation of myeloproliferative diseases**
3. **Assessment of hyperviscosity states**
4. **Evaluation for suspected erythrocytosis**

B. CBC provides information about **bone marrow function.**

1. A **decrease in cell counts** signifies defective production, peripheral destruction, blood loss, or sequestration.
2. An **increase in cell counts** signifies bone marrow hyperfunction either independent (hematologic malignancies) or in response to a peripheral stimulus.

III. **Performance Characteristics**

A. **Electric impedance** (one of the basic technologies in automatic analyzers) directly measures hemoglobin (Hg), mean corpuscular volume (MCV), and erythrocyte count. The following parameters are **calculated:**

1. **Hematocrit (Hct)** = red blood cell (RBC) count × MCV
2. **Mean corpuscular hemoglobin concentration (MCHC)** = Hb/Hct
3. **Mean corpuscular hemoglobin (MCH)** = Hb/RBC count
4. **Red cell distribution width (RDW)**
5. **Platelet distribution width (PDW)**

B. **Sample requirements**

1. Purple top tube with ethylenediamine tetra-acetic acid as anticoagulant
2. The tubes should be filled and immediately inverted to block coagulation.
3. Care should be taken to avoid:

a. Excessive anticoagulation, which leads to dilution errors
b. Hemolysis due to traumatic venipuncture

c. Dilution by drawing blood above an intravenous line
d. Delay of more than 4 (maximum 8) hours, which may affect certain parameters

IV. Interpretation of Results

A. **Hct and Hb** rise and fall together. Either is sufficient for serial assessment of disease processes such as anemia and erythrocytosis.

1. A **decrease in Hb is termed anemia** and an **increase is termed polycythemia** (see Chapter 43).
2. Patients in **volume-depleted states and shock** may have normal or high Hct or Hb despite decreased red cell mass.
3. **Lipemia** may spuriously elevate Hb.

B. **RBC count** forms the basis for calculating the Hct, MCH, and MCHC.

1. The RBC count may help in **differentiating iron-deficiency anemia from thalassemias.**
   a. In **iron-deficiency anemia,** the decrease in RBC count is proportional to the decrease in Hb.
   b. In **thalassemias,** the RBC count may be normal or even increased relative to Hb.
2. A **spurious decrease in the RBC count** is seen when red cells are very small and may be counted as platelets. **Red cell autoagglutination** (a condition seen in cold agglutinin disease) also results in a spurious decrease in the RBC count, but with a marked elevation of MCV and impossibly high values for the calculated MCHC.
3. A **spurious elevation in the RBC count** is seen with severe leukocytosis.

C. **RBC indices and reticulocyte count**

1. **RBC indices** include MCV, MCH, and MCHC. They help to determine cell size, individual cell Hb, and overall Hb concentration, respectively.
   a. **MCV is the average volume of erythrocytes.** It is used to morphologically classify anemias into normocytic, macrocytic, and microcytic (see THE ANEMIAS section of this chapter).
   b. **MCH and MCHC are rarely used clinically.** MCHC is elevated in spherocytosis.
2. **RDW** is the coefficient of variation or the standard deviation of the red cell histogram. It shows the variation in the red cell size. Whenever there is great variation in cell size, the RDW is increased. This is seen in conditions such as iron-deficiency anemia, folate and B_{12} deficiency anemias, hemoglobinopathies, posttransfusion states, myelodysplastic syndromes, immune hemolysis, cold agglutinins, and chronic lymphocytic leukemia (CLL).
3. **Reticulocytes** are young red cells normally released by the bone marrow to the peripheral blood count. Their count—a measure of erythrocyte production—is normally 1%–2% of circulating erythrocytes. The reticulocyte count may be increased with the decrease in red cell life span (normally 120 days), provided the bone marrow is able to increase the

production of RBCs. They are detected by their ability to stain with special stain. New analyzers obtain reticulocyte counts automatically.

D. White blood cell (WBC) count

1. **Leukocytosis** is defined as an increase in WBCs above $11.3 \times 10^9/L$.

   a. **Differential counts** (subpopulations of WBCs): Changes in absolute counts are more important than values expressed as a percentage of the total WBC count. In addition, morphologic alterations of white cells are also indicators of disease states.

   b. **Neutrophilic leukocytosis** (i.e., granulocytosis), an increase in neutrophils above $7.5 \times 10^9/L$, is usually associated with some degree of "shift to the left," which means an increased number of bands. It is associated with bacterial infections, most commonly suppurative infections such as abscess, empyema, meningitis, trauma, hemorrhage, and infarction. The most important distinction is between infectious and noninfectious causes. Among the latter, inflammatory states and myeloproliferative diseases are of greatest concern along with malignancy.

   c. **Leukemoid reaction** is defined as a WBC count greater than 50,000 or a differential count with more then 5% metamyelocytes. Even more immature cells may be seen on the peripheral blood smear, but blasts are rare. Leukemoid reaction may be seen with very severe bacterial infections, with extensive bone marrow replacement by tumor, in severe hemolysis and tissue destruction such as in burns or massive infarctions, and with corticosteroid treatment.

   d. **Lymphocytosis** is defined as an increase in lymphocytes above $3.4 \times 10^9/L$. It may be associated with normal WBC or decreased granulocyte counts, hence it is generally a relative (%) decrease. An absolute increase occurs in pertussis, infectious mononucleosis, cytomegalovirus (CMV), infants with adenovirus, and sometimes hepatitis. Besides viral infections, absolute lymphocytosis is seen in toxoplasmosis, CLL, and sometimes with trauma.

   e. **Monocytosis,** an increase in monocytes above $0.6 \times 10^9/L$, may be seen in tuberculosis, subacute bacterial endocarditis, and chronic monocytic leukemia (CML).

   f. **Eosinophilia,** an increase in eosinophils above $0.6 \times 10^9/L$, is found in allergic and inflammatory states, parasitosis, Hodgkin's disease, and myeloproliferative diseases. It is also caused by certain drugs, and in assessing organ transplant rejection.

   g. **Basophilia,** an increase in basophils above $0.3 \times 10^9/L$, is a significant finding in CML.

   h. **Bandemia,** an increase in bands above 2% of WBCs, is an early sign of infection.

2. **Leukopenia** is a decrease in WBCs below $4.4 \times 10^9/L$.

   a. **Neutropenia (i.e., granulocytopenia)** is a decrease in neutrophils (granulocytes) below $1.6 \times 10^9/L$, and is seen as the result of chemotherapy, radiation therapy, drugs, hematologic malignancies, and systemic lupus erythematosus.

    b. Lymphopenia, a decrease in lymphocytes below 0.9×10^9/L, is common in acute infections, malaria, HIV, and chronic infections such as tuberculosis, histoplasmosis, and brucellosis.

3. Approach to abnormal WBC counts

    a. If a decrease or increase in the total WBC count reflects a **mild change in all white cell populations** rather than a distinct change in a simple group of leukocytes, it may have no clinical significance.

    b. Are the WBC changes related to an acute event (e.g., fever, infection, hemorrhage, necrosis, burns), **or are they an unexpected finding on routine examination?**

    c. Are the WBC abnormalities isolated, or are they associated with changes in other cell lines (e.g., RBCs, platelets)?

    d. Are the WBC changes observed only in the mature forms, or are they associated with the presence of immature cells of the same subpopulation?

    e. When observing manual results (% differentials), is the low percentage of neutrophils due to **true neutropenia,** or is it related to an increase in other populations (e.g., lymphocytosis, monocytosis)?

    f. Is the high percentage of neutrophils due to **true neutrophilia,** or is it related to lymphopenia?

The Anemias

Liberto Pechet

  I. Definition. Anemia is a **reduction in Hb and Hct,** leading to a decrease in the oxygen supply to peripheral tissues.

 II. Overview. The incidence of anemia is hard to determine since it is a ubiquitous finding. It varies geographically and with socioeconomic conditions.

III. Causes. Ninety percent of anemias are due to iron deficiency, acute blood loss, or inflammatory diseases.

  A. Anemias can best be classified and treated based on the red cell size.

    1. RDW provides a useful measurement of the variation in size of red cells (normal = 11.6–13.7 fL), indicating the presence of anisocytosis when elevated.

    2. MCV (normal = 83–101 fL) and **reticulocyte count** constitute the primary approach to classifying anemias.

    3. Once the general category of anemia is determined, further, more complex laboratory tests or bone marrow biopsy may be indicated to ascertain the cause.

  B. Common causes of anemias

    1. Acute

      a. Bleeding

      b. Hemolysis

2. Chronic

   a. Deficiencies (e.g., iron, folic acid, vitamin B_{12})
   b. Congenital conditions (e.g., hemoglobinopathies, hereditary spherocytosis)
   c. Neoplasia
   d. Renal disease
   e. Chronic inflammatory conditions
   f. Myelodysplastic syndromes

IV. How to Confirm the Diagnosis

   A. **History.** Note family history of anemia, jaundice, and splenomegaly.
   B. **CBC.** Obtain a CBC, including red cell indices, white cell differential, examination of the peripheral blood smear, and reticulocyte count.
   C. **Define type of anemia.** Once the suspicion of anemia is confirmed by finding a reduction in Hb and Hct, define the type of anemia by following the algorithms in Figures 41–1, 41–2, and 41–3. The first line of investigation is to uncover an underlying disease, gastrointestinal condition, or excessive menstrual bleeding.

V. Variants

   A. **Microcytic anemias** (see Figure 41–1) are anemias characterized by low MCV (i.e., below 83 fL) and hypochromia, easily identified by examination of the peripheral blood smear.

   1. **Etiology** (also see section VI): Iron-deficiency anemia, which is characterized by decreased iron stores, is the most common type of microcytic anemia. The **most common causes of iron-deficiency anemia** include:

      a. **Gastrointestinal blood loss** (usually chronic)

         (1) Colon tumors (cancer, polyps)
         (2) Peptic ulcers
         (3) Inflammatory bowel disease and severe malabsorption
         (4) Gastric cancer
         (5) Presence of *Helicobacter pylori* in the stomach (mechanism unknown)
         (6) Intestinal parasites

      b. **Urogenital bleeding**

         (1) Uterine cancer or myomas
         (2) Chronic menorrhagia
         (3) Bladder cancer or hemorrhagic cystitis
         (4) Hypertrophy of the prostate

      c. **Inadequate diet**

         (1) Poor diet in women who are menstruating
         (2) Repeated pregnancies with inadequate iron supplements
         (3) Prolonged breast-feeding of babies without iron supplements
         (4) Patients with anorexia nervosa or on fadist diets that are low in iron

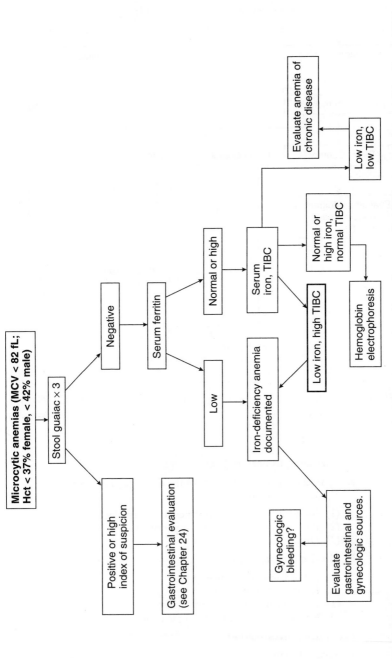

FIGURE 41–1. Algorithm for the diagnosis of microcytic anemias. *Hct* = hematocrit; *MCV* = mean corpuscular volume; *TIBC* = total iron-binding capacity.

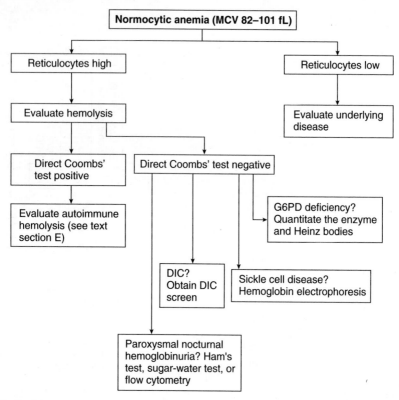

■ **FIGURE 41–2.** Algorithm for the diagnosis of normocytic anemias. *DIC* = disseminated intravascular coagulation; *G6PD* = glucose-6-phospate dehydrogenase; *MCV* = mean corpuscular volume.

2. **History and physical findings**

   a. **Symptoms** commensurate with the degree of anemia and the rapidity of development.

      (1) Increasing weakness, shortness of breath, lack of energy
      (2) Pica (compulsive chewing, especially ice)
      (3) Dysphagia

   b. **Physical findings** include:

      (1) Pallor without jaundice
      (2) Enlarged spleen (although rare)
      (3) Koilonychia (spoon-shaped nails)
      (4) Absence or flattening of tongue papillae

3. **Laboratory investigation**

   a. **Serum ferritin**

      (1) **If serum ferritin is low** (< 12 μg/L), the diagnosis is con-

250
▲

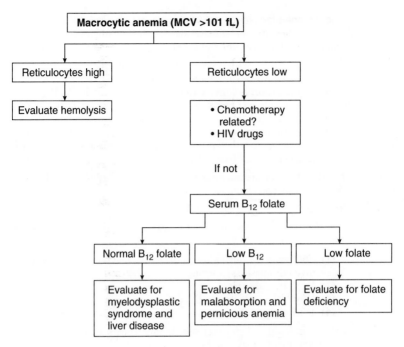

■ **FIGURE 41–3.** Algorithm for the diagnosis of macrocytic anemia. *MCV* = mean corpuscular volume.

firmed, and there is no need to obtain serum iron or total iron-binding capacity (TIBC). Proceed with investigation of the cause.

(2) **If serum ferritin is normal or borderline** ($< 45 \mu g/L$), obtain serum iron and transferrin reported as TIBC.

b. **Serum iron and TIBC**

(1) **If the serum iron is very low and the TIBC is elevated** (with the ratio serum iron to TIBC $< 16\%$), the diagnosis is confirmed.

(2) **If the serum iron and TIBC are normal,** an iron deficiency can be excluded in most cases.

(3) **If the serum iron and TIBC are low,** the anemia is most likely associated with chronic disease.

(4) **If the serum iron is high and the TIBC is normal,** the most likely diagnosis is thalassemia (see page 255).

c. **Bone marrow biopsy.** If the diagnosis is still in doubt, obtain a bone marrow biopsy for Prussian blue stain.

(1) It will be negative in iron deficiency.

(2) If iron is present in bone marrow macrophages, diagnosis of iron deficiency is excluded.

B. Normocytic anemias (see Figure 41–2) are most often secondary to an underlying nonhematologic disease, such as chronic inflammation, malignancy, renal disease, and hemolysis (i.e., shortened red cell survival)

1. **Anemia associated with a chronic disease** will show normal to slightly reduced MCV (in inflammatory conditions MCV = 75–90 fL); normal red cell morphology, with only mild variation in RDW, inadequate reticulocyte response, and increased serum ferritin; reduced serum iron and TIBC; and low erythropoietin in renal failure.

2. **Hemolytic anemias:** Because the hemolytic anemias may be either normocytic or microcytic (and occasionally even macrocytic), they will be described separately (see V E).

C. Macrocytic anemias are anemias with larger than normal red cell size (MCV > 101 fL) [see Figure 41–3].

1. **Etiologies**

   a. In the United States, the **most common causes** of macrocytosis are seen in patients:

      (1) Following (or during) chemotherapy, or HIV meds, or with a myelodysplastic syndrome
      (2) With liver disease
      (3) With folate or vitamin B_{12} deficiency
      (4) With thyroid disease

   b. Vitamin B_{12} deficiency increases in incidence with age.
   c. Aplastic anemia may also be macrocytic.

2. **Types of macrocytic anemias**

   a. **Megaloblastic anemias**

      (1) **Peripheral blood findings**

         (a) Oval macrocytes, poikilocytosis, high RDW, small teardrop cells
         (b) Inadequate reticulocytes for the degree of anemia
         (c) Moderate leukopenia with large granulocytes, many with hypersegmented nuclei (at least five cells with five lobes or even one with six lobes)
         (d) Mild thrombocytopenia

      (2) **Bone marrow biopsy**

         (a) Marked erythroid hyperplasia with frank megaloblastic red cell precursors
         (b) Giant metamyelocytes
         (c) Large megakaryocytes with hyperploid nuclei
         (d) Increased iron stores
         (e) Inability to morphologically differentiate vitamin B_{12} deficiency from folate deficiency

      (3) **Serum**

         (a) High lactate dehydrogenase
         (b) Elevated indirect bilirubin

   b. **Vitamin B_{12} (cobalamin) deficiency**

(1) Etiology

  (a) A dietary cause may be found in vegans (although this is very rare).

  (b) Decreased absorption may be a cause due to absence of intrinsic factor. Examples include pernicious anemia, total or extensive partial gastrectomy, intestinal bacterial overgrowth (blind loop syndrome), ileum resection, regional enteritis, and pancreatic insufficiency. Histamine$_2$ antagonists, proton pump inhibitors, and *H. pylori* infection may aggravate the deficiency.

  (c) A diagnosis of vitamin B$_{12}$ deficiency is not the equivalent of pernicious anemia, which has to be positively ruled in.

(2) History and physical findings

  (a) Very gradual development of symptoms reflecting progressive anemia

  (b) Paresthesias, physical and mental sluggishness

  (c) Decreased vibratory and position sense (subacute combined degeneration of dorsal and lateral columns)

  (d) Yellowish skin; vitiligo; sore beefy red, smooth, tender tongue; high output heart failure (commensurate with the degree of anemia)

(3) Laboratory investigation

  (a) If serum vitamin B$_{12}$ is very low to absent (i.e., < 100 pg/ml), a deficiency is confirmed.

  (b) If serum vitamin B$_{12}$ is borderline (between 100–350 pg/ml) and the suspicion is high, obtain serum methylmalonic acid (normal: 70–270 nM) and total homocysteine (normal: 5–14 μM). If both are increased, the diagnosis of cobalamin (vitamin B$_{12}$) deficiency is confirmed.

  (c) When pernicious anemia is suspected, the following additional tests are available:

   ▦ Antiparietal cell antibodies are present in the serum of 90% of patients with pernicious anemia.

   ▦ Blocking ant-intrinsic factor antibodies are present in 50%–60% of patients with pernicious anemia, and in 96% of black women with pernicious anemia.

   ▦ The Schilling test, rarely performed today, remains an option.

c. Megaloblastic anemias due to folate deficiency

(1) Etiologies

  (a) Secondary to a diet deficient in folate, especially in the presence of alcoholism, liver disease, chronic hemolysis, or pregnancy

  (b) Malabsorption (e.g., gluten enteropathy, tropical sprue)

  (c) Phenytoin administration

(2) History and physical findings. Clinically, folate deficiency is not associated with neurologic manifestations.

(3) **Laboratory investigation:** Serum folate level below 3 ng/mL and normal serum B_{12} level; red cell folate < 100 µg/L indicates folate deficiency (normal: 166–640 µg/L); see also V C 2 a

d. Other macrocytic anemias

(1) Anemia of chronic liver disease
(2) Myelodysplastic syndrome
(3) Down's syndrome
(4) Hypothyroidism

D. Acquired aplastic anemia is pancytopenia resulting from failure of the bone marrow to produce all three hematopoietic lineages. In this condition, the bone marrow is replaced by fat cells, with only occasional islands of hematopoiesis, especially early in the disease.

E. Hemolytic anemias

1. **Definition:** Hemolytic anemias result from an increase in the rate of RBC destruction (or a decrease in the rate of RBC survival).

2. **Etiologies**

   a. Acute causes (usually acquired): Most commonly immune mechanisms due to autoantibodies or drugs
   b. Chronic causes (usually congenital): Hemoglobinopathies, enzymopathies, or membrane defects
   c. Chronic hemolysis may be associated with acute exacerbations.

3. **When to suspect hemolysis**

   a. History. Patients with a family history of anemia, anemia since early childhood, or early gallstones; patients taking certain drugs; if the history is negative, suspect immune hemolysis
   b. Physical findings. Fluctuating jaundice and dark urine, normal-colored stools
   c. Laboratory findings

   (1) High reticulocyte counts
   (2) Low MCV with elevated MCHC
   (3) Spherocytes or deformed cells on peripheral blood smear
   (4) Splenomegaly

4. **Confirm suspicion of hemolysis**

   a. Evaluate the reticulocyte count and serum bilirubin (total and unconjugated).
   b. Check for a low Hb and an elevated lactate dehydrogenase.

5. **Types.** Once hemolysis is confirmed by elevated reticulocyte count and elevated indirect bilirubin, define the type of hemolytic anemia, either by site of RBC destruction or by the cells' defect.

   a. By site of destruction

   (1) **Intravascular:** Mechanical injuries, paroxysmal nocturnal hemoglobinuria
   (2) **Extravascular** (i.e., RBC destruction in macrophages): Congenital and immune anemias, hypersplenism
   (3) **Intramedullary** (ineffective erythropoiesis): Thalassemias

(partially), myelodysplastic syndrome (partially), and megaloblastic syndromes

b. By defect (see VI and VII)

VI. Intrinsic Red Cell Defects (usually congenital)

A. Hemoglobinopathies. More than 1000 mutations involve the globin gene; they result from amino acid substitution or abnormalities of synthesis. Hemoglobinopathies are diagnosed by Hb electrophoresis in most cases. The most common types in the United States are **sickle cell disease** and **thalassemia syndromes.**

1. **Sickle cell disease** predominantly presents in populations of African ancestry.

   a. Homozygous

   (1) **Sickle cell anemia** (homozygous SS) is a severe anemia that starts in childhood (after 2–3 months of age).

   (2) **Laboratory findings**

   (a) Hb electrophoresis shows predominant Hb S in combination with severe anemia.

   (b) Fetal Hb may modify the severity of sickle cell anemia, resulting in higher red cell counts and improved symptoms.

   (c) In the classic picture of sickle cell anemia, the peripheral blood smear shows sickle cells and severe poikilocytosis, anisocytosis (reported as an increased RDW), polychromasia (increased reticulocytes), nucleated RBCs, target cells, Howell-Jolly bodies (reflect autosplenectomy), and slight elevation in serum bilirubin.

   b. Heterozygous

   (1) **Sickle cell trait** is generally an asymptomatic condition, except when the affected person is exposed to severe deoxygenation. The diagnosis is important mostly for genetic counseling.

   (2) **Laboratory findings:** Normal blood counts, RBC morphology, and Hb elevation show less than 45% Hg S; sickled cells appear after incubation with sodium metabisulfite; screening by solubility test

   c. Combinations with Hg C trait or β-thalassemia minor (occasionally with α-thalassemia minor) are more severe than each trait alone.

2. **Thalassemias** are a group of chronic, inherited **microcytic anemias** characterized by abnormalities in either the α or β chain.

   a. Homozygous

   (1) **β-thalassemia major (Cooley's anemia)** is the homozygous form (both β chains affected), consisting of 2 α and 2 γ chains. It is more common in Mediterranean populations but is found in African-Americans.

   (2) **Laboratory findings.** Severe anemia, microcytosis, reduced MCHC, severe elevation in RDW and poikilocytosis, markedly hypochromic RBCs, target cells, nucleated RBCs, basophilic

stippling of RBCs; high serum iron; increasing transferrin saturation and serum ferritin with repeated transfusions (iron overload); in addition to Hg electrophoresis, genetic polymerase chain reaction (PCR)-based tests may be obtained when indicated.

b. Heterozygous

  (1) **β-thalassemia minor or trait** is the heterozygous form of thalassemia; patients are asymptomatic.
  (2) **Laboratory findings:** Hg 10–13 g/dL, MCV 60–70 fL, basophilic stippling of RBCs, target cells, normal or even slightly elevated red cell count; Hg electrophoresis. The benchmark for diagnosis is increased Hb A_2, which can be detected in almost all cases if appropriate techniques are used.

c. α-thalassemia is a defective α chain synthesis with a complex inheritance involving the α chains of Hg on two loci/genes on each chromosome. This is in contrast to β chains of Hg, which have only one gene/locus on each of the two chromosomes. It is prevalent in persons of Southeast Asian ancestry. The laboratory diagnosis of the four types of α-thalassemia is complex but can be assessed by genetic analysis. Generally, Hg A_1 and A_2 are decreased.

B. Hereditary spherocytosis is a congenital, red cell membrane defect resulting from reduced or abnormal red cell cytoskeletal membrane and transmembrane components.

  1. History: Chronic anemia, mild jaundice, cholelithiasis, and splenomegaly
  2. Laboratory findings: Spherocytes on peripheral blood smear, increased red cell osmotic fragility, elevated MCHC, decreased MCV, decreased serum haptoglobin, reticulocytosis, negative direct Coombs' test

C. Enzymopathies are anemias caused by abnormalities in red cell metabolism resulting from enzyme deficiencies.

  1. Glucose-6-phosphate dehydrogenase (G6PD) deficiency

    a. Etiologies

      (1) African-Americans (type A). Enzymopathies can be caused by a sex-linked congenital decrease in G6PD. Patients are symptomatic only upon exposure to oxidants.
      (2) Mediterranean ancestry (type B). When enzymopathies are present in subjects of Mediterranean ancestry, the anemia is more severe and continuous, with fatalities occurring after exposure to oxidants, particularly fava beans.

    b. Laboratory findings

      (1) The peripheral blood when stained with special stains shows Heinz bodies.
      (2) G6PD is decreased in red cells when quantitated by commercially available kits because reticulocytes have normally

increased levels of G6PD and may result in falsely normal or elevated enzyme levels.

(a) In type A, the assay should be postponed for at least 6 weeks after a hemolytic episode.

(b) The enzyme levels decrease with the cells' age.

2. **Pyruvate kinase deficiency** is a **chronic, nonspherocytic anemia.** It can cause severe neonatal jaundice in some cases. Red cell counts normalize in adults. Diagnosis is made by quantitation of the enzyme in red cells.

D. Paroxysmal nocturnal hemoglobinuria is an acquired stem cell membrane defect resulting in intravascular hemolysis, followed by leukopenia, thrombocytopenia, and thrombotic episodes, including Budd-Chiari syndrome.

1. **History:** The patient may often report red urine in the early morning. Paroxysmal nocturnal hemoglobinuria may evolve into aplastic anemia, and it may also progress into acute leukemia.

2. **Laboratory findings:** Anemia (with normal red cell morphology), neutropenia, thrombocytopenia, iron deficiency, low or absent leukocyte alkaline phosphatase and low serum haptoglobin, hemosiderinuria, positive sucrose hemolysis (screening) or Ham acid hemolysis (confirmatory), flow cytophotometry (the recommended diagnostic test): lymphocytes lack CD48, CD52, CD58, or CD59

VII. Extrinsic Red Cell Membrane Defects (usually acquired)

A. Autoimmune hemolytic anemia (AIHA) occurs as a result of the development of warm or cold autoantibodies directed against RBCs. The diagnostic hallmark for this group of anemias is the presence of a positive antiglobulin test (Coombs' test).

1. **Warm-reactive AIHA**

a. **Etiology:** About 60% of cases are idiopathic, and the rest are secondary to lymphoma and leukemias, other neoplasia, autoimmune disorders (systemic lupus erythematosus), and viral infections including HIV and drugs.

b. **Laboratory findings:** Severe decrease in Hg and Hct, elevated reticulocyte count; microspherocytes; polychromatophilic and nucleated red cells on peripheral blood smear; increased indirect bilirubin; elevated urine and fecal urobilinogen; positive direct immunoglobulin G (IgG) antiglobulin (Coombs' test)

2. **Cold-reactive AIHA** is secondary to immunoglobulin M (IgM) antibodies that react best at cold temperatures (0–4°C). The hemolysis is either intravascular or extravascular.

a. **Etiology:** The most common causes are infections (*Mycoplasma pneumoniae,* infectious mononucleosis) and lymphomas. The idiopathic form, also called **cold agglutinin disease,** is seen most commonly in the elderly.

b. **Laboratory findings:** Anemia (severity depends on cold agglutinin titer); anomalous high MCV and MCHC, and low Hct (artifacts due to RBC clumping at room temperature); RBC clumping on peripheral blood smear; high reticulocyte count; positive anticomplement (C3) Coombs' test; positive IgM anti-I or anti-i cold-reacting antibodies. Cold agglutinin titers in excess of 1:1000 are diagnostic.

3. **Drug-induced hemolytic anemias:** The most common drugs involved include sulfa drugs, quinine, quinidine, ribavirin, high-dose penicillins, cephalothin sodium, and streptomycin.

B. Mechanical hemolysis

1. **Overview:** Mechanical hemolysis is the result of physical damage to RBCs leading to fragmentation and intravascular hemolysis.

   a. **Microangiopathy** is an endothelial cell injury in small blood vessels. It is seen in disseminated intravascular coagulation, thrombotic thrombocytopenic purpura, hemolytic uremic syndrome, disseminated malignancy, malignant hypertension, and vasculitis.

   b. **Macroangiopathy** is an RBC injury from malfunctioning valvular prosthesis, severe cardiac valve deformities, or aortic atheromatous.

2. **Laboratory findings:** Greater than 5/1000 red cells are deformed (schistocytes); d-dimer and fibrinogen degradation products (FDPs) are elevated if disseminated intravascular coagulation is present; elevated plasma Hg and urine hemosiderin; decreased plasma haptoglobin; anemia commensurate with severity of underlying process; varying degrees of thrombocytopenia

VIII. Special Considerations

A. Situation when anemia may be missed: Anemia may be missed in patients with parallel decrease in plasma volume as seen in the early stage of acute hemorrhage or with severe dehydration.

B. Situations in which the Hct and Hg may appear increased: When the plasma volume is contracted, but the red cell mass is normal, polycythemia should be considered.

C. The **low red cell indices** of thalassemia trait variants may be misinterpreted as iron-deficiency anemia.

D. Normal indices may be misleading in cases of **dimorphic anemias** (combined microcytic and macrocytic). The very high RDW or biphasic histogram is the clue.

E. A **normal or elevated ferritin value** does not exclude iron deficiency. It may be falsely elevated in patients with active liver disease or chronic inflammatory conditions.

F. The normal steady state of a patient with **thalassemia minor** (Hct around 36) may appear as severe anemia in the third trimester of pregnancy (Hct 30–32) because of expansion in the plasma volume.

SUGGESTED READING

Pechet, L: Anemias and Other Red Cell Disorders. In Noble J (ed): *Textbook of Primary Care Medicine*, 2nd ed. St. Louis, MO: Mosby Year Book, 1996, pp. 722–734.

42

Serum Protein Electrophoresis and Immunofixation

Robert B. Zurier

I. **Overview.** Serum proteins subjected to an electrical field separate into five zones (or bands), identified as albumin, α 1, α 2, β, and γ-globulin fractions. Immunoglobulins fall primarily in the γ-globulin zone, although some migration into the β and α regions occurs. **Zone electrophoresis** can be applied to other fluids, including cerebrospinal fluid and urine. The test is semiquantitative.

II. **Characterization and Quantification of Immunoglobulins**

   A. **Structure.** Immunoglobulins are glycoproteins secreted by terminally differentiated B lymphocytes or plasma cells following encounters with specific antigen. These cells produce five classes (isotypes) of immunoglobulin; the molecular structure of each consists of two identical heavy polypeptide chains (α, δ, ε, γ, μ) that bind two identical light chains (κ and λ) to form a Y-shaped monomeric protein.

   B. **Methodology** consists of a two-step procedure:

   1. **Proteins are separated electrophoretically in a gel.**
   2. **Monospecific antibodies are added to the gel surface,** resulting in immune complex formation and immunoprecipitation. The gel is stained; multiple intense bands result from oligoclonal immunoglobulins in normal specimens, or an intense narrow band is formed by a monoclonal immunoglobulin.

III. **Clinical Use.** Serum protein electrophoresis is useful only in limited clinical contexts, such as in cases of suspected myeloma or cryoglobulinemia. Otherwise, the information obtained is usually nonspecific and contributes little to the diagnosis.

   A. **Multiple myeloma** (see Chapter 43) results in hypergammaglobulinemia of a specific class of immunoglobulins. Hypogammaglobulinemia of recent onset in an adult also justifies a search for myeloma, especially for the possibility of light chain disease. For this diagnosis, examination of Bence Jones protein in urine is useful.

   1. **Serum protein electrophoresis** detects the clonal immunoglobulin as a narrow spike of homogeneously migrating immunoglobulin molecules.
   2. **Immunofixation,** a technique with better resolution, identifies the isotype of light and heavy chains. It can be used also for identification of monoclonal light chains in urine.

   B. **Cryoglobulinemia** is characterized by **immunoglobulins that undergo reversible precipitation in the cold.**

1. **Technique.** Blood must be allowed to clot at 37°C. Serum is removed and kept at 4°C. Cryoglobulins yield precipitates within 1–7 days and can then be quantitated and characterized by immunoprecipitation.
2. **Causes.** Cryoglobulins are found in **infections, autoimmune diseases, lymphoproliferative disorders, liver diseases,** or may be **"essential"** (i.e., idiopathic).
3. **Types.** There are three types of cryoglobulins:
    a. Type 1: Monoclonal
    b. Type 2: Mixed monoclonal
    c. Type 3: Mixed polyclonal
4. About 50% of patients with cryoglobulins have **mixed cryoglobulinemia.** Of these, about half have a **lymphoproliferative disease** or **autoimmune vasculitis.** Most patients do not develop a specific disease.

IV. Indications for Ordering Tests

A. Serum Protein Electrophoresis

1. **Hypergammaglobulinemia** (noticed on chemical determination of serum globulins)
2. **Paraproteinemias:** Whenever there is clinical suspicion or clinical findings of:
    a. Multiple myeloma or light chain disease
    b. Amyloidosis
    c. Heavy chain disease (although rare)
    d. Lymphoma (4.5% of diffuse lymphomas are "secretory")
    e. Hypoproteinemia
    f. Malnutrition
    g. Nephrotic syndrome
    h. Protein-losing enteropathies
    i. Hypobuminemia
    j. Liver disease (e.g., cirrhosis and diffuse acute hepatodegenerative disorders)
    k. Inflammatory disorders
    l. Alpha-1 antitrypsin deficiency

B. Immunofixation

1. High clinical suspicion of a monoclonal gammopathy
2. Ambiguous results by serum protein electrophoresis

SUGGESTED READING

Heren DF, Warren JS, Lowe JB: Strategy to diagnose monoclonal gammopathies in serum: High resolution electrophoresis, immunofixation, and kappa/lambda quantification. *Clin Chem* 32:2196, 1988.

43

Diagnostic Approach to Hematologic Disorders
Liberto Pechet, Fauzia Khan, and Sandra Senno

Disorders Resulting in Excessive Bleeding
Liberto Pechet

I. **Definition.** Excessive bleeding is defined as **bleeding beyond physiologic expectations.**

    A. **Spontaneous hemorrhage** is always abnormal, except for occasional, self-limiting epistaxis.

    B. **Excessive surgical, traumatic, or menstrual bleeding** is also considered abnormal.

II. **Incidence.** The incidence of inherited bleeding disorders varies with each particular congenital abnormality; some are as common as 1 in 100 people (e.g., von Willebrand's disease), while others are extremely rare (e.g., a deficiency of clotting factors V, II, X, I). The incidence of hemophilia A is 1 in 10,000 people, and the incidence of hemophilia B is 1 in 100,000 people.

III. **Common Causes**

    A. **Congenital causes**

        1. **Plasma defects** (e.g., clotting protein deficiency, usually single defect)

        2. **Platelet abnormalities**

            a. **Congenital thrombocytopenias are rare.** Examples include Bernard-Soulier syndrome and thrombocytopenia-absent radius (TAR) syndrome.

            b. **Thrombocytopathies** result from abnormal function of platelets.

    B. **Acquired causes**

        1. **Plasma coagulation abnormalities** are usually multiple. (An exception is acquired circulating anticoagulants.)

        2. **Platelet disorders**

            a. **Quantitative:** Thrombocytopenias

            b. **Qualitative:** Thrombocytopathies

IV. **When to Suspect an Underlying Bleeding Problem**

    A. **Spontaneous bleeding.** Whenever a patient presents with spontaneous bleeding, particularly if there have been similar episodes in the past, and/or if there is a family history of a known coagulopathy, or at least of un-diagnosed spontaneous, repeated bleeding in another family member, an underlying bleeding disorder should be suspected.

        1. It is important to establish the diagnosis of a bleeding tendency **prior to surgery.**

    2. Particular attention should be paid to patients with renal or liver disease.

B. Excessive bleeding. Whenever a patient bleeds more than expected for the degree of trauma or surgery, an underlying bleeding disorder should be suspected.

V. How to Confirm the Diagnosis

A. History. Interview the patient in detail with respect to personal bleeding history and gynecologic history for women.

B. Physical examination. Check for petechiae and ecchymosis (see Chapter 40).

    1. Mucosal bleeding suggests a platelet disorder or von Willebrand's disease.

    2. Visceral bleeding is seen more commonly in coagulopathies.

C. Laboratory investigations

    1. Suspected congenital defects in clotting

        a. Factor VIII (hemophilia A) or **factor IX** (hemophilia B) **deficiency**

            (1) Prolonged partial thromboplastin time (PTT) with normal prothrombin time (PT) and thrombin time (TT)

            (2) Clotting factors VIII and IX decrease by 0%–1% in the most severe cases.

            (3) All other individual clotting factors are normal. (It is not necessary to test other clotting factors once the diagnosis is established by finding a very low factor VIII or IX and a positive family history of excessive bleeding.)

        b. Factor XI

            (1) Prolonged PTT with normal PT and TT

            (2) Clotting factor XI generally does not decrease severely.

            (3) Factors VIII and IX will be normal.

        c. Factor XII, high-molecular-weight kininogen, and prekallikrein deficiencies

            (1) Prolonged PTT with normal PT and TT; no clinical bleeding

            (2) A decrease (usually not profound) may occur in any one of these factors; specific assays are available.

        d. Suspected inhibitors

            (1) In most cases, the inhibitors are antibodies directed against factors VIII or IX, especially in patients who are heavily treated for hemophilia.

            (2) Lack of correction of PTT after incubation of a mixture of one-half normal plasma and one-half patient's plasma

            (3) Lack of shortening of PTT or of increase in factors VIII or IX, respectively, after infusion of clotting factor concentrate

        e. Von Willebrand's disease may need to be differentiated from hemophilia A (Figure 43–1). The condition is divided into subtypes.

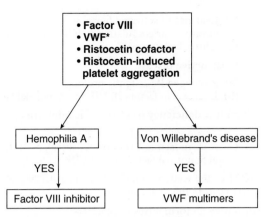

■ **FIGURE 43–1.** Algorithm for the laboratory differential diagnosis of hemophilia A and von Willebrand's disease. *VWF* = von Willebrand factor.
*Omit ristocetin cofactor and VWF antigen if there is a confirmed family history of hemophilia A.

    (1) Type I: Quantitative deficiency of plasma von Willebrand factor (VWF); prolonged PTT and bleeding time [neither is a reliable test for diagnosis]; abnormal ristocetin-induced platelet aggregation and ristocetin cofactor; decrease in factor VIII and VWF antigen; decrease in all multimers of the molecule

    (2) Type II: Selective deficiency of plasma high-molecular-weight VWF multimers; decrease in VWF antigen; decrease in factor VIII

        (a) Type IIa: Decrease in large and intermediate multimers; prolonged bleeding time and PTT in severe cases; abnormal ristocetin-induced platelet aggregation and ristocetin cofactor

        (b) Type IIb: Synthesis of abnormal large multimers with high affinity for platelets; characteristically, platelets aggregate with low concentration of ristocetin (in normal specimens, this concentration results in no aggregation); mild thrombo-cytopenia

    (3) Type III: Rare, but most severe, with very low levels of VWF and factor VIII

2. Suspected acquired clotting defects

    a. Liver disease: Perform chemistry and serology tests to determine the type of liver disease, and specific coagulation assays.

        (1) Parenchymal disease

            (a) Prolonged PT > PTT

            (b) Decrease in clotting factors V (most specific), VII, II, X, IX, I, and antithrombin in advanced disease; normal factor VIII

(c) Evidence of activated fibrinolysis and disseminated intravascular coagulation (DIC) in severe cases

(d) Thrombocytopenia

(2) Obstructive disease

(a) Prolonged PT, slightly prolonged PTT

(b) Decrease in factors II, VII, IX, X; normal factors V and VIII

b. **Vitamin K deficiency or effect of K inhibitors**

(1) Prolonged PT > PTT, normal TT

(2) Decrease in factors VII (most sensitive), X, II, IX, and proteins C and S; normal factors V and VIII

c. **DIC** (see the section on DISORDERS RESULTING IN EXCESSIVE CLOTTING in this chapter)

3. Quantitative abnormalities of platelets

a. **Thrombocytopenia**

b. **Other specific conditions** (which can be confirmed with laboratory studies)

(1) Suspected neoplasia or hematologic malignancy

(a) Bone marrow aspirate and biopsy

(b) Flow cytometry and histochemical studies (for the precise diagnosis of hematologic malignancies)

(2) Myelosuppression: If the cause is known, no specific studies are indicated.

(3) Immune thrombocytopenic purpura (ITP)

(a) Idiopathic: If there is no obvious cause, test for platelet antibodies. The results are credible if a high platelet antibody titer is reported.

(b) Obtain serology for HIV, in cases where HIV is suspected.

(c) Rule out autoimmune disorders by checking antinuclear antibodies, anticardiolipin antibodies, and lupus inhibitors.

(d) Rule out a lymphoproliferative disorder.

(e) Rule out the use of drugs that may produce platelet antibodies.

(f) Rule out history of blood transfusion in the previous 7 to 10 weeks by checking the platelet antigen (Pl^{A1}).

(4) Neonatal thrombocytopenia

(a) If there is a history of ITP in the mother, perform a laboratory workup of ITP in the mother and newborn [see V C 3 b (3)].

(b) Check maternal platelet alloantibodies, if sensitization with platelet antibodies during gestation is suspected.

(5) Hypersplenism: Determine the cause of the enlarged spleen.

(6) Mechanical destruction: Establish the primary cause (severe valvular disease or atheromas).

4. Qualitative abnormalities of platelets

a. **Platelet aggregation studies**

b. **Flow cytometry** of platelet membrane receptors

c. **Bleeding time** is the least reproducible, and rarely recommended.

5. Congenital platelet defects (follow laboratory investigations as described in V C 4). In certain cases, electron microscopy or special studies may be obtained in research laboratories.

Disorders Resulting in Excessive Clotting

Liberto Pechet

I. **Definition.** Thrombophilia (i.e., a hypercoagulable state) is the **tendency to have recurrent or acute, multiple, severe thrombosis.**
II. **Causes and Types** (Table 43–1)
III. **How to Confirm the Diagnosis** (Figure 43–2)

A. **History.** Ascertain previous history of venous or arterial thrombosis at a young age, unusual locations of thrombosis, and similar history in the family.

B. **Laboratory investigations.** Because no simple single screening assay is available, **evaluation of a suspected case** requires a battery of tests.

1. **Inherited thrombophilia**

   a. **Types of assays**

      (1) Functional (clotting or enzymatic)
      (2) Immunologic (antigen quantitation)
      (3) Genetic

   b. **Diagnostic approach** (see Figure 43–2 and Table 43–2)
   c. **Effects of anticoagulants**

      (1) **Heparin**

         (a) Does not interfere with immunologic or genetic tests
         (b) May affect antithrombin and functional factor II

      (2) **Oral anticoagulants** (vitamin K antagonists)

         (a) Patients should be off anticoagulants for 10 days before functional tests are performed for protein C and protein S.
         (b) Antithrombin is not affected by oral anticoagulants.
         (c) The genetic test and a modified activated protein C-resistance functional assay are not affected.

2. **Acquired thrombophilia**

   a. **Diagnostic evaluation of DIC**

      (1) DIC is a pathophysiologic mechanism secondary to a wide variety of conditions caused by simultaneous activation of the coagulation and fibrinolytic pathways resulting in hypercoagulability and hyperfibrinolysis.
      (2) DIC accompanies sepsis, acidosis, leukemia, neoplasms, certain obstetrical accidents, and hemolytic transfusion reactions.
      (3) **Laboratory findings:** The recommended DIC screen consists of d-dimers, fibrin degradation products (FDPs), and anti-thrombin.

TABLE 43–1. Inherited and Acquired Thrombophilic States

Acquired Thrombophilia	Hereditary Thrombophilia

Disseminated intravascular coagulation (DIC)
Cancer (Trousseau's syndrome)
Antiphospholipid antibodies
Lupus anticoagulant
Pregnancy and puerperium
Amniotic fluid embolism
Oral contraceptive use
Myeloproliferative disorders
Nephrotic syndromes
Heparin-induced thrombocytopenia
Surgery (abdominal; gynecologic, especially for cancer; orthopedic for knee, hip, or multiple fractures)
	Established:
	    Antithrombin deficiency
	    Protein C deficiency
	    Protein S deficiency
	    Factor V Leiden mutation (APC-R)
	    Abnormal prothrombin (factor II)
	    Increased lipoprotein a
	    Hyperhomocystinemia
	
	Suspected:
	    Elevated PAI-1
	    Abnormal fibrinogen
	    Elevated clotting factors VIII, VII, VWF, XI, IX
	    Heparin cofactor II deficiency
	    Abnormal thrombomodulin
	    Plasminogen deficiency
	    Tissue plasminogen activator deficiency

ACP-R = activated protein C-resistance; PAI-1 = plasminogen inhibitor 1; VWF = von Willebrand factor.

    (a) Elevation of d-dimers in a **latex agglutination test,** a relatively less sensitive test than enzyme-linked immunosorbent assay (ELISA) d-dimer, is the most specific assay.

    (b) FDPs are sensitive but not specific for DIC (the assay reflects activated fibrinolysis).

    (c) A decrease in antithrombin parallels the severity of the condition.

    (d) **Prothrombin fragments 1–2** and **fibrinopeptide levels** may be superior to d-dimers, FDPs, and antithrombin, but are not presently available in most clinical laboratories.

  b. Diagnostic evaluation for antiphospholipid antibody

    (1) A baseline PTT is necessary.

    (2) If the PTT is prolonged for no obvious reason or if there is a strong clinical suspicion, obtain antiphospholipid (anticardiolipin) antibodies and a lupus anticoagulant assay (commercial kits are available).

3. Venous thrombosis (or suspected acquired venous thrombophilia)

  a. A baseline PT and PTT are necessary if anticoagulation is started.

  b. Compression ultrasonography (duplex) of lower extremities and venography may be required in special situations or for follow-up of therapy.

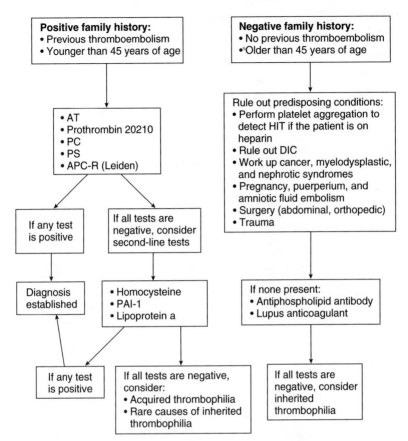

■ **FIGURE 43–2.** Algorithm for the laboratory workup for thrombophilia. *APC-R* = activated protein C-resistance, *AT* = antithrombin; *DIC* = disseminated intravascular coagulation; *HIT* = heparin-induced thrombocytopenia; PAI-1 = plasminogen inhibitor 1; PC = protein C; PS = protein S.

    c. Antiphospholipid antibodies and lupus anticoagulant may be positive in the antiphospholipid antibody syndromes.

    d. A negative d-dimer [if the assay is very sensitive, such as obtained with ELISA methodology (see III B 4)] makes the diagnosis unlikely.

4. Pulmonary embolism

    a. Sensitive automated ELISA d-dimer: In assays with a usual cut-off of 500 ng/mL, values < 500 ng/mL are considered negative and rule out pulmonary embolism.

    b. A negative or low probability ventilation-perfusion ($\dot{V}\dot{Q}$) scan or a negative spiral computed tomography (CT) scan, in conjunction

TABLE 43–2. The Laboratory Findings in Inherited Thrombophilia

Condition	Functional Test	Antigen Concentration	Genetic Test
Venous thrombophilia			
	Antithrombin:		
	Normal	Not necessary	
	Decreased	Recommended*	
	Protein C:		
	Normal	Mandatory	
	Decreased	Optional	
	Protein S:		
	Normal	Mandatory	
	Decreased	Optional	
	APC-R:		
	Normal		Factor V Leiden mutation
			Prothrombin mutation 20210
			Recommended*
	Factor II		
	Abnormal		Recommended†
Arterial thrombophilia			
	Homocysteine (fasting):		
	Increased		Recommended
	Lipoprotein a:		
	Increased		
	PAI-1:		
	Increased		

*Test should be ordered if the results of functional assays are ambiguous.
†Test should be ordered when family studies are undertaken.

with a negative sensitive ELISA d-dimer, makes the diagnosis of venous thrombosis with pulmonary embolism unlikely.

c. Pulmonary angiography is recommended only in difficult diagnostic situations.

SUGGESTED READING

Khan F, Pechet L, Snyder LM: The laboratory of hypercoagulability. *J Thrombosis Thromboly-sis* 5:269–276, 1998.

Khan F, Snyder LM, Pechet L: The laboratory of coagulation. A review of present laboratory techniques. *J Thrombosis Thrombolysis* 5:83–88, 1998.

Kholi A, Khan F, Snyder ML, et al: Hemostasis laboratory: Assays for platelet function and von Willebrand disease. *J Thrombosis Thrombolysis* 6:159–167, 1998.

Yu M, Nardella A, Pechet L: Screening tests of disseminated intravascular coagulation. Guidelines for rapid and specific diagnosis. *Crit Care Med* 28:1777–1780, 2000.

Non-Hodgkin's Lymphoma and Hodgkin's Disease

Fauzia Khan

I. Definitions

  A. Non-Hodgkin's lymphoma is a clonal lymphoproliferative disease characterized by proliferations of transformed B and T cells.

  B. Hodgkin's disease is a lymphoproliferative disease characterized by abnormal binucleated or multinucleated cells with distinct nucleoli (i.e., Reed-Sternberg cells). Hodgkin's lymphoma is divided into two types:

    1. Classic Hodgkin's disease, with additional subdivisions

    2. Lymphocyte-predominant nodular-type Hodgkin's disease

II. Diagnosis

  A. Physical examination will generally reveal the presence of painless, asymptomatic lymphadenopathy.

  B. Biopsy of an abnormally enlarged lymph node or suspicious mass is usually the first diagnostic step (see Chapter 38).

    1. **Histology** provides information about the cells' type and tissue architecture.

    2. **Molecular examination** determines gene rearrangements and is considered more important in non-Hodgkin's lymphoma than in Hodgkin's disease.

    3. **Fine-needle aspiration (FNA)** provides information only about cell type—not about architecture. It is rarely useful in determining the type of lymphoma.

  C. Bone marrow biopsy determines if the bone marrow is involved by lymphoma; if positive, the patient is in advanced-stage disease (stage 4). Bilateral iliac crest bone marrow biopsy is recommended for staging Hodgkin's disease; unilateral bone marrow biopsy is recommended for staging non-Hodgkin's lymphoma.

  D. Laboratory investigation

    1. A **complete blood count (CBC),** with white cell differential and platelet counts, is required.

    2. **Eosinophilia** may accompany both non-Hodgkin's and Hodgkin's lymphoma.

    3. **Liver function tests** are required.

    4. β_2-**microglobulin** and **lactate dehydrogenase** are indicators of disease activity and confer prognostic information.

  5. **Uric acid levels** may be elevated and raises a red flag for a hyper-
     uricemic syndrome.
  6. **Calcium levels** may be elevated and requires further study to deter-
     mine the cause.

E. Imaging

  1. **Chest radiography** is useful both for diagnosis and screening and for
     assessing the result of therapy.
  2. **CT scans** of the chest, abdomen, and pelvis provide more detailed
     information that is sometimes missed on plain films.
  3. **Magnetic resonance imaging** (MRI) is useful in special cases (e.g.,
     neurologic, bone, and suspected bone marrow involvement) and pro-
     vides information that may be missed by biopsy.
  4. **Gallium scan** provides baseline information and is a particularly good
     tool for assessing the results of therapy.

F. Special tests are indicated when there is suspicion of any of the following
causes:

  1. HIV
  2. Human T-cell lymphoma virus 1
  3. Epstein-Barr virus (EBV)
  4. Hepatitis B and C

SUGGESTED READING

Harris NL: Hodgkin's lymphomas: Classification, diagnosis, and grading.[Review]. *Semin Hematol* 36:220–232, 1999.

Acute Leukemias

Liberto Pechet

  I. Definition. The acute leukemias are **rapidly developing hematologic
  malignancies that involve the early hematologic precursors in the bone
  marrow.** They can be divided by the stem cell where they originate into acute
  nonlymphocytic leukemia (ANLL) and acute lymphocytic leukemia (ALL).
  II. Classification. ANLL can be classified by the mode of onset.

  A. De novo ANLL has no antecedent hematologic disease and is not preceded
  by chemotherapy or radiation therapy. This type of leukemia is "primary"
  and usually responds more favorably to therapy.
  B. Secondary ANLL follows another hematologic condition or exposure to
  chemicals (e.g., benzene) or is preceded by chemotherapy or radiation
  therapy.

  III. Laboratory Investigation. Specific diagnosis and lineage assignment can be
  achieved in 70% of cases by studying the bone marrow and peripheral blood

smear morphology. The accuracy increases to 90% when supplemented with cytochemical, immunophenotypic (by flow cytometry), and cytogenetic (determination of karyotype) methods.

A. CBC

1. Leukocytosis

   a. The white blood cell (WBC) count is elevated at presentation in 80%–90% of cases, but may initially be normal or low.

   b. Most cells are immature, although a few mature or intermediate forms may be present.

   c. Immature cells and blasts, or uniform, monotonous mature cells may be present.

2. Thrombocytopenia and **anemia** may be profound.

B. Bone marrow aspirate and biopsy

1. Morphology: Hypercellularity, with many immature, bizarre cells (> 30% of all nucleated cells) may be present, with a marked decrease or absence of normal bone marrow hematopoietic cells.

2. Chromosomes: Abnormal karyotypes, studied by chromosome cultures or by fluorescence in situ hybridization assays, can be found in the majority of cases. The chromosome characteristics bear a direct relationship to the diagnosis of the subtype of leukemia and to prognosis.

3. Phenotypic studies performed by flow cytometry are highly discriminant for the subtype of leukemia.

4. Studies of hemostasis are frequently necessary because certain types of ANLL, especially promyelocytic leukemia, are associated with proteolytic activation of the clotting and fibrinolytic mechanisms.

IV. Variants

A. ANLL. The eight subtypes are described by the letter M followed by a numerical subscript—from M_0 through M_7.

B. ALL. The three subtypes are described by the letter L followed by a numerical subscript—from L_1 to L_3.

SUGGESTED READING

Appelbaum FR: Molecular diagnosis and clinical decisions in adult acute leukemias. *Semin Hemat* 36:401–410, 1999.

Myeloproliferative Disease

Liberto Pechet

I. Definition.

Myeloproliferative disease is characterized by **clonal tri-lineage bone marrow myeloid hyperplasia,** resulting in excessive proliferation of granulocytic, monocytic, erythroid, and megakaryocytic precursors (Table 43–3).

TABLE 43–3. Classification of Myeloproliferative Diseases

Condition	Major lineages involved
Chronic myelogenous leukemia (CML)	Granulocytes
Chronic myelomonocytic leukemia (proliferative, that is >12,000 white cells per μL)	Monocytes and granulocytes
Agnogenic myeloid metaplasia (AMM)	All lines and fibroblasts in bone marrow
Polycythemia vera	Red cells, granulocytes and platelets
Essential thrombocythemia	Platelets
Unclassified myeloproliferative disease	Usually all lines

II. Variants

A. Chronic myelogenous leukemia

1. **Description:** Chronic myelogenous leukemia is expressed predominantly by the proliferation of granulocytic elements. It is a biphasic disease with an initial, chronic phase, followed by transformation into acute leukemia after 3–5 years. With the advent of new pharmacologic agents, such as Gleevec (i.e., a specific protein kinase inhibitor), the outlook in cases of chronic myelogenous leukemia is greatly improved.

2. **Laboratory findings**

   a. **Peripheral blood counts**

      (1) The WBC count shows severe leukocytosis (50,000–300,000 per μL at the time of diagnosis).

      (2) Segmented neutrophils, metamyelocytes, and myelocytes predominate, with < 12% blasts.

      (3) Eosinophilia and basophilia are common, with occasional hybrid (basophilic and eosinophilic) granules in the same cell.

      (4) Monocytes, often abnormal in appearance, are increased, but are not > 2% of the WBC count.

   b. The **bone marrow** is very hyperplastic, with all white cell precursors present, and < 5% myeloblasts in the chronic phase.

   c. **Leukocyte alkaline phosphatase** (LAP) is decreased or absent in granulocytes; it may reappear or even increase in the accelerated phase.

   d. **Chromosomes:** The Philadelphia chromosome or its variants is present in > 98% of cases of chronic myelogenous leukemia. The Philadelphia chromosome is the result of a translocation between chromosomes 9 and 22, t (9;22). Duplication of the Philadelphia chromosome or additional karyotypic abnormalities (e.g., trisomy 8 or 19, loss of chromosome Y, 17q+) develop in the accelerated phase.

e. Serum **uric acid** is elevated.

B. Agnogenic myeloid metaplasia (AMM)

1. **Description:** AMM is characterized by extramedullary proliferation of granulocytic elements, megakaryocytes, and red cell precursors with progressive bone marrow failure, replacement of bone marrow by fibrosis, and progressive splenomegaly. Symptoms of abdominal pressure followed by early satiety and left upper quadrant pain develop due to splenomegaly.

2. **Laboratory findings**

   a. **Peripheral blood counts:** There is a leukoerythroblastic picture, with teardrop and nucleated red cells, immature myeloid elements, and increased eosinophils and basophils.

   b. **Platelets:** Thrombocytosis appears initially in 50% of patients. Eventually, progressive thrombocytopenia develops with large, bizarre platelets, circulating single-lobed megakaryocytes, and defective platelet function (demonstrable by platelet aggregation studies).

   c. **Bone marrow aspirate** is difficult to obtain because of fibrosis. The biopsy marrow is initially hypercellular with patchiness of hematopoietic cellularity and reticulin fibrosis, and shows:

      (1) Increased megakaryocytes (in clusters) with dysplastic morphology (micro- and macromegakaryocytes)

      (2) Progressive fibrosis with increased reticulin

      (3) A progressive decrease in white and red cell lines

      (4) Dilated sinusoids containing intravascular hematopoiesis

   d. **Karyotype:** Abnormalities are present in 50%–60% of cases, but none are specific. The Philadelphia chromosome is absent.

   e. **Hyperuricemia** frequently accompanies AMM.

   f. **LAP** may be elevated or normal, but it is rarely decreased.

3. **Imaging studies**

   a. **Bone radiographs** show increased bone density and increased bony trabeculae. They do not offer findings necessary for diagnosis.

   b. **MRI** can assess the degree of bone marrow replacement by fibrosis, with important diagnostic value.

C. Polycythemia vera

1. **Description:** Polycythemia vera is characterized by an increase in red blood cell (RBC) mass, granulocytes, and platelets.

2. **When to suspect polycythemia vera:** The condition has to be differentiated from other myeloproliferative diseases, particularly chronic myelogenous leukemia and AMM (see Table 43–3) and also from nonclonal disorders associated with an increase in RBCs (i.e., erythrocytosis), such as seen with pulmonary insufficiency, hypoxia, and congestive heart failure (CHF). Note that in cases of secondary erythrocytosis, the WBC and platelet counts are normal.

3. **Laboratory findings**

a. **Peripheral blood counts:** There is an increase in all formed elements.

b. **Bone marrow aspirate:** The morphology is relatively normal, showing hyperplasia but without a disproportionate increase in immature cells. There are clusters of megakaryocytes.

c. **LAP** is usually high (a distinction from chronic myelogenous leukemia).

d. **Serum iron and ferritin levels** are usually decreased.

e. **Uric acid and vitamin B$_{12}$ levels** are elevated.

f. **Erythropoietin levels** are normal or very low.

g. CBC mass studies may be necessary.

D. Essential thrombocythemia

1. **Description:** Essential thrombocythemia is a clonal, chronic, hematopoietic disorder, characterized by a pronounced and sustained increase in the number of megakaryocytes and platelets. It leads to thrombosis and hemorrhage.

2. **Laboratory findings**

a. **Peripheral blood counts:** Thrombocytosis is present, usually 1–3 × 10^6 per μL. There is a moderate increase in granulocytes (10–15,000 per μL) and a modest increase in RBCs.

b. **Peripheral smear:** Platelets are increased with many clumps and abnormalities in shape, size, and structure. There are megakaryocytic fragments. White cells are relatively normal, except for a mild increase in eosinophils and basophils. Red cells have normal morphology.

c. Both **bone marrow aspirate** and **biopsy** are moderately hyperplastic, with no increase in immature forms, but a great increase in megakaryocytes and platelets, many of which are in clumps. There is no fibrosis and normal iron stores.

d. **Karyotype:** The Philadelphia chromosome is absent.

e. **LAP** is elevated in as many as 40% of cases.

f. **RBC mass** is normal.

g. Spurious in vitro **increases in serum K, acid phosphatase, and inorganic phosphorus** may be found, all due to thrombocytosis and clotting.

SUGGESTED READING

Dickstein JI, Vardiman JW: Issues in the pathology and diagnosis of the chronic myeloproliferative disorders and the myelodysplastic syndromes. *Am J Clin Pathol* 99:513–525, 1993.

Myelodysplastic Syndromes

Liberto Pechet

I. **Definition.** The myelodysplastic syndromes are **clonal abnormalities of hematopoiesis presenting with uni- or multilineage cytopenias.**

II. Diagnosis

A. History. Onset is usually insidious. Symptoms are related most commonly to chronic progressive anemia, infections, or hemorrhages.

B. Laboratory findings

1. **Peripheral blood count** shows pancytopenia.
2. **Bone marrow biopsy** and **aspirate** are hyperplastic in most cases.

   a. **Red cell line:** The red cell line may be involved alone in refractory anemia or refractory anemia with ring sideroblasts, presenting with dysplastic (megaloblastic) features in the absence of vitamin B_{12} or folate.

   b. **White cell line:** The white cell line shows dysplastic features in granulocyte and monocyte lineage and increased blasts except in refractory anemia or refractory anemia with ring sideroblasts.

   c. **Megakaryocytes:** Dysplastic features, micro- and mononuclear megakaryocytes, or cells with multiple small nuclei separated by strands of nuclear material are present.

3. **Karyotypes:** Chromosome studies are essential in the diagnosis of myelodysplastic syndromes.

   a. **Primary myelodysplastic syndrome:** The karyotype is abnormal in 40%–60% of cases; most common abnormalities are seen in chromosomes 5, 7 (deletions, monosomies), and 8 (trisomy).

   b. **Secondary myelodysplastic syndrome:** The karyotype is abnormal in > 80% of cases. Those abnormalities best documented in therapy-related myelodysplastic syndrome are monosomy 7, 5q-, trisomy 8, and monosomy 5, 20q-. Frequently, complex abnormalities are present.

SUGGESTED READING

Kouides PA, Bennett JM: Morphology and classification of the myelodysplastic syndromes and their pathologic variants. *Semin Hemat* 33:95–110, 1996.

Chronic Lymphocytic Leukemia

Liberto Pechet

I. Definition. Chronic lymphocytic leukemia (CLL) and its variants are **chronic lymphoproliferative diseases resulting from accumulation of clonal, immunologically incompetent lymphocytes in the bone marrow, blood, spleen, and lymph nodes.** CLL is one of the most indolent forms of leukemia, but it is nearly always fatal if not cured by intensive chemotherapy with stem cell support.

II. Diagnosis

A. History. CLL is diagnosed accidentally in 40% of patients during routine examination or admission for pneumonia or other infection.

B. Laboratory findings

1. **Peripheral blood counts:** The following findings should prompt the investigation of CLL or other chronic lymphoproliferative diseases.

   a. **WBC count** from 20,000 to > 200,000 per μL with from 70% to > 95% of the lymphocytes appearing mature without visible nucleoli
   b. **Lymphocytosis** with absolute counts > 5,000 (in most cases > 15,000) per μL accounts for leukocytosis

2. **RBC count:** The RBC count shows normochromic, normocytic, anemia in advanced cases, with spherocytes when accompanied by a positive Coombs hemolytic process in 25% of cases.

3. **Platelets:** Thrombocytopenia is present and can be due to immune mechanisms (any stage), hypersplenism, or marrow replacement (advanced stage).

4. **Bone marrow:** The bone marrow is hypercellular with increased mature-appearing lymphocytes.

5. **Flow cytometry:** The phenotype of peripheral blood and bone marrow lymphocyte is **CD_5 positive.**

6. **Hypogammaglobulinemia** is more severe with advancing disease.

7. **β_2-microglobulin:** A high level denotes poor prognosis.

SUGGESTED READING

Pangalis GA, Angelopoulou MK, Vassilakopoulos TP, et al: B-chronic lymphocytic leukemia, small lymphocytic lymphoma, and lymphoplasmacytic lymphoma, including Waldenstrom's macroglobulinemia: A clinical, morphologic, and biologic spectrum of similar disorders. *Semin Hemat* 36:104–114, 1999.

Plasma Cell Dyscrasias

Sandra Senno

I. **Definition.** Plasma cell dyscrasias are characterized by **proliferation and clonal expansion of differentiated B lineage cells, in most cases plasma cells.** The monoclonal immunoglobulins (Ig) produced are referred to as paraproteins or monoclonal gammopathies. The letter M refers to a single spike that is (usually) discovered on serum protein electrophoresis.

   A. **Multiple myeloma,** a clonal proliferation of plasma cells, is the most typical and common plasma cell dyscrasia.
   B. **Monoclonal gammopathy of unknown significance,** an indolent variant, is much more common. Because there are no symptoms, this condition is generally diagnosed accidentally when an elevation in serum globulins is discovered.
   C. **Waldenstrom's macroglobulinemia** is another variant that has a predominance of lymphocytoid plasma cells and IgM gammopathy.

II. Diagnosis

A. **History.** In a middle-aged to elderly patient with symptoms of anemia, hypercalcemia, or hyperviscosity, check for a history of bone pain or symptoms of progressive renal failure.

B. **Physical findings** are nonspecific but secondary to progressive anemia of renal failure. Occasionally, there are pathologic fractures.

C. **Laboratory findings**

1. **Blood studies** may show normochromic anemia without clear etiology, serum hypergammaglobulinemia, very elevated sedimentation rate, hypercalcemia, and proteinuria.

2. **Serum protein electrophoresis** shows a monoclonal spike; it should be followed by **immunofixation** for better delineation.

3. **Quantitation of serum immunoglobulins** (IgG, IgA, and IgM) is needed to establish the severity of the condition and as a tool for follow-up.

4. **Urinary Bence Jones protein** should be tested for the presence of light chains. If a screening test is positive, it should be followed by quantitation of light chains on a 24-hour urine collection.

5. **Blood urea nitrogen/creatinine and serum calcium levels** may be elevated with advanced disease.

6. **Bone marrow biopsy** is required to assess the number and distribution of normal and abnormal plasma cells.

7. **β_2-microglobulin** is an excellent prognostic indicator; it predicts short survival if elevated.

8. **Serum viscosity** is useful, especially if Waldenstrom's macroglobulinemia or IgA myeloma has been diagnosed, or if there are clinical signs of hyperviscosity (e.g., unexplained bleeding, mental changes).

D. **Imaging**

1. **Skeletal radiography survey** (metastatic series) will uncover osteolytic lesions.

2. **MRI studies** of the bone marrow, as well as the skeleton, may provide more detailed information.

SUGGESTED READING

Malpas J, Bergsagel D, Kyle R, et al (eds): *Myeloma: Biology and Management.* New York: Oxford University Press, 1988.

Iron-Storage Diseases

Liberto Pechet

I. **Definition.** Iron-storage diseases are **conditions in which the storage of body iron is excessive.** Because humans eliminate only minimal amounts of iron (except for menstruating females and during pregnancy), any excessive intake of iron, either intestinal or by transfusions, results in iron overload.

A. Hemosiderosis refers to an increase in the tissue content of macrophages, at least initially, and is usually secondary to excessive iron input. When the total body iron exceeds 11 g (normal is 4 g), iron is deposited also in parenchymal cells.

B. Hemochromatosis (i.e., hereditary hemochromatosis) is a metabolic abnormality of iron metabolism, resulting from an autosomal recessive abnormality. It is manifested by excess iron in parenchymal cells and involves the liver, heart, pancreas, joints, and central nervous system (CNS) [i.e., the hypothalamus]. Hemochromatosis is the result, in most cases, of an HLA-linked abnormal gene, which interferes with the normal control of iron absorption. As a result of the mutation, three times the normal amount of iron is absorbed by the intestine.

II. When to Suspect an Iron-Storage Disease

A. Hemosiderosis will develop with certainty in all patients whose survival depends on continuous red cell transfusions (> 100 transfused units). It is also seen in heavy wine drinkers, patients with liver cirrhosis especially if secondary to alcohol abuse, and in patients with high dietary iron intake.

B. Hemochromatosis should be suspected in individuals with:

1. A family history of hemochromatosis
2. Unexplained cardiomyopathy, liver disease, diabetes, and arthritis; increasing pigmentation of the skin; or hypogonadotropic hypogonadism
3. An incidental laboratory finding of high iron saturation or ferritin

III. Diagnosis

A. Laboratory findings

1. **Transferrin saturation:** An elevated transferrin saturation is considered a reliable indicator (i.e., the iron divided by TIBC = transferrin saturation). The threshold for additional investigations varies among investigators between $> 42\%$ and $> 62\%$. For female patients, it is now recommended to set a threshold of 50% transferrin saturation; for males, the threshold is set at $> 55\%$.

   a. The patient should fast before undergoing the test.
   b. The transferrin saturation is elevated even in children with hemochromatosis.
   c. Serum iron is invariably elevated.

2. **Serum ferritin:** An iron-storage disease should be suspected when serum ferritin is $> 200 \, \mu g/L$ in women and $> 300 \, \mu g/L$ in men. Plasma ferritin rises to a maximum concentration of 4000 $\mu g/L$ as the body iron burden increases (further elevations may be seen as the result of additional morbid factors).

3. **Liver chemistries** will reveal mild elevations, given the nature of this chronic, infiltrative process. **Blood sugar levels** and **cardiac function** are recommended investigations to assess the degree of organ impairment.

4. **Genetic tests** (for the C2824 and H63D mutations) are recommended

to confirm the diagnosis of hemochromatosis when transferrin saturation is elevated.

B. Liver biopsy is recommended for all patients with high transferrin saturation or ferritin concentrations > 300 ng/mL. It is used to quantitate tissue iron and examine the extent of hepatic damage.

C. MRI: Hepatic signal intensity and transverse relaxation time decrease with iron loading.

SUGGESTED READING

El-Serag HB, Inadomi JM, Kowdley KV: Screening for hereditary hemochromatosis in siblings and children of affected patients. *Ann Intern Med* 132:261–269, 2000.

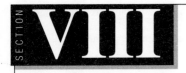

Infectious Diseases

44

Fever of Unknown Origin

Jennifer S. Daly and Richard H. Glew

I. **Definition.** Fever of unknown origin is an **illness characterized by rectal temperature > 38.3°C (> 101°F) on more than 3 occasions, over 3 weeks or longer, with no diagnosis reached after 1 week of inpatient or thorough outpatient investigation.**

II. **Etiologies.** Infection, autoimmune disease, and neoplasia account for most cases. The commonly cited differential diagnoses include:

A. **Infectious causes**

1. **Systemic infections**

a. **Infective endocarditis** (pathogens include viridans group streptococci, *Haemophilus*, and related organisms) and **Q fever** (*Coxiella burnetii*)

b. **Atypical mononucleosis-like illness** due to cytomegalovirus (CMV), Epstein-Barr virus (EBV), toxoplasmosis, brucellosis, secondary syphilis, or primary HIV-1 infection

c. **Miliary tuberculosis**

d. **Protozoal infections,** such as babesiosis and malaria

e. **Borreliosis,** including Lyme disease (*Borrelia burgdorferi*) and relapsing fever (*Borrelia recurrentis*, other species)

f. **Immunocompromised patients,** due to old age, diabetes, alcoholism, cancer, drug abuse, HIV, burns, and immunosuppressive and autoimmune disorders

g. **Whipple's disease** (*Tropheryma whippleii*)

h. **Disseminated fungal disease** (e.g., histoplasmosis, coccidioidomycosis)

i. **Chronic or recurrent meningococcemia**

2. **Localized infections**

a. **Hepatobiliary tract** (recurrent cholecystitis, cholangitis, empyema of the gallbladder, viral hepatitis)

b. **Visceral abscess** (liver abscess, tubo-ovarian abscess, pancreatic abscess)

c. **Intra-abdominal abscess** (periappendiceal abscess, peridiverticular abscess, subhepatic or subphrenic abscess, pelvic or retroperitoneal abscess, psoas abscess)

    d. Urinary tract (pyelonephritis, renal carbuncle, perinephric abscess, prostatitis or prostatic abscess)

    e. Osteomyelitis, especially vertebral osteomyelitis or disk space infection in the elderly, or injection drug use

    f. Sinusitis

    g. Dental (periapical abscesses)

    h. Intestinal tract (yersiniosis)

    i. Giardiasis

    j. Amebiasis (colonic ameboma)

    k. Tuberculosis or typhlitis

B. Neoplasia

1. **Tumors** with fever as a symptom include:

    a. Non-Hodgkin's lymphoma

    b. Hodgkin's disease [relapsing, periodic fever pattern (Pel-Ebstein fever)]

    c. Hypernephroma (renal cell carcinoma)

    d. Hepatoma or carcinoma metastatic to liver

    e. Colon carcinoma

    f. Preleukemia (especially monocytic leukemia)

2. **Complications**

    a. Mechanical sequelae of solid tumor (i.e., obstruction, fistula, infection)

    b. Sequelae of treatment (surgery, radiation) [i.e., fistula, obstruction leading to infection]

C. Inflammatory diseases

1. **Medication reaction:** Clues include rash, eosinophilia, little pulse response to fever, relatively well-appearing, history of atopy and use of prescription medications or over-the-counter medications.

2. **Connective tissue diseases:** Systemic lupus erythematosus, rheumatoid arthritis, Still's disease (i.e., juvenile rheumatoid arthritis), Reiter's syndrome, Behçet's syndrome, polyarteritis nodosa, giant cell arteritis, polymyalgia rheumatica, and acute rheumatic fever can all present with fever.

3. **Granulomatous diseases:** Wegener's granulomatosis, sarcoidosis, and granulomatous hepatitis can cause fever.

4. **Inflammatory bowel disease** (especially Crohn's disease) is often accompanied by fever.

D. Miscellaneous

1. Pulmonary embolism (recurrent, small emboli)

2. Alcoholic hepatitis

3. Familial Mediterranean fever

4. Cardiac myxoma

5. Hematoma

6. Factitious: In this case, the patient appears well, has no weight loss, is affable or theatrical, and has a normal pulse. An electronic thermometer

is most reliable. Also feel the patient's skin and check the urine temperature.

III. Clinical Evaluation

A. History

1. **Symptoms.** Assess severity, tempo, acuity, and duration of symptoms. Note any weight loss or disability.
2. **Past medical history**
   a. Assess prior evaluations, including tests, medications, and treatment.
   b. Inquire about prior surgery, exposure to blood products, system review, allergies, and medications.
3. **Family and social history**
   a. **Familial diseases,** such as familial Mediterranean fever, gallbladder disease, cancer, and connective tissue disorders, should be noted.
   b. **Common exposure** should be noted, such as recent febrile illnesses in family, social setting, and relatives or close friends with tuberculosis.
   c. **Travel** (or residence), especially in exotic locales, is important to ascertain.

B. Physical examination

1. **Skin:** Check for petechiae, splinter hemorrhages, and rash.
2. **Eyes:** Examine for fundi, and look for Roth spots, hemorrhages, and iritis.
3. **Lymph nodes** should be palpated, especially the supraclavicular and epitrochlear.
4. **Rectal:** Examine for prostatitis, prostatic abscess, and colon cancer.
5. **Abdomen:** Check for splenomegaly or a mass (e.g., tumor, abscess).
6. **Genitalia:** Perform a pelvic examination in women and an external genitalia examination in men.
7. **Repeat physical examination** for missed findings and transient signs (e.g., rash of juvenile rheumatoid arthritis) or evolving findings.

C. Laboratory investigations. In general, perform the easiest, least morbid tests first, focusing on clinical clues.

1. **Routine tests**
   a. Complete blood count (CBC), including differential white count
   b. Erythrocyte sedimentation rate (ESR)
   c. Urinalysis and urine culture
   d. C-reactive protein
   e. Liver chemistries
   f. Antinuclear antibody
   g. Blood cultures
   h. Serologies, per history, such as for EBV, CMV, *Brucella*, *Toxoplasma*, syphilis, *Borrelia*, cat-scratch disease (*Bartonella*), or HIV
   i. Antinuclear cytoplasmic antibody and angiotensin-converting enzyme (ACE) level, especially if ESR and C-reactive protein are high
2. **Special considerations**
   a. If the patient has a **headache,** order computed tomography (CT) or

magnetic resonance imaging (MRI) of the head, or perform a lumbar puncture.

b. If the patient has **elevated liver chemistries,** perform serologies as follows:

  (1) Check serologies for viral infections, such as hepatitis A, B, and C
  (2) Check serologies for CMV
  (3) Check serologies for EBV (infectious mononucleosis)

c. Consider liver biopsy with special stains, cultures for aerobic and anaerobic organisms, acid-fast bacilli, and *Bartonella* and *Brucella* species.

3. Imaging studies need to be directed by the history and physical examination findings.

  a. Chest radiography: In miliary tuberculosis, millet seed granulomata may take weeks to appear. Disseminated histoplasmosis, pulmonary coccidioidomycosis, lymphoma, and other lesions may be identified.

  b. CT scan: Look for lymphoma, renal cell carcinoma, and hepatoma. Chest CT is preferable to abdominal CT for diagnosing lymphoma, miliary tuberculosis, and disseminated fungal infections.

  c. Nuclear medicine scans are of little utility.

  (1) Gallium, indium[111], and white blood cell (WBC) scans are insensitive and nonspecific.

  (2) A **hepato-iminodiacetic acid scan** may be used to detect occult, chronic, recurrent cholecystitis and common duct stricture.

4. Biopsy: Following Sutton's law, pursue clinical clues or abnormalities discovered via imaging or laboratory studies. If no clues are discovered, consider blind biopsies, especially of the bone marrow and liver.

SUGGESTED READING

DeKleijn EM, et al: Fever of unknown origin (FUO): A prospective multicenter study of 167 patients with FUO, using fixed epidemiologic entry criteria. *Medicine* 76:392–414, 1997.

45

Tuberculosis
Jennifer S. Daly and Michael Mitchell

I. **Definition.** Tuberculosis is an **infection with *Mycobacterium tuberculosis*.**

II. **Overview.** *M. tuberculosis* may cause active or latent infection. When the infection is latent, the diagnosis can be confirmed by a positive tuberculin skin test (formerly called the Mantoux test). Because the skin test is not specific for infection with *M. tuberculosis,* its use should be limited to patients in whom the diagnosis of tuberculosis is being considered or patients with a high risk of exposure to tuberculosis. In the high-risk groups, a positive skin test generally indicates tuberculosis infection; therefore, patients of any age should be considered for preventive treatment. Patients with HIV infection may not exhibit typical symptoms, may have a normal chest radiograph despite pulmonary disease, and may not develop the typical granulomatous reaction in tissue.

III. **Clinical Evaluation**

A. **History and physical examination**

1. Patients should be questioned about and examined for the following symptoms:

   a. Cough
   b. Fever
   c. Chills
   d. Weight loss
   e. Pleuritic chest pain

2. Note any organ that may be affected, including bones and joints, eyes, organs in the central nervous system (CNS), organs in the genitourinary system, and lymph nodes.

3. Patients may be asymptomatic.

B. **Laboratory testing and evaluation.** The Centers for Disease Control and Prevention (CDC) recommends that for any patient admitted to a healthcare facility with a possible diagnosis of tuberculosis, a smear of a respiratory specimen should be prepared and read within 24 hours. Ideally, concentrated smears should be used.

1. **Specimen collection:** Specimens should be transported to the laboratory in sterile containers within 2 hours of collection.

   a. **Respiratory specimens:** Pulmonary infection is the most commonly suspected mycobacterial disease. Three successive first-morning deep-coughed specimens are recommended for evaluation. Sputum induced by inhalation of warm saline mist and bronchoscopically obtained specimens are also excellent for diagnosis. Sensitivity for diagnosis of smear is around 80% and culture around 95%.
   b. **Urine:** Three first-morning voiding specimens are recommended if tuberculosis of the genitourinary system is a diagnostic consideration.

   c. **Cerebrospinal fluid:** For mycobacterial testing, 3–10 ml of spinal fluid should be obtained. Sensitivity of a single smear is < 5%–10% and culture is around 50%–80%.

   d. **Other fluids and tissue:** For mycobacterial testing, 3–10 ml of fluid should be obtained. The detection of mycobacterial infection is significantly improved (around 80%) by submission of infected tissue (e.g., pericardial or pleural biopsy).

   e. **Blood:** The detection of mycobacteria has been dramatically improved by the use of the lysis centrifugation (Dupont Isolator) technique or broth-based, continuous monitoring systems. In AIDS patients, *M. tuberculosis* or atypical mycobacteria is usually high grade and detectable with a single blood specimen.

2. **Direct examination:** Mycobacterial cell walls contain long-chain fatty acids (mycolic acids) that form a thick, waxy outer layer around bacterial cells. This layer makes mycobacterial cells resistant to Gram stain. A carbol fuchsin (Kinyoun or Ziehl-Neelsen) or auramine-rhodamine (fluorochrome)-based staining procedure can be used to demonstrate mycobacteria directly.

3. **Mycobacterial culture:** Several commercially available systems automate the detection of mycobacterial growth in broth culture, resulting in marked reduction in the time needed to detect positive cultures. Cultures are incubated for **as long as 8 weeks** before reporting a negative result.

4. **Mycobacterial identification and rapid testing:** Rapid DNA probe tests are available for confirmation of the identity of an organism from a positive culture, but as yet they are not reliable enough and are too expensive to use to screen sputum smears. These molecular probes, using rRNA sequences from *M. tuberculosis*, *M. avium-intracellulare*, and the nonpathogenic (but frequently isolated) *M. gordonae* can be used to test suspicious colonies, with final results available within several days of colony isolation. Other species are generally identified by Public Health or Reference Laboratories. Identification by routine biochemical testing may take 2–4 weeks after isolation in primary culture. The CDC recommends identification of *M. tuberculosis* within 21 days after specimen collection.

5. **Mycobacterial susceptibility testing:** Because of the increased rate of resistance to antimycobacterial drugs, all *M. tuberculosis* isolates must have susceptibility testing performed. The final results should be available **within 28 days** after specimen submission according to CDC recommendations.

C. **Chest radiograph.** All tuberculin-positive individuals should have a chest radiograph. Patients with abnormal chest radiograph need sputum examination. Patients with symptoms or sign of specific end-organ disease need specific laboratory testing of material from the affected area.

SUGGESTED READING

Christie JD, Calihan DR: The laboratory diagnosis of mycobacterial diseases. *Clin Lab Med* 15:279, 1995.

46

Primary HIV Infection in the Adult
Pauline Himlan, Raul Davaro, and Jennifer S. Daly

I. **Definition.** Primary HIV type I (HIV 1) infection can be **asymptomatic** or **produce a characteristic syndrome, which may have severe constitutional or neurologic signs and symptoms during seroconversion.**

II. **Overview.** During the initial 2–6 weeks of primary infection, standard diagnostic testing with enzyme-linked immunosorbent assay (ELISA) may be falsely negative. Diagnosis of acute HIV-1 disease is extremely important because of the potential benefit of early interventions with potent antiretroviral regimens. Acute symptomatic primary antiretroviral syndrome is a marker for more rapid disease progression.

III. **Cause.** HIV 1 is most commonly found in the United States; HIV 2 is found in Africa.

IV. **When to Suspect the Diagnosis**

    A. History

        1. **Risk factors** include men who have sex with men, injection drug users, sexual activity without consistent use of barrier protection, sexual contact with injection drug users, and "crack" cocaine use.

        2. **History of sexually transmitted diseases** (STDs) should be noted.

    B. Symptoms and objective findings

        1. Adult presenting with mononucleosis-like illness

        2. Maculopapular rash, fever, fatigue, pharyngitis, lymphadenopathy, headache, myalgia, or arthralgia

        3. Acute meningoencephalitis

V. **How to Confirm the Diagnosis**

    A. Use **ELISA** to test for HIV antibody. If the test is positive, confirm the diagnosis by using the **Western blot assay** for specific antibodies.

    B. If ELISA remains negative during the first 4 weeks, the diagnosis may be established with demonstration of quantitative plasma HIV RNA polymerase chain reaction (PCR) titers of 10^2–10^6 or HIV p24 antigen (if available) > 20 pg/ml.

VI. **Assessment of Adults Known to Be HIV Infected**

    A. History. Obtain a complete history in any patient with a positive ELISA and confirmatory Western blot assay.

        1. **History of HIV infection**

            a. Ask about opportunistic infections, neoplasms, previous testing, constitutional symptoms, antiretroviral treatment, and prophylaxis.

            b. Determine risk factors for HIV infection (so as to modify behavior).

        2. **History of exposure to tuberculosis:** Note the date, the result of the last tuberculin skin test, and history of antituberculosis treatment.

    3. Travel history
    4. History of animal contacts

B. Physical examination. A complete examination is required.

    1. Evaluate the skin, eyes, oral cavity, and genitalia.
    2. Perform a neurologic examination, including the mini-mental status examination (see Figure 50–1 in Chapter 50, DEMENTIA).

C. Initial laboratory testing

    1. CD4 cell count: Establish immunologic status with an absolute and relative CD4 cell count. A complete blood count (CBC) including platelet count and differential is part of the T-cell subsets.
    2. HIV viral load: Establish virologic status with an HIV viral load.
    3. Routine chemistries: Obtain the following tests:

        a. Serum creatinine and blood urea nitrogen (for kidney function)
        b. Liver enzymes, alkaline phosphatase, total bilirubin (for liver)
        c. Total protein and albumin (for liver function)
        d. Blood sugar
        e. Cholesterol/fasting triglycerides
        f. Amylase
        g. Creatine phosphokinase (CPK)

    4. Serologic evaluation: Check for syphilis serology [rapid plasma reagin (RPR) or automatic reagin test], toxoplasmosis immunoglobulin G (IgG) antibody, hepatitis B surface antigen and antibody, hepatitis B core antibody, and hepatitis C antibody.

D. Subsequent testing

    1. Quantitative HIV by RNA establishes 5·PPD viral load, predicts progression to AIDS, and allows the clinician to monitor therapeutic response to antiretroviral therapy.

        a. A baseline viral load is considered the initial test followed by repeat testing at 2 weeks.
        b. The determination should be obtained after 4 weeks of immunizations or intercurrent infections to avoid false readings.
        c. Testing should be performed by the same laboratory and drawn at the same time of day.
        d. The response to newly started antiretroviral therapy should be assessed at 4 weeks (look for ≥ 1 log decrease) and then every 12–16 weeks.

    2. CD4+ cell count should be repeated every 4–6 months to assess immune status, to predict prognosis and response to treatment, and for prophylaxis of opportunistic infection.
    3. CBC with differential. In HIV-infected individuals, anemia, leukopenia or neutropenia, and thrombocytopenia are common. Obtain a CBC with differential during the initial evaluation and then every 3–4 months unless the patient receives bone marrow toxic drugs or is compromised at the outset.
    4. Chemistries should be performed to monitor the effects of multiple medications on the liver, kidney, lipid metabolism, and insulin resistance.

SUGGESTED READING

US Preventive Services Task Force: *Guide to Clinical Preventive Services*, 2nd ed. Baltimore: Williams & Wilkins, 1996.

47

Tick Bites
Peter Dain

I. Background. Hard ticks (Ixodidae) are by far the most likely types to parasitize human beings and transmit disease. As tick bites are essentially painless, it is often only the immune reaction following the bite that leads patients to seek medical attention.

II. Evaluation

A. History and physical examination

1. **Rash:** The tick inoculum may cause a papular pruritic area of local irritation or the development of persistent nodules of up to several centimeters in diameter (i.e., granulomas). Infectious organisms transmitted by the tick may cause other lesions as well.

   a. **Lyme disease** is characterized by an erythematous lesion that expands to a diameter of at least 5 centimeters, with a well-demarcated circumferential erythematous border and partial central clearing, sometimes with an area of induration or even necrosis near the center (erythema migrans).

   b. **Rocky Mountain spotted fever** is characterized by macules up to one-half centimeter in diameter that arise on the ankles and wrists, and later spread to proximal extremities and the trunk. The patient usually has a fever and other constitutional symptoms.

2. **Fever, headache, nausea, and malaise:** If related to the tick bite, these symptoms should resolve within 24–36 hours of removal of the arthropod.

3. **Weakness** begins at least 2 days after attachment of a pregnant female tick in human tick paralysis. The weakness is classically ascending and flaccid. Primary proximal weakness and ataxia have also been noted in some cases.

4. **Geographic exposure:** Frequenting woodlands or grasslands in endemic areas is a predisposing factor for a tick bite.

5. **Climate:** Tick exposure generally occurs only in temperate times of the year.

B. Laboratory assessment

1. **Initial workup** should include a complete blood count (CBC) with differential, looking for leukopenia, thrombocytopenia, anemia, and immature white blood cells (WBCs) [Table 47–1].

2. **Alkaline aminotransferase (ALT)** and **aspartate aminotransferase (AST)** can screen for hepatic involvement. Serum albumin is often low in Rocky Mountain spotted fever.

3. **Other studies** should be done based on clinical suspicion.

   a. **Evaluation of cerebrospinal fluid:** If the patient has a stiff neck or central nervous system (CNS) changes, the cerebrospinal fluid should be evaluated. Antibody levels to *Borrelia* in cerebrospinal fluid

TABLE 47–1.   Disease Association with Abnormal Lab Values

Lab Value	Associated Disease
Leukopenia	Human ehrlichiosis
Thrombocytopenia	Human ehrlichiosis
Elevated transaminases (AST, ALT)	Human ehrlichiosis
Prolonged PT/INR	Rocky Mountain spotted fever (late stage)
Low serum albumin	Rocky Mountain spotted fever (late stage)
Peripheral blood smear: Intra-erythrocytic ring is formed that has tetrads of mero-zoites that resemble Maltese crosses. The affected erythrocytes lack pigment granules.	Babesiosis
Peripheral blood smear: Neutrophils and monocytes with Ehrlichiae visible in cytoplasmic vacuoles.	Human ehrlichiosis

ALT = alkaline aminotransferase; AST = aspartate aminotransferase; INR = international normalized ratio; PT = prothrombin time.

are **not** required to diagnose Lyme neuroborreliosis because if they are present, serum antibodies are generally seen as well.

   b. **Lyme titers:** If infection is suspected to have occurred within the past month, immunoglobulin M (IgM) and immunoglobulin G (IgG) acute and convalescent titers are recommended. **Western Blot assay** is used as a supplemental test for any positive or indeterminate results.

   c. **Rocky Mountain spotted fever serology:** Immunofluorescence assay and latex agglutination are both reliable tests that can be performed about a week after the onset of illness. A solid-state enzyme immunoassay is also available. **Immunohistologic evaluation** of a punch biopsy of the skin rash is the only useful diagnostic test early in the disease course.

4. **Peripheral blood smear:** Evaluate for suspected babesiosis in red blood cells (RBCs), and human granulocytic ehrlichiosis in neutrophils. Poor sensitivity (7%) makes searching monocytes for human monocytic ehrlichiosis not worthwhile.

5. Correlate the species of tick, type of rash, physical examination findings, and laboratory values with specific tick-borne diseases.

SUGGESTED READING

Brown SL, et al: Role of serology in the diagnosis of Lyme disease. *JAMA* 282:62–66, 1999.

48

Diagnostic Approach to Common Infectious Diseases

Michael Mitchell and Jennifer S. Daly

General Aspects

Michael Mitchell

I. General Issues in Infectious Diseases

A. Specimen collection for microbiology

1. **Swabs** for culture are adequate for a limited number of specimen types (i.e., skin, mucous membranes, genital mucosa, anal crypts) because swabs can only pick up a small volume of material. Also, some pathogens may "stick" in the swab and not get to the media.

   a. Swabs can be used for other specimens only if the amount of material is very small.

   b. Submit one swab for every test needed.

2. **Special swap transport kits** are available for certain pathogens (e.g., chlamydia, gonorrhea). The charcoal in some kits may interfere with Gram stain interpretation.

3. **Syringes** are not a desirable way to transport medium. If they are used, excess air should be carefully expelled, and the syringes should be hand-carried to the laboratory to prevent leakage.

4. **Transport conditions** must maintain the viability of pathogens within the specimen. Several conditions must be controlled:

   a. Delay of greater than 2 hours may result in the death of fastidious organisms or overgrowth by contaminating flora. If delayed transport is expected, the specimen should be chilled or placed in an appropriate bacteriostatic transport system.

   b. Extremes of temperature and desiccation should be avoided.

   c. Saline solutions

      (1) Some of the saline solutions available contain a bacteriocidal agent and should not be used.

      (2) Smaller biopsy specimens may be placed in a nonbacteriostatic saline solution (e.g., Ringer's lactate solution).

      (3) Specimens that have been placed in formalin are unacceptable for culture.

   d. Specimens submitted in anaerobic transport kits are acceptable for aerobic, mycobacterial, and mycology culture.

II. **Detection Methods.** Three strategies are generally used to identify infectious agents: direct detection of the pathogen or its microbial products, documentation of specific immune response in the patient, and detection by culture.

A. **Direct methods for identification.** Rapid, direct diagnostic tests may be broadly specific (Gram stain or Kinyoun stain), narrowly specific (*Pneumocystis carinii* pneumonia, monoclonal, or rRNA sequence probe), or nonspecific (methylene blue).

1. **Gram stain** (direct visual detection): Although the Gram stain is less sensitive than culture for detecting microorganisms, it is still the most useful rapid test in microbiology laboratories. Bacteria present in quantities of $> 10^3$ to 10^4 colony-forming unit (cfu)/ml can be detected by Gram stain examination. Requests for Gram stain should include requests for bacterial and other relevant cultures.

   a. **Indications:** Gram stains are useful to assess the quality of clinical specimens.

   b. **Special considerations:** Gram-positive bacteria whose cell walls have been damaged by antimicrobial therapy, host response, or other damaging effects may appear Gram negative by stain.

2. **Potassium hydroxide (KOH) wet mount.** Staining of fungal elements by Gram stain may be variable. The cell wall carbohydrate of fungi resists degradation by 10% KOH, which lyses host cells. KOH wet mounts, therefore, provide a reasonably reliable, direct detection method for fungi.

3. The **capsular polysaccharide antigen direct test** for cryptococcal meningitis is a very reliable test with sensitivity well above 90%. The antigen "titer" may be helpful in predicting ultimate prognosis and in monitoring success of therapy. Cryptococcal antigen testing has replaced the India ink examination in most laboratories.

4. **Nucleic acid probes** are now available to aid in the diagnosis of many infections. A nucleic acid probe is a sequence of either DNA or RNA that binds to nucleic acid sequences. This test has a very high specificity, and thus, can identify the causative agent.

   a. **Indications**

      (1) The Gen-Probe Pace II system detects rRNA in urethral or cervical swab specimens (*Neisseria gonorrhoeae* and *Chlamydia trachomatis*).

      (2) The use of nucleic acid amplification is especially useful when applied to the detection of **unculturable agents** or pathogens that grow slowly in culture, such as mycobacteria.

   b. **Special considerations:** False-positive results are possible when the probes are not specific for the pathogenic species.

B. **Detection by serologic method.** Infection may be inferred by documenting specific antibody or cell-mediated immune response. Serologic testing may be used for diagnosis of acute infection or as a test for immune status.

1. **Acute versus past infection:** For most infections, differentiating acute from past infection is important, but it may be difficult. A fourfold or greater increase in antibody titer between acute and convalescent (2–4

weeks later) serum specimens is strong evidence of acute infection. Acute and convalescent serum specimens should be run at the same time to ensure that any difference in titer is not due to run variation of the assay. Serologic tests are not helpful in making initial therapeutic decisions because results may not be available until well into the convalescent phase of infection.

2. **Immunoglobulin M (IgM) antibodies:** The detection of specific IgM antibodies may be useful as an adjunctive test for early documentation of acute infection. IgM antibodies are usually detectable within 7 days and peak at 2–3 weeks. IgM antibodies are especially useful in documenting infection in newborns because IgG antibodies could have crossed the placenta from the mother.

3. **False-negative reactions** may occur if the serum sample was taken too early or too late in the course of disease when antibody levels are undetectable. Furthermore, immunocompromised patients may be unable to elicit an antibody response despite intensive exposure to antigen.

4. **False-positive reactions** due to "cross-reactive" antibodies may occur as a result of host exposure to a related or a completely unrelated organism that shares the test antigen. "Cross-reactive" antibodies may be more prevalent during times of inflammation when Ig levels are high.

5. **Amount of specific antibodies:** A measure of the amount of specific antibody present in the specimen is usually determined by testing serial dilution of serum. The titer reported is the greatest dilution that gives a positive test reaction. Many assays are now performed using an immuno-enzyme format; therefore, the amount of signal in the test is a measure of the amount of specific antibody in the specimen. Positive results are defined as signals unequivocally greater than background.

6. **Serodiagnosis** is useful for the following diseases.

   a. **Cat-scratch disease:** Enzyme immunoassay (EIA) for IgM and IgG should yield sensitivity and specificity approximately 95% or higher.

   b. **Cytomegalovirus (CMV):** A majority of adults have measurable antibodies against CMV. IgM antibodies may indicate primary or reactivation infection. Viral culture is recommended to provide unequivocal evidence of CMV infection.

   c. *Ehrlichia* **disease** can be diagnosed by a fourfold rise in titer or a single high titer ($\geq$ 1:128). False-positive results are avoided by using immunoblot or species-specific testing.

   d. **Epstein-Barr virus (EBV):** The monospot test for heterophile antibodies is reliable for the confirmation of acute infectious mononucleosis in adults, with sensitivity around 90%. In children younger than 4 years of age, patients with chronic disease, or patients with syndromes other than acute mononucleosis, testing directed against EBV-specific antigens is available. Early antigen (EA), viral capsid antigen (VCA), and EB-associated nuclear antigen (EBNA) appear sequentially and may be useful in differentiating uninfected patients from patients with acute or past infections. The use of diffuse versus restricted patterns of EA may help to define reactivation of infection as well as EBV-related Burkitt's lymphoma and nasopharyngeal carcinoma.

e. ***Helicobacter pylori* disease.** Antibodies (IgG) against *H. pylori* are sensitive and specific in patients with gastritis. Asymptomatic patients may be seropositive. Detection of *H. pylori* antigen in stool is emerging as a sensitive and specific marker of acute *H. pylori* disease.

f. **Legionellosis.** Legionella culture and urinary antigen testing (serogroup 1 only) should be considered for all cases of suspected legionellosis. Serology shows good specificity (> 95%), but low sensitivity when paired sera are tested (60%–80% of patients show no, or delayed, seroconversion).

g. **Measles** (i.e., rubeola): In subacute sclerosing panencephalitis, serum and cerebrospinal fluid IgG antibody titers are high.

h. **Mycoplasma pneumonia:** Because neither culture nor molecular methods are widely available, serologic testing is often ordered to support a clinical diagnosis of mycoplasma pneumonia. Sensitivity and specificity are relatively poor.

i. **Group A streptococci:** For infection in patients with nephritis or rheumatic fever, both antistreptolysin O and antideoxyribonuclease (DNAse) B should be ordered. Peak titers occur around 3 weeks after acute infection. IgG and IgM antibodies can be measured, usually by immunofluorescent antibody (IFA) or EIA techniques. Seroconversion, or demonstration of a fourfold increase in IgG titer, suggests recent infection.

j. **Toxoplasmosis:** A capture-EIA test for IgM may help with diagnosis. Low IgM titers may be clarified by repeating the test after several weeks.

k. **Varicella-zoster virus** (i.e., chickenpox): IgG, IgM, or IgA can be detected using several techniques.

C. **Detection of bacterial pathogens by culture.** The presence of an isolate does not mean it is causing infection; clinical correlation may be necessary.

1. **Special issues related to anaerobic pathogens**

   a. Samples must be transported to the laboratory quickly (ideally within 1 hour) under conditions that protect the specimen from oxygen, which diffuses into large pieces of tissue slowly.

      (1) Most specimens (e.g., biopsy, urine, sputum) should be transported in sterile jars as is done for routine aerobic cultures.

      (2) Other specimens should be transported in transport systems designed specifically for anaerobic specimens.

   b. Do not refrigerate specimens for anaerobic isolation, even if transport is delayed, because of the deleterious effect of cooling on some anaerobic pathogens.

   c. ***Nocardia* isolates** require incubation of cultures for 1–2 weeks. These infections are best detected using fungal and mycobacterial culture. A modified acid-fast bacilli (AFB) stain should be requested when *Nocardia* infection is suspected.

   d. Alert the laboratory if infection due to ***Actinomyces*** is suspected. Special processing is needed for sensitive detection of infections due to these organisms.

2. **Specimens unsuitable for routine anaerobic culture** (Table 48–1)

TABLE 48–1. Specimens Unsuitable for Routine Anaerobic Culture

Urine (except for suprapubic aspirates)

Vaginal, urethral, or cervical swabs

Throat or upper respiratory specimens

Superficial skin or mucosal specimens

Specimens containing stool

Lower respiratory specimens (except for those collected by direct abscess aspiration, open biopsy, or protected bronchial brush)

III. Detection of Fungal Pathogens

A. **Specimen collection.** In general, specimens are collected and transported for bacterial culture, with the following exceptions:

1. For **dermatophyte infections,** clean the affected area with alcohol before sampling. Affected hair, nails, and debris from under the nail are submitted in a clean vial. Skin or scalp scales can be removed by scraping with the side of a glass slide.

2. **Vaginal or oral thrush** is most efficiently diagnosed by Gram stain or wet mount of scrapings. Fungal culture adds little to the direct examination.

3. **Blood cultures** are rarely positive for invasive molds like *Aspergillus.* Sampling the infected tissue is more reliable for diagnosis. The Isolator (Wampole Laboratories), or other system optimized for fungal isolation, should be used when fungal sepsis is suspected.

B. **Fungal infections.** Fungal cultures are planted on special media to optimize isolation of fungal pathogens and inhibit bacterial contamination. The fungi most commonly isolated from urine are *Candida* and *Torulopsis* species. These genera will usually grow on routine bacterial cultures within 48 hours of incubation. Fungal cultures of urine, therefore, may be finalized within 72 hours of incubation unless another pathogen is suspected. The quantitation of fungi in urine does not have the same predictive value as bacterial quantitation. Therapeutic decisions should be made considering other culture and clinical data. For example, is the culture mixed? Is the patient diabetic? Does the patient have a structural abnormality, obstruction, or recent surgery of the urinary tract?

1. *Candida albicans:* A presumptive rapid identification of *C. albicans* can be made on the basis of a positive germ tube test.

2. *Cryptococcus neoformans*: Encapsulated yeast can be presumptively identified as *C. neoformans* on the basis of several rapid assays. A rapid urease assay is performed by inoculating urea agar with a heavy suspension of test organism. Urea-positive isolates may be identified as

Cryptococcus species. Also, *C. neoformans* can be presumptively identified by several rapid tests that demonstrate phenol oxidase activity.

IV. Detection of Parasitic Pathogens (see also Chapter 18, DIARRHEA, V A)

A. Specimen collection for enteric parasites

1. The majority of enteric parasitic infections can be diagnosed using the routine ova and parasites (O&P) examination.

2. **Transporting stool specimens:** If stools can be transported to the laboratory within 1–2 hours of collection, a clean container with a tight-fitting lid may be used. For specimens requiring longer transport, preservative kits are needed. In general, three samples taken every other day are adequate for diagnosing parasitic causes of diarrhea.

3. **Detection of pinworm infection** (i.e., *Enterobius vermicularis*): Collect eggs with clear cellophane or a "pinworm paddle." The sticky surface is applied to the perianal area during the night. Four to six specimens should be examined before the testing is considered negative.

4. **Caveats for specimen collection**

   a. Stool taken from the toilet or from toilet paper is unacceptable for O&P examination.

   b. Do not submit stool from patients who have been exposed to barium within the previous 14 days.

   c. On the requisition slip, note specifically if *Cryptosporidium, Isospora, Giardia, Cyclospora,* and *Microsporidium* are suspected clinically. These parasites may require special testing.

   d. Wet mounts for vaginal or urine samples (to rule out *Trichomonas vaginalis*) may only be available during weekday shifts. Plan sampling accordingly if a specific diagnosis is needed.

B. Identification of enteric parasites. Most parasites are identified by morphology and staining characteristics.

1. A wet mount for motile forms is examined for fresh stool specimens.

2. Preserved specimens are used to prepare stained smears and concentrated wet mounts.

3. Detection by EIA or monoclonal antibody staining is available for some parasites.

C. Detection of blood parasites. Parasites other than *Plasmodium malariae* are rarely detected in the United States.

1. **Suspected cases.** Examination of stained blood smears is the best method for documenting *Plasmodium* infection. Specimens should be collected on each of 3 successive days, every 6–8 hours (until positive) for optimal detection.

   a. Freely flowing capillary blood (e.g., by earlobe puncture) is ideal if good quality thin and thick smears can be prepared at the bedside.

   b. Alternatively, ethylenediamine tetraacetic acid (EDTA) anticoagulated blood can be used. Thin and thick smears should be prepared as soon as possible; therefore, only parasites and white blood cells remain. The thick smear is particularly useful in patients with low-level parasitemia.

2. Follow-up. Blood should be examined in treated patients after 3–6 days to assess the effectiveness of therapy. If trypanosomes or microfilariae are suspected, examination of buffy coat smears is recommended. *Trypanosoma* infection is diagnosed the same way as malaria.

D. Detection of viral pathogens. Viral infection can be diagnosed by serology, antigen detection, or molecular techniques (see I A, B). Some viruses can be detected by viral culture. Always note on the requisition slip the viral agent suspected.

1. Specimen collection for virology: The sensitivity of viral culture often wanes with increasing time after onset of illness. Therefore, culture should be performed as early in the illness as possible. Generally, only one sample, source, admission, or visit is needed for diagnosis.

  a. Specimens collected on swabs for viral culture should be placed in transport media and transported on wet ice to the laboratory.

  b. Calcium alginate swabs should not be used for detection of herpes simplex virus (HSV).

  c. Tissue, fresh-voided urine, stool, and other fluids may be transported on wet ice without transferring into transport media.

  d. Every attempt should be made to deliver the specimen to the laboratory during routine working hours so that cell cultures can be inoculated as soon as possible.

  e. The ideal specimen should not be taken from the "apparently" infected site.

2. Identification of viral pathogens

  a. Clinical specimens are inoculated onto several eukaryotic cell lines prepared from different kinds of tissues (e.g., rhesus monkey kidney, human diploid fibroblasts). Virus growth in cell culture is usually detected by the appearance of a cytopathic effect, or a disruption or change in the normal morphology of the cell line.

   (1) Presumptive identification of the type of virus present can often be made by the timing of the cytopathic effect, the types of cell lines that permit viral growth, and the appearance of the "cytopathic cells."

   (2) Infected cells produce hemadsorbing glycoproteins on their outer membranes that can be detected by the addition of guinea pig red blood cells to the culture.

   (3) Definitive identification usually involves staining infected cells from the culture with antibodies specific for the viral pathogen.

  b. Clinical virology laboratories will commonly isolate:

   (1) Herpes viruses (e.g., HSV, CMV, varicella-zoster virus)
   (2) Enteroviruses [e.g., enteric cytopathic human orphan (ECHO) virus, coxsackie virus, polio]
   (3) Adenovirus
   (4) Influenza and parainfluenza
   (5) Respiratory syncytial virus
   (6) Measles and mumps virus

   c. Rapid viral detection for influenza, parainfluenza, respiratory syncytial virus, and adenovirus may be available using fluorescently tagged monoclonal antibodies to stain respiratory specimens. Also, specific tagged monoclonal antibodies may be available to stain vesicular lesions for HSV and varicella-zoster virus (more sensitive and specific than the Tzanck test).

Bacteremia

Michael Mitchell

I. Definition. Bacteremia is the **presence of bacteria in the blood.**

  A. Causes of bacteremia. The most common organisms causing bacteremia are *Staphylococcus aureus,* coagulase-negative staphylococci, and enterococci.

  B. Types of bacteremia. Three types of bacteremia are generally recognized: continuous, intermittent, and transient.

    1. Continuous bacteremia. Patients with endocarditis, endovascular infection, and overwhelming sepsis have continuous bacteremia. Because the concentration of bacteria in the blood may vary, the most important factor in detection is the **volume** of blood cultured.

    2. Intermittent bacteremia. Patients experiencing breakthrough bacteremia associated with deep abscesses, pyelonephritis, or other localized infections may have intermittent bacteremia. The volume of blood cultured is the most critical factor in these patients; however, some clinicians also find it valuable to draw cultures "just before" or during the upswing of the fever curve.

    3. Transient bacteremia, in which bacteria occasionally enter the vascular system, is considered insignificant.

II. Collection of Specimens. Routine blood cultures have included one aerobic and one anaerobic bottle. Most aerobic isolates are able to grow in the anaerobic bottle, and many anaerobes will grow in the aerobic broth.

  A. Fungemia is more common than anaerobic bacteremia in most settings, but less predictable clinically. Some laboratories have recently moved to using two aerobic bottles for routine blood cultures (to improve detection of unsuspected fungemia), and the anaerobic bottle only if anaerobic sepsis is suspected.

  B. Septic episodes. In the evaluation of septic episodes in critically ill patients with vascular catheters, draw at least two blood cultures by a **percutaneous peripheral vein or artery puncture.** Catheter-associated sepsis may be suspected in such patients in whom no other cause can be identified. The distal segment of a central venous catheter may be clipped with sterile scissors and submitted for culture. Arterial and peripheral intravenous catheters have rarely been associated with sepsis, so submission of these for culture is discouraged.

  C. Diagnosis. About 99% of significant bacteremias will be diagnosed if two or three blood cultures are submitted during the initial sepsis workup. Sequential (back-to-back) sampling of two of the cultures in sepsis syndromes is acceptable. It is critical, however, that each blood culture be taken from a separate, properly performing venipuncture.

1. **Reculturing:** Unless there is a significant change in clinical status, wait 72 hours before reculturing to allow the initial culture results to become available. If the results are negative but the diagnosis is clinically indicated, resume with three cultures submitted over 24 hours.
2. **Daily cultures:** The practice of ordering "daily cultures" for febrile patients is not cost-effective and should not be done. Likewise, single blood cultures should never be performed. Because the agents of sepsis are often components of the patient's own normal flora (especially in immunocompromised patients), differentiating true bacteremia from contamination usually requires the examination of two or three separate blood cultures.
3. **Fever of unknown origin:** Patients with fever of unknown origin are an exception to the rule. In these cases, draw two separate blood cultures on the initial day of evaluation, and draw a second set the following day.

III. **Methods of Detection.** Recent technical advances have improved blood culture methods.

A. **Automated systems** have been developed that can detect growth by CO_2 production, change in the pH of the culture broth, or change in the headspace pressure of positive blood culture bottles. Positive blood cultures are identified much earlier with automated systems than systems that use traditional detection.

B. **Prolonged incubation.** Slow-growing, fastidious pathogens, like the HACEK (*Haemophilus, Actinobacillus, Cardiobacterium, Eikenella*, and *Kingella*) organisms, may require prolonged incubation (14–21 days) and blind subculture for efficient detection. Cultures taken from patients who have recently received antibiotics may also require prolonged incubation.

Common Bacterial Infections of Skin and Soft Tissue

Jennifer S. Daly

I. Definitions

A. **Cellulitis** is a bacterial infection of the skin and skin structure that is characterized by erythema, warmth, and edema. It may extend into the subcutaneous fat to the level of the fascia.

B. **Impetigo** is a localized superficial infection of the skin that is characterized by vesicles and pustules forming under the most superficial layer of the skin (i.e., the stratum corneum). Vesicles may be bullous or nonbullous and are restricted to the epidermis.

C. **Erysipelas** is a superficial cellulitis of the dermis that spreads along the dermal lymphatics.

D. Folliculitis is inflammation of the ostium of a hair follicle.
E. Furuncles and carbuncles are infections of the hair follicle that extend into the dermis.

1. Individual lesions are furuncles.
2. A mass of coalescing furuncles with pus draining from multiple follicular orifices is called a carbuncle.

F. Abscesses are painful, tender, fluctuant, erythematous nodules, often with a pustule on top.
G. Fasciitis is inflammation and infection that centers in the superficial fascia.
H. Myositis is an infection that involves muscle.
I. Necrotizing and gangrenous cellulitis, fasciitis, and myositis are severe infections that involve the skin, skin structure, and even fascia and muscle. These infections produce necrosis (tissue death) and require surgical debridement as well as antibiotic therapy.

II. Common Pathogens

A. *Staphylococcus aureus*
B. *Streptococcus pyogenes* (group A beta-hemolytic streptococcus)
C. Mixed bowel flora (necrotizing fasciitis)

III. Special Considerations

A. All bites—anaerobes
B. Cat bites—*Pasteurella multocida*
C. Dog bites—*Staphylococcus intermedius*
D. Human bites—human mouth flora including *Eikenella corrodens*
E. Traumatic wounds—*Clostridium perfringens*
F. Foot wound (especially through a sneaker)—*Pseudomonas aeruginosa*
G. Fresh water wounds—*Aeromonas* species
H. Fish-associated wounds—*Erysipelothrix schenckii*

IV. When to Suspect a Bacterial Infection

A. **History.** Clinical symptoms include fever, chills, and previous trauma.
B. **Physical examination.** Clinical signs include warmth (color), swelling (tumor), erythema (rubor), pain (dolor), and drainage of purulent materials (pus).
C. **Clinical evaluation and therapy.** Based on the clinical signs and symptoms and the extent of the body part involved, the practitioner decides whether to give oral or intravenous antibiotics.

V. How to Confirm the Diagnosis

A. **Aerobic cultures.** Obtain aerobic cultures of the drainage, or incise and drain the lesion to obtain cultures of pus.
B. **Blood cultures.** Obtain blood cultures for patients with systemic signs and symptoms requiring intravenous antibiotics (see the BACTEREMIA section in this chapter).
C. **Radiographs.** Perform radiographs to rule out osteomyelitis if an infection is present for weeks, or to rule out a foreign body or fracture if there is a history of trauma.

VI. Differential Diagnosis. The differential diagnoses may include osteoarthritis with a Baker's cyst (popliteal cyst), deep venous thrombosis, insect or venomous bites, contact or allergic dermatitis, viral exanthem, trauma, hematoma, autoimmune processes such as vasculitis, and erythema nodosum.

SUGGESTED READING

Miller M: *A Guide to Specimen Management in Clinical Microbiology,* 2nd ed. Washington, DC: ASM Press, 1999.

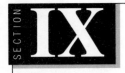

Neurology

49

Delirium
Robert Lebow

I. **Definition.** Delirium is defined as an **acute confusional state that is characterized primarily by disordered attention and disorganized thinking.** There is often a change in cognition, such as memory disturbance or disorientation, which may include a disturbance of the sleep-wake cycle. The onset is usually within hours or days, and the course often fluctuates. Some practitioners also consider autonomic hyperactivity as a necessary condition for the diagnosis of delirium.

II. **Overview**

    A. **Causes.** The most common causes of delirium are found outside the central nervous system (CNS). These include:

        1. Systemic illness (infection most frequently)
        2. Metabolic derangements
        3. Toxins
        4. Drug use or withdrawal

    B. **Approach.** The primary evaluation should rule out immediate life-threatening conditions before proceeding with a more detailed evaluation.

III. **Differential Diagnosis** (Table 49–1 and Figure 49–1). Psychosis and dementia do not necessarily cause delirium, but they need to be considered as comorbid conditions in the patient presenting with mental status changes.

    A. **Psychosis.** The symptoms of psychosis tend to be long-standing, usually occurring in a patient with a known diagnosis.

    B. **Dementia** is a risk factor for delirium and may coexist with delirium. The onset of dementia is slower (i.e., over the course of months or years), and the patient is usually alert.

IV. **Clinical Evaluation**

    A. **History**

        1. **Preceding events**

           a. In a patient with delirium, the history of preceding events, pre-existing illness, and drug use is of paramount importance, and every

TABLE 49–1. Common Causes of Delirium

Disorder	Causes
CNS disorders	Neoplasm (frequently with acute hemorrhage) Subarachnoid hemorrhage Cerebrovascular accident Postictal state Trauma Meningoencephalopathy (e.g., acute meningitis, HSV, Wernicke's syndrome)
Systemic illnesses	Cardiopulmonary compromise (e.g., low output, low perfusion, impaired oxygenation) Hypertensive encephalopathy Metabolic derangements (e.g., hypoxia, hepatic or renal insufficiency, thiamine deficiency, acid-base disturbances, electrolyte disturbances) Anemia Endocrinologic disorders (e.g., thyroid abnormalities, adrenal abnormalities, hypoglycemia, hypercalcemia, pituitary apoplexy) Infection (e.g., sepsis, pneumonia, urinary tract infection) Inflammation (giant cell arteritis)
Drugs	Alcohol (intoxication or withdrawal) Illicit drugs (e.g., heroin, cocaine) Medications (including withdrawal states), particularly sedatives or hypnotics, opioids, psychotropic agents, over-the-counter medications (e.g., diphenhydramine), and cholinergic agents
Industrial chemicals	Heavy metals, carbon monoxide, insecticides, and cyanide
Primary psychiatric illness	Psychosis
Beclouded dementia	Delirium in a patient with dementia
Sensory deprivation	As encountered in an ICU

CNS = central nervous system; HSV = herpes simplex virus; ICU = intensive care unit.

attempt should be made to obtain a reliable history from relatives, caregivers, and the primary care physician.
   b. Inquire about head injury, headache, nausea or vomiting, neck stiffness, fever, loss of consciousness, or seizure.
2. Medications: Inquire about medication use (including over-the-counter and prescription medications, and illicit drugs) and the

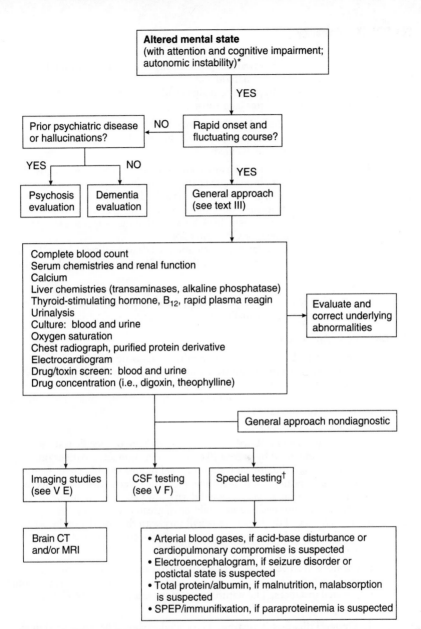

FIGURE 49–1. Algorithm for the evaluation of altered mental state. *CSF* = cerebrospinal fluid; *CT* = computed tomography; *MRI* = magnetic resonance imaging; *SPEP* = serum protein electrophoresis.

*This approach assumes a nonfocal neurologic examination and lack of meningeal signs. If either is present, immediate pursuit of neuroimaging and possible lumbar puncture is indicated.

†These tests may contribute valuable information, but should be limited to circumstances where the history, physical examination, or available data raise an indication. For example, an anion gap would prompt an arterial blood gas.

possibility of withdrawal states (especially from steroids, alcohol, benzodiazepines, and narcotics).

3. **Disease states:** Inquire about signs and symptoms of associated or causative disease states (see Table 49–1).

B. **Physical examination.** As delirium may be the presenting symptom of a myriad of medical conditions (especially in the elderly), the examination should be thorough and detailed.

1. **Skull fracture:** A careful assessment should be made for any signs of skull fracture (e.g., bruising over the eye; raccoon eyes, which is characterized by bruising over the mastoid; Battle's sign).

2. **Meningeal irritation:** Check for signs of meningeal irritation.

3. **Focal neurologic signs:** Check for signs that may suggest a stroke, subdural hematoma, or CNS infection.

4. **Substance abuse:** Particular attention needs to be directed toward identifying signs of substance withdrawal (e.g., pinpoint pupils, needle marks).

5. **Metabolic decompensation:** Check for signs of metabolic decompensation (e.g., cardiac, pulmonary, renal, or hepatic insufficiency; endocrinologic abnormalities).

V. Diagnostic Approach

A. **"Coma cocktail."** Concurrent with initial diagnostic testing, a "coma cocktail" is frequently administered that includes glucose (draw blood glucose first) with thiamine, naloxone, and flumazenil. These agents are best administered sequentially to identify the metabolic cause, and they are also of therapeutic value.

B. **Test recommendations**

1. The sequence of test ordering and the selection of specific tests are largely influenced by pretest likelihood. For instance, a patient on anticoagulant therapy with signs of head trauma would benefit from coagulation studies and neuroimaging. The elderly patient discovered with a pulmonic infiltrate would derive low yield from neuroimaging, whereas a sepsis evaluation would be of greater relevance.

2. The efficacy of diagnostic tests will vary with the population being studied (e.g., elderly, febrile patient, immunocompromised patient, patient with evidence of substance abuse).

C. **Laboratory studies** can be divided into two categories including general diagnostic testing and those tests indicated in the setting of focal symptoms or selected instances. The nature of delirium as a symptom renders it uniquely dependent on diagnostic studies.

1. **General diagnostic testing:** These studies should be considered in all patients presenting with delirium, especially when the cause is not apparent on initial evaluation. This does not imply that each test is indicated in all patients. Clinical judgment, influenced by the presenting history and physical examination, will guide prudence in test ordering. Studies include:

   a. A complete blood count (CBC)
   b. Glucose, sodium, potassium, calcium, and magnesium

   c. Blood urea nitrogen/creatinine
   d. Hepatic enzymes (e.g., transaminases, alkaline phosphatase)
   e. Prothrombin time (PT)
   f. Rapid plasma reagin (RPR)
   g. Thyroid-stimulating hormone (TSH)
   h. Drug and toxin screen
   i. Urinalysis
   j. Chest radiograph
   k. Electrocardiogram (ECG)
   l. Blood and urine culture
   m. Neuroimaging

      (1) A strong recommendation for neuroimaging is indicated for the following cases:

         (a) Head trauma
         (b) Known or suspected malignancy
         (c) Abnormal focal neurologic examination (including neck stiffness)
         (d) Known coagulopathy
         (e) Immunocompromised condition
         (f) Prior to cerebrospinal fluid sampling

      (2) In the emergent setting, a computed tomography (CT) scan without contrast is sufficient.
      (3) In the setting of a presumed non-CNS cause for delirium, neuroimaging may be reasonably withheld, unless there are other compelling indications.

   n. Cerebrospinal fluid evaluation

      (1) This test should be considered when causes outside the CNS are unlikely or have been reasonably excluded.
      (2) It should also be undertaken when primary CNS disease processes are likely (e.g., infection, malignancy, immunocompromised conditions).

 2. Additional studies: In the patient with focal symptoms or suggestive diagnoses, see Table 49–2. This is not intended as an exhaustive list.

TABLE 49–2. Studies Recommended in the Patient with Focal Symptoms or Suggestive Diagnoses

Arterial blood gas	Electroencephalogram
B_{12} level	Echocardiography
Folate level	Purified protein derivative
HIV serology	Erythrocyte sedimentation rate (ESR)
Lyme serology	Serum protein electrophoresis
Heavy metal screen	Vascular imaging (e.g., carotid duplex,
Methemoglobin	magnetic resonance angiography)
Abdominal radiographs	Ammonia level

Workup must be governed by the history, physical examination, and clinical probabilities.

SUGGESTED READING

Greene HL, Johnson WP, Lemcke D (eds): *Acute Behavior Change in Decision Making in Medicine: An Algorithmic Approach*, 2nd ed. St Louis: Mosby, 1998.
Lipowski ZJ: *Delirium—Acute Confusional States*. New York: Oxford, 1990.

50

Dementia

Majaz Moonis

I. **Definition.** Dementia is characterized by **loss of memory and two other cognitive domains that cause impairment in functions of activities of daily living.**

II. **Differential Diagnosis** (Table 50–1)

A. **Alzheimer's disease** is the most common cause of dementia (65% of cases) and is characterized by a progressive decline in cognitive function, including memory. The examination should reveal no focal neurologic deficits and no other causes of dementia. Short-term memory is affected early in the course of illness, while immediate recall and remote recall are retained. Hippocampal atrophy on magnetic resonance imaging (MRI) and biparietal hypoperfusion on single-photon-emission computed tomography (SPECT) or positron emission tomography (PET) scans are characteristic. Cerebrospinal fluid may show reduced Aβ 42 and elevated tau protein.

B. **Lewy body dementia** is the second most common cause of dementia. It should be suspected when there are prominent hallucinations (especially visual), recurrent falls, extrapyramidal signs (with tremor being uncommon), and sensitivity to neuroleptics (symptoms worsen with therapy).

C. **Frontotemporal dementia.** Memory may not be affected early in the process. A patient will present with behavioral disturbances, social disinhibition, and incontinence. Early primitive release reflexes (e.g., suck, snout, palmomental) may be present.

D. **Multi-infarct dementia** is characterized by a history of strokes, hypertension, nocturnal confusion, and incontinence. There tends to be a stepwise progression, although sudden deterioration may occur. Focal neurologic signs may be present. Computed tomography (CT) and MRI show evidence of infarcts and extensive white matter changes.

E. **Vasculitis.** The dementia is usually a manifestation of multiple organ involvement, frequently with a multi-infarct-like presentation.

F. **Granulomatous angiitis of the nervous system (GANS)** is characterized by multifocal neurologic deficits, seizures, and headaches with lack of systemic involvement. Leptomeningeal biopsy is diagnostic.

G. **Normal pressure hydrocephalus** is characterized by a chronic progressive course. The triad of ataxia, incontinence, and dementia should raise suspicion. CT shows ventricular dilation out of proportion to cortical atrophy.

H. **Infectious dementias.** Except for prion disorders, the cerebrospinal fluid will evidence abnormalities.

I. **Neoplasm.** Frontal and temporal tumors may present with cognitive decline. Secondary hydrocephalus (characterized by headaches, visual obscurations, focal signs, and rapid worsening) may be causative.

TABLE 50–1. Differential Diagnosis of Dementia

Symptom	Condition
Degenerative types	Alzheimer's disease Lewy body dementia Frontotemporal dementia Multisystem atrophy Dementia with Parkinson's disease Huntington's disease Wilson's disease
Vascular	Subdural hematoma Multi-infarct dementia Vasculitis, including granulomatous angiitis of the nervous system (GANS)
Normal pressure hydrocephalus	
Infective	Syphilis Neuroborreliosis HIV Chronic meningoencephalitis Herpes simplex encephalitis Prion disorders
Neoplasm	Frontal, temporal tumors
CADASIL (cerebral autosomal dominant arteriopathy with subcortical infarcts and leukoencephalopathy)	Chromosome 19 encodes a signaling protein; may be associated with migraines, stroke, and vascular dementia
Toxic and drug induced	
Heavy metal poisoning	Lead, arsenic, mercury
Nutritional	B_{12} deficiency Niacin deficiency Thiamine deficiency Protein calorie malnutrition
Metabolic	Hypothyroidism Hepatic and uremic encephalopathy Addison's disease Cushing's disease
Mitochondrial encephalopathies	

Paraneoplastic syndromes, such as limbic encephalitis, may present with dementia.

J. Psychosis. The absence of significant psychosis, which is usually associated with a more rapid decline, is a good prognostic sign.

K. Pseudodementia. Features that suggest **pseudodementia** include:

1. Ability to carry out activities of daily living
2. Early, marked emotional incontinence
3. History of depression, substance abuse, or suicide attempts
4. Flat affect, easy tearfulness, and no attempt to take the mini-mental status examination (III A 2) [i.e., patients with dementia usually answer incorrectly; patients with pseudodementia do not answer at all]
5. An absence of dementia on psychometric testing

III. Clinical Approach

A. History

1. A **detailed history** should be obtained from as many individuals involved with the patient as possible and should include:

   a. Onset and progression of the cognitive impairments
   b. Psychosis and neuroleptic sensitivity
   c. History of headaches and visual obscurations that may suggest conditions with elevated cerebrospinal fluid pressure, such as obstructing hydrocephalus or tumors
   d. Stepwise deterioration, early incontinence, and focal deficits (vascular causes)
   e. History of any nutritional deficits and metabolic conditions
   f. History suggestive of prion dementia, including subacute dementia, gait difficulties, extrapyramidal and pyramidal signs, metamorphopsia, and blindness
   g. History of cancer or risk factors for cancer
   h. The functional status of the patient
   i. A detailed drug history

2. The **mini-mental status examination** should be used in the initial assessment (Figure 50–1).

B. Physical and neurologic examination. As cognitive decline is a feature of a myriad of medical conditions, the examination must be thorough and detailed.

1. **The presence of papilledema or loss of venous pulsations** suggests elevated intracranial pressure (e.g., hydrocephalus, subdural hematoma, tumors).
2. **Focal neurologic findings** on examination suggest a structural cause (vascular, neoplastic, traumatic, subdural hematoma).
3. **The presence of chorea or parkinsonism** should prompt consideration of Huntington's disease, Parkinson's disease, or Wilson's disease.

IV. Diagnostic Evaluation (Figure 50–2)

A. Reversible causes of dementia. Evaluate the patient for reversible causes of dementia.

Mini Mental State Examination—Sample Items

I   Orientation (1 point for each correct response; 10 possible points):

  • What is the date, year, month, day of the week?

II Registration (1 point for each correct response; 3 possible points):

  • Ask the patient to name 3 objects (i.e., car, lake, house).

III Language (9 possible points):

  • Naming—Point to 2 items, such as a watch or pen, and ask the patient to name the items (1 point for each).

  • Reading—On a piece of paper, write the sentence "Close your eyes." Ask the patient to read the sentence and do what it says (1 point if they close their eyes).

■ **FIGURE 50–1.** Mini Mental State Examination – Sample items. The full Mini Mental State Examination is available through Psychological Assessment Resources (PAR), Inc.

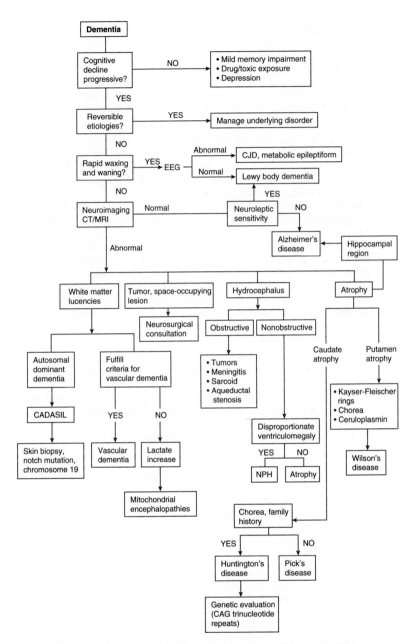

■ **FIGURE 50–2.** Algorithm for the workup of patients with dementia. *CADASIL* = cerebral autosomal dominant arteriopathy with subcortical infarcts and leukoencephalopathy; *CJD* = Creutzfeldt-Jakob disease; *CT* = computed tomography; *EEG* = electroencephalogram; *FH* = family history; *MRI* = magnetic resonance imaging; *NPH* = normal pressure hydrocephalus; *SDH* = subdural hematoma.

1. For all patients, obtain a complete blood count (CBC), liver chemistries, renal studies, thyroid-stimulating hormone (TSH), B_{12} level, rapid plasma reagin (RPR), erythrocyte sedimentation rate, and chest radiograph.
2. Other tests should be done as clinically indicated. The diagnostic yield is quite variable depending on the population studied. In the dementia population, the overall likelihood of finding a reversible cause is low.

B. **Imaging.** At a minimum, all patients should get a CT scan of the head (preferably an MRI) to assess for subdural hematoma, vascular etiologies, normal pressure hydrocephalus, and tumors. Although the yield may be low (5%–30%), imaging is a valuable tool given the importance of identifying reversible causes of dementia.

C. **Electroencephalogram** is indicated in cases of suspected epileptiform encephalopathy, Creutzfeldt-Jakob disease, and herpes simplex encephalitis with periodic complexes.

D. **Lumbar puncture** is indicated when the following conditions are suspected: normal pressure hydrocephalus, acute and chronic infections, prion dementia (protein 14-3-3 in the cerebrospinal fluid confirms the diagnosis), and difficult cases of Alzheimer's disease (e.g., elevated tau, reduced Aβ 42 protein). There may also be utility in other conditions such as autoimmune disease and suspected malignancy.

E. **Selected investigations**

1. **Suspected paraproteinemia** (in the presence of other systemic symptoms): Serum and urine protein electrophoresis, skeletal survey, and bone marrow biopsy
2. **Suspected vasculitis:** Antinuclear antibody (ANA), rheumatoid factor (RF), cytoplasmic antineutrophilic cytoplasmic antibody, and chest radiograph
3. **Dementia in the setting of cancer or suspected cancer**

   a. Paraneoplastic antibodies include:

      (1) Anti-Hu (seen in small cell lung cancer and associated with limbic encephalitis)
      (2) Anti-Yo (seen in ovarian and breast cancer and associated with cerebellar brain-stem syndrome)
      (3) Anti-Ri (seen in breast cancer and associated with opsoclonus myoclonus)
      (4) Anti-Ma/Ta (seen in testicular cancer and other malignancies)

   b. If the patient is not known to have an underlying neoplasm, age- and gender-specific health screening is recommended.
   c. Cerebrospinal fluid cytology, in instances where the patient is known to have a malignancy or where carcinomatous meningitis is suspected, has a diagnostic yield of 10%–20%.

4. **Dementia with chorea:** Huntington's disease, Wilson's disease, and neuroacanthocytosis are diagnostic considerations. Genetic testing for CAG trinucleotide repeats, ceruloplasmin, and wet smear for red cell acanthocytes, respectively, should be considered.

5. **Suspected CNS vasculitis.** Brain and leptomeningeal biopsy may be useful in establishing the diagnosis in prion disorders (e.g., Creutzfeldt-Jakob disease).

SUGGESTED READING

Fleming K, Adams A, Petersen R: Dementia: Diagnosis and evaluation. *Mayo Clin Proc* 70: 1093–1107, 1995.

51

Headache
Howard Sachs

I. Overview

A. The **primary headache disorders include migraine, tension-type, and cluster** (comprising more than 90% of headache diagnoses). These disorders can be diagnosed by history and physical examination alone, without the need for further diagnostic studies.

B. Headache, in some instances, may be the **harbinger of a life-threatening condition.** The clinician's goal is to identify those life-threatening conditions while maintaining a judicious approach to diagnostic testing.

II. Headache Classification.
In 1988, the International Headache Society published a classification scheme for headache (Table 51–1). They classified headache into 13 major categories, with 129 subcategories.

A. **Types and symptoms.** Many patients experience more than one type of headache, and there is overlap of symptoms among the headache classes.

B. **Duration.** Headaches that are present for more than a few months are rarely associated with intracranial pathology.

C. **Drug therapy.** Response to drug therapy does not establish a diagnosis. Specifically, a subset of patients with episodic tension-type headache will respond to migraine treatment, as will some patients with secondary headache disorders.

D. **Migraine headache.** The criteria for diagnosis of migraine headache include:

1. **Recurrent attacks**
2. **Duration of 2 to 72 hours**
3. **Characteristic features:** Unilateral, throbbing, moderate to severe, aggravated by physical activities
4. **Associated symptoms:** Nausea, vomiting, photophobia, phonophobia
5. **Composite criteria:** Whereas tension-type headache can share individual features, the composite criteria are suggestive of the diagnosis.
6. **Migraine aura** is a transient neurologic symptom that may precede a migraine. The symptoms are frequently visual in nature (scintillating scotoma), but may also be somatosensory (paresthesia), motor, or speech related.

E. **Tension-type headache.** It is useful to think of three types of tension headaches: chronic, episodic, and those that occur in patients with migraine headache. The latter two types may be difficult to distinguish from migraine headache. The criteria for diagnosing tension-type headache can be summarized to include:

1. **Frequent episodes**
2. **Duration of 30 minutes to 7 days**

TABLE 51–1. International Headache Society Classification of Headache

1. **Migraine**

1.1. Migraine without aura

1.2 Migraine with aura

1.3 Ophthalmoplegic migraine

1.4 Retinal migraine

1.5 Childhood periodic syndromes that may be precursors to or associated with migraine

1.6 Complications of migraine

1.7 Migrainous disorder not fulfilling above criteria

2. **Tension-type headache**

2.1 Episodic tension-type headache

2.2 Chronic tension-type headache

2.3 Tension-type headache not fulfilling above criteria

3. **Cluster headache and chronic paroxysmal hemicrania**

3.1 Cluster headache

3.2 Chronic paroxysmal hemicrania

3.3 Cluster headache-like disorder not fulfilling above criteria

4. **Miscellaneous headaches not associated with structural lesion**

4.1 Idiopathic stabbing headache

4.2 External compression headache

4.3 Cold stimulus headache

4.4 Benign cough headache

4.5 Benign exertional headache

4.6 Headache associated with sexual activity

5. **Headache associated with head trauma**

5.1 Acute posttraumatic headache

5.2 Chronic posttraumatic headache

6. **Headache associated with vascular disorder**

6.1 Acute ischemic cerebrovascular disorder

6.2 Intracranial hematoma

6.3 Subarachnoid hemorrhage

6.4 Unruptured vascular malformation

6.5 Arteritis

6.6 Carotid or vertebral artery pain

6.7 Venous thrombosis

6.8 Arterial hypertension

6.9 Headache associated with other vascular disease

7. **Headache associated with nonvascular intracranial disorder**

7.1 High cerebrospinal fluid (CSF) pressure

7.2 Low CSF pressure

7.3 Intracranial infection

continued

TABLE 51–1. International Headache Society Classification of Headache (*Continued*)

7.4 Intracranial sarcoidosis and other noninfectious inflammatory diseases	10.2 Hypercapnia
	10.3 Mixed hypoxia and hypercapnia
7.5 Headache related to intrathecal injections	10.4 Hypoglycemia
	10.5 Dialysis
7.6 Intracranial neoplasm	
	10.6 Headache related to other metabolic abnormality
7.7 Headache associated with other intracranial disorder	
8. Headache associated with substances or their withdrawal	**11. Headache or facial pain associated with disorder of cranium, neck, eyes, ears, nose, sinuses, teeth, mouth, or other facial or cranial structures**
8.1 Headache induced by acute substance use or exposure	11.1 Cranial bone
8.2 Headache induced by chronic substance use or exposure	11.2 Neck
8.3 Headache from substance withdrawal (acute use)	11.3 Eyes
	11.4 Ears
8.4 Headache from substance withdrawal (chronic use)	11.5 Nose and sinuses
8.5 Headache associated with substances but with uncertain mechanism	11.6 Teeth, jaws, and related structures
	11.7 Temporomandibular joint disease
9. Headache associated with noncephalic infection	**12. Cranial neuralgias, nerve trunk pain, and deafferentation pain**
9.1 Viral infection	12.1 Persistent (in contrast to tic-like) pain of cranial nerve origin
9.2 Bacterial infection	12.2 Trigeminal neuralgia
9.3 Headache related to other infection	12.3 Glossopharyngeal neuralgia
	12.4 Nervus intermedius neuralgia
10. Headache associated with metabolic disorder	
10.1 Hypoxia	12.5 Superior laryngeal neuralgia

continued

TABLE 51–1. International Headache Society Classification of Headache (*Continued*)

12.6 Occipital neuralgia	12.8 Facial pain not fulfilling criteria in groups 11 or 12
12.7 Central causes of head and facial pain other than tic douloureux	**13. Headache not classifiable**

Olesen J: Headache Classification Committee of the International Headache Society. Classification and diagnostic criteria for headache disorders, cranial neuralgia, and facial pain. *Cephalgia* 8(suppl 7): 1–96, 1988.

    3. Characteristic features: Pressure or tightness, mild to moderate intensity, bilateral location, not aggravated by physical activity

    4. Lack of associated symptoms (see II D 4)

F. Cluster headache is a syndrome characterized by severe head and facial pain accompanied by various autonomic abnormalities.

    1. Patients are prone to **recurrent symptoms** during episodes of cluster headache.

    2. Duration of 1 to 3 months, during which time the patient experiences **daily episodes lasting 60–90 minutes.** Infrequently, patients may have a chronic variant, where the "cluster" may last longer than a year.

    3. Characteristic features: The usual headache is described as lancinating, sharp, or burning occurring in an oculofrontal, oculotemporal, or retro-orbital distribution. It is generally described as unilateral, and attacks frequently awaken patients from sleep.

    4. Associated symptoms (occurring in as many as 85% of patients) include ipsilateral lacrimation, conjunctival injection, rhinorrhea, nasal congestion, and partial Horner's syndrome (i.e., miosis, ptosis).

G. Analgesic rebound headaches occur in patients who use analgesics on a near daily basis. Overuse of the medication perpetuates and escalates the headache pattern.

H. Bacterial meningitis. In the setting of bacterial meningitis, headache is typically severe, bilateral, and associated with photophobia, nausea, and vomiting. An altered mental status (e.g., confusion, drowsiness) may accompany the headache. Fever is frequently present as well as signs of meningeal irritation.

I. Subarachnoid headache. The characteristic feature of subarachnoid headache is the severe rapidity (like a blow to the head or neck) with which it presents. The headache comes on in a matter of seconds. Subarachnoid headache accounts for approximately 1% of all headaches presenting to the emergency department. Commonly cited reasons for misdiagnosis of subarachnoid headache include failure to appreciate the full spectrum of clinical presentation, failure to appreciate the limitations of computed tomography (CT), and failure to perform and interpret the results of lumbar puncture.

J. Intracranial neoplasm. Cerebral tumors are usually located in a hemisphere and give rise to neurologic symptoms early in the course of illness.

Headache may be the primary complaint in 20%–50% of patients presenting with intracranial neoplasm.

K. **Meningiomas** generally cause localized headaches. The headache is progressive over time (weeks to months).

L. **Giant cell arteritis.** The diagnosis of giant cell (temporal) arteritis should be considered in patients 50 years or older with complaints of headache. Additional diagnostic criteria include the presence of jaw claudication, temporal artery abnormality on clinical examination (e.g., tenderness, decreased pulsation, or scalp tenderness/nodules), an elevation of the erythrocyte sedimentation rate (ESR) [50 mm/hr by the Westergren method], and an abnormal temporal artery biopsy. The headache is often described as a deep, burning pain, sometimes with a throbbing quality. In 30% of cases, the ophthalmic arteries may be involved, leading to blindness from retinal ischemia.

M. **Subdural hematoma** results from rupture of the bridging veins between the dura mater and the arachnoid lining. It may result from relatively minor head trauma, which the patient may not recall. The frequency increases with age. Risk factors include anticoagulation and alcohol abuse. The headache is usually mild in intensity, persistent, and localized to the side of the hematoma. Confusion and impaired memory are frequently present.

N. **Carotid artery dissection** frequently arises in the setting of trauma. The classic triad is unilateral headache, ipsilateral partial Horner's syndrome (i.e., ptosis, miosis), and contralateral symptoms of cerebral ischemia. Headache may be the first or only symptom of the dissection. It usually presents acute-subacute with associated facial pain.

III. **Clinical Evaluation** (Figure 51–1)

A. **History** is directed toward identifying diagnostic features, precipitants, previous evaluation, and treatment regimens. The history should include:

1. **Onset and duration:** Nocturnal awakening, worst time of day (e.g., morning), rapidity of onset, "warning" headache (occurring days or weeks previously)

2. **Quality** (severity of pain, throbbing) and **location** (bilateral versus unilateral, localized, neck or jaw pain)

3. **Precipitating features:** Chewing, light, sound, odors, trauma, caffeine use or cessation, foods or fasting, alcohol, environmental exposures (e.g., carbon monoxide), relation to exertion, stress, menstrual cycle, recent lumbar puncture

4. **Relieving features:** Sleep or inactivity, use of medications and frequency, pacing/activity (cluster)

5. **Associated/prodromal features:** Weight loss, nausea, vomiting, visual disturbances, seizures, numbness, weakness, tearing, nasal congestion, flushing, neck ache, fevers, postnasal drip, depressive symptoms, sleep disturbance, paresthesia, speech disturbance

6. **Other:** Age, family history of headache or central nervous system (CNS) disease, medication use [especially oral contraceptive pills (OCPs), anticoagulants, monoamine oxidase (MAO) inhibitors, or chronic ergotamine use]

7. **Red flag symptoms:** Specific symptoms that may indicate a more serious underlying cause include:

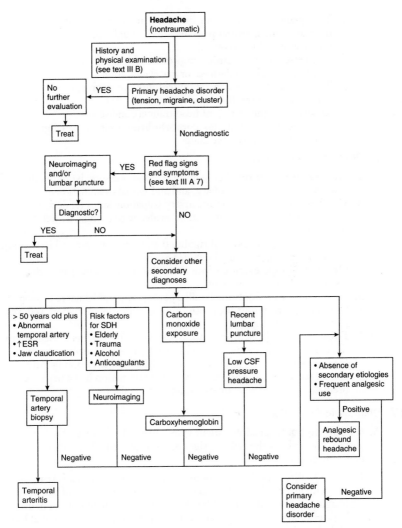

■ **FIGURE 51–1.** Algorithm for workup of patients with headache. *CSF* = cerebrospinal fluid; *ESR* = erythrocyte sedimentation rate; *SDH* = subdural hematoma.

    a. The **first or worst headache** of the patient's life, particularly if the onset was rapid

    b. A **change** in the frequency, severity, or clinical features of the usual attack

    c. A **new onset of headache** in middle age or later, or a significant change in a long-standing headache pattern

    d. The occurrence of a **new or progressive headache** that lasts for days

     e. The precipitation of head pain with maneuvers associated with
increased intracranial pressure (e.g., coughing, sneezing, bending,
exercise, sexual intercourse)

     f. The presence of **systemic symptoms,** such as myalgia, fever, malaise,
weight loss, scalp tenderness, or jaw claudication

     g. The presence of **associated neurologic symptoms,** including
confusion, memory loss, apathy, decreased level of consciousness
(especially in the setting of head trauma), and seizure

     h. The presence of **high-risk comorbidities,** especially malignancy or
an immunocompromised state

B. Physical examination

     1. General examination: Temperature; blood pressure; lymph node
assessment; cardiac, pulmonary, and abdominal examinations

     2. Head examination: Temporal artery palpation, sinus tenderness,
temporomandibular joint palpation, evidence of trauma, dental
tenderness

     3. Neck examination: Nuchal rigidity (i.e., signs of meningeal irritation),
range of motion, paraspinal tenderness

     4. Ophthalmologic examination: Fundi for hemorrhage, papilledema,
visual field/acuity assessment

     5. Neurologic examination: Pupillary reactions, cranial nerve assessment
(e.g., for ophthalmoplegia, ptosis, miosis), motor examination, reflexes,
plantar responses, gait

     6. Focal neurologic examination: In one study of patients presenting to
the emergency department with headache, a focal neurologic examination had a positive predictive value of 39% in determining intracranial pathology. A normal neurologic examination had a negative
predictive value of 98% in excluding intracranial findings.

IV. Diagnostic Evaluation

     A. Neuroimaging. In an adult patient whose headache follows a benign
pattern (i.e., it lacks the red flag signs and symptoms), the positive yield of
neuroimaging is low.

     **1. The Quality Standards Subcommittee of the American Academy
of Neurology** published a practice parameter on the use of neuroimaging in the evaluation of headache in patients with normal neurologic examinations. In this publication, they concluded a total yield of
pathology in patients with migraine headaches to be 0.4% and non-
migraine headaches to be 2.4%.

     2. Indications for neuroimaging include "red flag symptoms" (see III A
7), focal neurologic signs or symptoms, altered mental status (especially
in the setting of head trauma), and fever with signs or symptoms of
meningeal irritation.

     3. Contrast-enhanced CT has a 95% accuracy rate in identifying the
presence of intracranial pathology, but drops to 85% in the absence of
contrast. Sensitivity for blood in the subarachnoid space on the day of
an aneurysmal bleed is approximately 90% compared to approximately
75% 2 days later.

     B. Cerebrospinal fluid evaluation is indicated when meningitis, encephalitis,
subarachnoid hemorrhage, and elevated intracranial pressure are diagnostic

considerations. When considering lumbar puncture in a patient with suspected subarachnoid hemorrhage, it is important to wait approximately 6 hours after the headache onset (if the patient is not seriously ill). This will enable the clinician to distinguish between a traumatic tap and bleed (i.e., the presence of xanthochromia) [see Chapter 54].

C. ESR. In cases where giant cell arteritis is suspected, a sedimentation rate is of clinical utility. The ESR should be elevated to > 50 mm/hr, although it is often > 100 mm/hr. It may be normal in 1%–2% of patients with giant cell arteritis. In cases with a high clinical suspicion, temporal artery biopsy should be performed. Whereas the ESR is a relatively sensitive finding (~92%), it has low specificity (48%).

D. Carboxyhemoglobin level should be obtained if carbon monoxide exposure is suspected.

E. Other studies. Carotid duplex/Doppler, cerebral angiogram, and leptomeninges biopsy are uncommonly used in the evaluation of headache. Specific circumstances [i.e., dissection, aneurysm, CNS vasculitis suspected] dictate their use.

SUGGESTED READING

Olesen J: Headache Classification Committee of the International Headache Society. Classification and diagnostic criteria for headache disorders, cranial neuralgia, and facial pain. *Cephalagia* 8(suppl 7):1–96, 1988.

Report of the Quality Standards Subcommittee of the American Academy of Neurology: The utility of neuroimaging in the evaluation of headache in patients with normal neurologic examinations. *Neurology* 44(7):1353–1354, 1994.

52

First Seizure in the Adult Patient

Catherine A. Phillips and Stephen B. Erban

I. **Definition.** A seizure is a **paroxysmal event characterized by excessive synchronous firing of cortical neurons.**

   A. **Partial seizure** is characterized by focal cortical involvement, with the clinical manifestations of the seizure reflecting the underlying region of the cortex involved.

   B. **Generalized seizure** is generalized at onset.

   C. **Secondarily generalized seizure.** Focal seizure activity may rapidly spread to become generalized; the focal onset may or may not be clinically evident.

II. **Overview**

   A. **Symptomatic seizures.** Seizures that have an identifiable cause are termed symptomatic seizures.

      1. Seizures acutely provoked by metabolic or toxic perturbation in a patient with an otherwise entirely normal brain are called **primary generalized** or **idiopathic seizures.**

      2. Seizures caused by an acute cerebral lesion are called **acute symptomatic seizures.**

      3. Seizures caused by a more chronic or subtle cerebral lesion are called **remote symptomatic seizures.**

      4. Seizures without an underlying metabolic or structural cause and that occur on a presumed genetic basis are called **primary generalized** or **idiopathic seizures.**

   B. **Epilepsy** is defined as the presence of recurrent, unprovoked seizures. A single seizure is not epilepsy.

   C. **Clinical presentations.** Seizures can have a number of different clinical presentations. An understanding of the variety of presentations is essential to the correct diagnosis.

      1. **Absence seizures.** Although absence seizures occur mostly in children who are otherwise entirely normal neurologically, they are not restricted to children. The seizures are characterized by motionless unresponsive staring that lasts for several seconds followed by immediate recovery. There is no warning or aura, and the child is often unaware that anything has happened. The seizures may occur many times per day. An electroencephalogram (EEG) classically shows a 3-second generalized spike and wave discharge.

      2. **Complex partial seizures** have a focal onset with enough cortical spread to impair consciousness at least partially. These seizures may be characterized by unresponsive staring for 1–2 minutes, and are sometimes associated with purposeless repetitive motor acts or

vocalizations called automatisms. Patients may fumble, mutter, cry out, have lip smacking or chewing movements, or may get up and wander around. An **aura,** or **simple partial seizure,** is a warning symptom that may either occur alone or precede the onset of a complex partial seizure. Common auras include a sense of déjà vu, nausea, a sense of dread or fear, visual distortions or hallucinations, and auditory or olfactory hallucinations. After a complex partial seizure, the patient is almost always confused or fatigued for at least several minutes.

3. **Generalized tonic-clonic seizures** (convulsions) may be either primary generalized events or secondarily generalized events.

   a. **Primary generalized seizures** occur abruptly without any warning.
   b. **Secondarily generalized seizures** may or may not have a clinically evident focal onset with either aura or focal clonic activity. These seizures may have atypical features such as unilateral clonic activity only or falling without associated clonic activity.

4. **Tonic seizures** are characterized by sudden rigid posturing of limbs or torso with loss of consciousness.

5. **Atonic seizures** or drop seizures involve the sudden loss of postural tone resulting in a head drop or abrupt fall to the ground with loss of consciousness. The event is very brief with rapid recovery. These seizures frequently occur in patients with diffuse brain injury and other types of seizures as well.

III. **Differential Diagnosis.** When evaluating a patient for possible seizure, it is essential to exclude nonepileptic paroxysmal events that may masquerade as seizures.

A. **Syncope** is often preceded by symptoms of "pancerebral" hypoperfusion, including lightheadedness or dizziness, nausea, flushing, and graying of vision. Patients usually fall limply. Tonic posturing and clonic movements may occur briefly ("convulsive syncope"). Urinary incontinence and tongue biting, although rare, may occur. Consciousness is usually regained quickly without postictal confusion.

B. **Transient ischemic attacks (TIAs)** usually produce "negative" symptoms (such as weakness, visual deficits, or numbness), while seizures usually result in "positive" symptoms (such as twitching of a limb or abnormal sensations). TIAs almost never produce sudden loss of consciousness. Recurrent neurologic events in an older patient with risk factors for cerebrovascular disease usually indicate TIAs, although if the events occur repetitively for longer than 3 weeks without progression seizures should be considered. The presence of a spike pattern on EEG suggests a chronic seizure disorder.

C. **Migraine** may begin with focal neurologic symptoms such as visual deficits or focal weakness, with subsequent development of unilateral headache; occasionally, the neurologic symptoms are not followed by headache ("migraine equivalent"). A past history of migraine headache or a family history of migraine can be helpful for diagnosis (see Chapter 51, II D).

D. **Psychogenic seizures** or pseudoseizures are involuntary events that resemble seizures clinically but are psychogenically induced, in essence representing a conversion disorder. These seizures can be very difficult to distinguish from epileptic seizures. Urinary incontinence, tongue biting, and injury can occur in both epileptic and nonepileptic seizures. Some behaviors that are more typically seen in psychogenic seizures include nonsynchronous thrashing of limbs, prolongation of the event for many minutes or hours, abrupt termination of the event without postictal confusion, active eye closure during the event, wailing or crying throughout the event, opisthotonic posturing, and pelvic thrusting. However, diagnosis based on behavioral observations alone is often incorrect. Simultaneous EEG monitoring during an actual event is sometimes required for definitive diagnosis.

E. Hyperventilation can cause symptoms that may be mistaken for seizures, particularly unilateral numbness or paresthesias. Having the patient hyperventilate for 5 minutes can usually reproduce these symptoms.

IV. Clinical Approach to the Patient with First Seizure (Figure 52–1)

A. It is essential to **determine if the event was in fact a seizure,** identify any underlying cause, and assess the likelihood of recurrence.

1. **Underlying brain disorder.** When evaluating a patient who has just had a first seizure, it is important to determine if there is evidence of an underlying brain disorder that might put the patient at risk for recurrent, unprovoked seizures. Alternatively, the seizure may have been precipitated by an environmental (e.g., sleep deprivation or acute head injury) or endogenous (e.g., hyponatremia) perturbation, without the presence of a more chronic underlying cerebral disturbance.

2. **Seizure precipitants** are factors that transiently lower the seizure threshold. These factors can trigger seizures in patients with epilepsy and can also acutely provoke seizures in nonepileptic patients. Some of the more common seizure precipitants are listed in Table 52–1.

3. **Recurrence.** Once the precipitating condition resolves (or is metabolized in the case of medications or toxins), seizures would not be expected to recur assuming a chronic cerebral disturbance is not present. It is important to remember that a definite cause is identified in less than half of all newly diagnosed cases.

B. History

1. **The seizure event:** A careful history is the cornerstone of diagnosis. Approximately 20% of cases are misdiagnosed as first seizure, most often as a result of inadequate history taking. A detailed description of the event must be obtained from both the patient, whose own recollection may be limited, and from witnesses, if possible. This should include a description of:

   a. **Behavior during the event:** In some cases, it may be better for a witness to mimic the patient's behavior, which can help distinguish subtle points such as a vibratory tremor versus clonic shaking.

   b. **Any warning symptoms or signs suggestive of an aura:** If a distinct symptom or a vague, indescribable sensation is present, ask about any prior occurrences. It is not uncommon to obtain a history of previous isolated auras that have never been brought to medical attention, indicating that the current seizure is a recurrent, not an isolated, event.

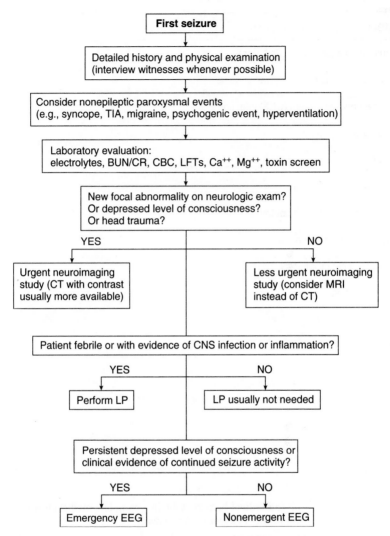

■ FIGURE 52–1. Diagnostic algorithm for the evaluation of first seizure in the adult patient. *BUN/CR* = blood urea nitrogen/creatine ratio; *CBC* = complete blood count; *CNS* = central nervous system; *CT* = computed tomography; *EEG* = electroencephalogram; *LP* = lumbar puncture; *MRI* = magnetic resonance imaging; *LFTs* = liver function tests; *TIA* = transient ischemic attack.

    c. Postictal phenomena: Postictal neurologic deficit such as hemiparesis or aphasia can indicate a focal seizure origin.
    d. Any possible triggers or precipitating factors (see Table 52–1).
2. Other patient history

TABLE 52–1. Seizure Precipitants

Acute head injury (within 24 hours)

Alcohol or sedative withdrawal

Central nervous system (CNS) infection

Eclampsia

Fever

Hepatic encephalopathy

Hypertensive encephalopathy

Hypo- and hyperglycemia

Hypo- and hypernatremia

Hypocalcemia

Hypomagnesemia

Medications

Sleep deprivation

Substance abuse (e.g., cocaine, amphetamines, marijuana)

Thyrotoxicosis

Uremia

---

a. **Complete medical history.** Obtain a complete medical history, focusing on any risk factors for seizure:

   (1) History of birth or perinatal trauma
   (2) Febrile seizures in infancy
   (3) Central nervous system (CNS) infection
   (4) Significant head injury (with loss of consciousness or associated symptoms suggesting a concussion)
   (5) Known cerebral insult such as stroke
   (6) Family history of seizures
   (7) History of developmental delay

b. **Medications:** Be certain to inquire about new medications or dose changes.

c. **Substance abuse:** Ask about the use or recent discontinuation of substances, especially alcohol, amphetamines, cocaine, or benzodiazepines.

    d. Lifestyle issues: Consider social, emotional, or professional issues that may influence the impact of the seizure on the patient.

C. Physical examination

  1. General examination

    a. It is important to identify any signs of a systemic illness or disorder that might be associated with seizure.

    b. If the examination is within several hours of the seizure, check for a **postictal neurologic deficit** (e.g., Todd's paralysis).

  2. Neurologic examination. Assess for any evidence of underlying cerebral dysfunction, either focal or generalized. Signs of permanent nervous system dysfunction may suggest the diagnosis of a symptomatic seizure (see II A).

V. Diagnostic Studies. The diagnostic evaluation should be done in a selective fashion seeking to confirm the clinical suspicions generated by the history and physical examination.

  A. Laboratory studies should include electrolytes, glucose, calcium, magnesium values, tests of kidney and liver function, and pulse oximetry. In actual practice, blood work is rarely useful in healthy adults, but it may have a higher yield in older patients. A toxicology screen should be obtained.

  B. Lumbar puncture should be done in a febrile patient with a new seizure, or if there is any other reason to suspect an infectious or inflammatory CNS process.

  C. EEG is a very useful aid in the diagnosis of seizures, and it assists in classifying the type of seizure (focal versus generalized). An EEG is not a substitute for clinical judgment, however, and the findings on EEG should not dictate the diagnosis.

    1. The likelihood of finding an epileptiform abnormality on EEG is highest in the first 24 hours after the seizure.

      a. The yield improves if the patient is sleep deprived and the EEG indicates light sleep.

      b. If the initial EEG is unhelpful, a repeat sleep-deprived study may be useful.

    2. Sharp waves and spikes are the classic EEG "thumbprint" of a seizure disorder, but these findings may also be seen in 1% of people who will never have an epileptic seizure.

    3. A normal EEG does not disprove the diagnosis of a seizure disorder. If the patient continues with a depressed level of consciousness after the initial seizure, or if there is clinical evidence of continued seizure activity, an EEG should be obtained urgently to determine if the patient is in status epilepticus.

  D. Imaging studies. Head computed tomography (CT) and brain magnetic resonance imaging (MRI) are useful in ruling out structural brain lesions that could cause seizures. When head CT is used, it should be performed with intravenous contrast.

    1. Sensitivity. The sensitivity of CT is 25%–30% compared to the > 80% sensitivity of MRI.

2. Indications

 a. Neuroimaging is needed urgently when seizures occur in the setting of head trauma, depressed level of consciousness or a new focal neurologic abnormality, or if the patient presents with a flurry of seizures or a prolonged seizure (longer than 5 minutes).

 b. CT is usually more readily available, on an urgent basis, than MRI. If imaging is not needed urgently, waiting for more definitive imaging with MRI should be considered.

3. Yield. The yield of a neuroimaging procedure is low in patients who have had a single generalized seizure without focal features, a normal neurologic examination, and a history of a potential seizure precipitant. Neuroimaging is not mandated in this setting, but many clinicians choose to obtain a study nevertheless.

SUGGESTED READING

Hauser WA, Annegers JF, Kurland LT: Incidence of epilepsy and unprovoked seizures in Rochester, Minnesota: 1935–1984. *Epilepsia* 34:453–468, 1993.

Sander JWAS, Sillanpaa M: Natural History and Prognosis. In Engel J, Pedley T (eds): *Epilepsy: A Comprehensive Textbook*. Philadelphia: Lippincott-Raven Publishers, 1997, pp 69–86.

53

Sleep Disorders
Stacia Sailer

I. **Overview.** Many people experience difficulties with sleep during their lifetime. Most cases are transient and are related to short illnesses, medications, stress, or scheduling. Other cases, however, involve chronic symptoms that adversely impact the patient's daytime function and health.

A. **Excessive daytime sleepiness (EDS)** is defined as an increased tendency to sleep during nonsleeping hours. The spectrum of EDS ranges from dozing off while idle to falling asleep during conversations and while driving.

1. Once it is determined that the patient sleeps a sufficient duration (i.e., approximately 7½–8 hr) and is not taking sedating medications, the focus shifts to disorders that disrupt or fragment sleep and cause EDS, such as:

a. Sleep-disordered breathing syndromes [e.g., obstructive sleep apnea (OSA)-hypopnea syndrome, upper-airway resistance syndrome]
b. Periodic limb movements during sleep (PLMS)
c. Narcolepsy
d. Idiopathic hypersomnia
e. Postviral hypersomnia
f. Posttraumatic hypersomnia

2. Symptoms of EDS correlate most closely with the degree of sleep fragmentation and the average number of transient electroencephalogram (EEG) arousals per hour (arousal index), except in the cases of narcolepsy and idiopathic hypersomnia where the disorders seem to be correlated with the regulation of sleep.

B. **Snoring and sleep-disordered breathing.** In 4%–9% of the middle-aged population, snoring is associated with significant sleep-disordered breathing, which has been shown to be a significant medical disorder. Intermittent upper-airway collapse or obstruction causes sleep disruption and fragmentation, and thus daytime sleepiness. The collapse or obstruction may be complete (apnea) or partial (hypopnea or respiratory event-related arousal), but the effects are the same. In addition to causing EDS, sleep-disordered breathing has been associated with increased morbidity and mortality and increased health-care utilization and costs.

C. **Restless leg syndrome (RLS) and PLMS**

1. **RLS** occurs in 4%–9% of the population, and the prevalence increases with age. RLS is characterized by an uncomfortable sensation in the legs, which occurs primarily at night when the patient is at rest. The sensation is relieved by movement. In some cases, the frequent need to move prevents the patient from falling asleep and may result in complaints of difficulties falling asleep (i.e., sleep initiation insomnia).

    2. PLMS. Approximately 60% of people with RLS also have involuntary leg jerks or twitches while they sleep. These leg jerks occur at regular intervals (e.g., every 30–60 seconds) and are associated with transient arousals, which may cause sleep fragmentation and EDS. In the absence of RLS, the diagnosis of PLMS requires an overnight polysomnogram.

    3. Both RLS and PLMS are associated with a number of medical conditions (e.g., iron-deficiency anemia, vitamins B_{12} and folate deficiencies), peripheral neuropathies, renal failure or dialysis, pregnancy, narcolepsy, and may be secondary to drugs [e.g., selective serotonin reuptake inhibitors (SSRIs), tricyclic antidepressants, alcohol].

D. Narcolepsy is a disorder that affects rapid eye movement (REM) sleep. Classic symptoms include EDS, irresistible sleep attacks, cataplexy (sudden loss of muscle tone while awake usually involving antigravity muscles and often occurring during intense emotion), hypnagogic hallucinations (dreams at sleep onset), and sleep paralysis (skeletal muscle paralysis at sleep onset).

E. Insomnia is described as the perception of inadequate sleep. Patients may complain of difficulties falling asleep (i.e., sleep initiation insomnia), difficulties staying asleep (i.e., sleep maintenance insomnia), or early morning awakenings.

    1. Underlying psychiatric disorder: Approximately 50% of patients who report insomnia have an underlying psychiatric disorder, which may include anxiety disorder or depression.

    2. Hyperarousal: Many patients with insomnia are thought to have a low arousal threshold. These patients frequently develop poor sleep habits (psychophysiologic insomnia) or use sleeping pills, which further exacerbate their symptoms.

    3. Other causes: It is useful to divide the other causes of insomnia into disorders associated with sleep initiation (e.g., RLS, psychophysiologic insomnia, delayed sleep phase syndrome, medication or caffeine abuse), disorders associated with sleep maintenance (e.g., EDS-related disorders, central sleep apnea, alcoholism, pain syndromes), and disorders related to early morning awakenings (e.g., depression, advanced sleep phase syndrome).

II. Clinical Evaluation (Figures 53–1 and 53–2)

A. History and physical examination. While the history and physical examination are not sensitive or specific enough to make a diagnosis or to determine the severity of sleep-disordered breathing, there are five clinical features that increase the likelihood of diagnosis. The presence of all five features is associated with a 70% chance of having OSA.

    1. Habitually loud snoring
    2. Witnessed apneas
    3. EDS
    4. History of hypertension
    5. A neck circumference $> 17''$ (men) or $> 16''$ (women)

B. How to confirm the diagnosis

    1. RLS and PLMS. The diagnoses of RLS and PLMS are made clinically based on the patient's history. Screening for anemia alone is

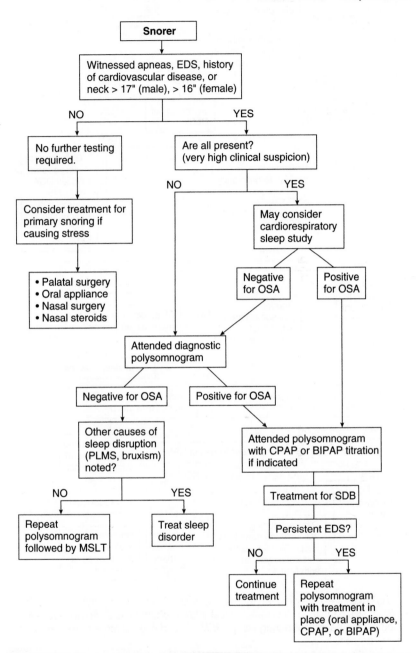

■ **FIGURE 53–1.** Algorithm for the workup of patients with excessive snoring. *BIPAP* = biphasic positive airway pressure; *CPAP* = continuous positive airway pressure; *EDS* = excessive daytime sleepiness; *MSLT* = multiple sleep latency test; *OSA* = obstructive sleep apnea; *PLMS* = periodic limb movements during sleep; *SDB* = sleep-disordered breathing.

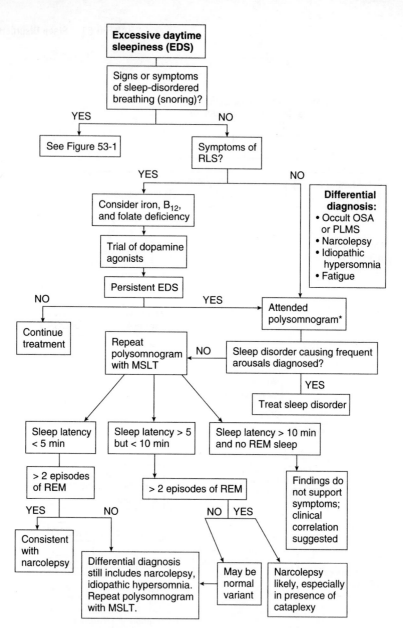

FIGURE 53–2. Algorithm for the workup of excessive daytime sleepiness (EDS). *MSLT* = multiple sleep latency test; *OSA* = obstructive sleep apnea; *PLMS* = periodic limb movement during sleep; *REM* = rapid eye movement; *RLS* = restless leg syndrome.

*If a patient presents with classic symptoms of narcolepsy (i.e., cataplexy, EDS, hypnagogic hallucinations, and sleep paralysis), does not snore, and does not have symptoms suggestive of RLS or PLMS, you may proceed with a polysomnogram and MSLT at this point. All other sleep disorders must be adequately treated before you can make a diagnosis of narcolepsy or idiopathic hypersomnia.

insufficient. Studies have demonstrated that underlying biochemical deficiencies are responsible for RLS, not the anemia per se.

    a. With **iron deficiency,** the central dopamine receptor becomes less "sensitive" given the presence of its iron moiety.

    b. In the case of **vitamin B_{12} or folate deficiency,** the resulting neuropathy is the problem, not the anemia.

    c. In addition to assessing for deficiencies (e.g., serum ferritin, vitamin B_{12}, folate), the history and physical examination should screen for **peripheral neuropathies, renal failure, pregnancy, narcolepsy,** and **medications or toxins.**

  2. Insomnia. The diagnosis of insomnia is made clinically, and the evaluation should include confirming the actual sleep schedule and time with a sleep log and using the history and physical examination to screen for medical and psychiatric disorders. Most patients have several contributing factors.

  3. Narcolepsy. The diagnosis of narcolepsy is made by confirming normal overnight sleep (i.e., by ruling out other causes of sleep disruption) and by using a polysomnogram followed by a multiple sleep latency test (MSLT) [see III A, B].

III. Diagnostic Evaluation

  A. Polysomnography. Attended overnight polysomnography is the gold standard for evaluating patients with complaints of EDS.

    1. Description: Polysomnography involves monitoring and staging sleep [i.e., by recording brain waves with EEG, eye movements with electro-oculogram (EOG), and chin movements with electromyogram (EMG)], breathing patterns (e.g., airflow, respiratory effort, pulse oximetry, heart rate), limb movements (e.g., of the legs and occasionally arms with EMG), and body position. Most patients are also monitored with remote audio and video recordings to observe for behaviors and seizures.

    2. Indications. Commonly cited indications for polysomnography include:

      a. EDS

      b. Snoring with witnessed apneas or symptoms of OSA

      c. Sleep maintenance insomnia associated with snoring

      d. Cases that are unresponsive to behavioral and psychiatric treatment

      e. Following upper-airway surgery or insertion of an oral appliance for treatment of OSA

      f. Persistent or recurrent EDS despite compliance with adequate continuous positive airway pressure or biphasic positive airway pressure

  B. MSLT. An MSLT is the accepted test to confirm a patient's daytime sleep tendency. The patient must be off all centrally acting medications for 2 weeks and have a "usual" consistent sleep pattern for 1 week before the test.

    1. Description: The test consists of a standardized series of naps at 2-hour intervals beginning 2–3 hours after awakening from an overnight polysomnogram.

   a. **Normal results:** A normal result is defined as sleep latency greater than 10 minutes and no episodes of REM.
   b. **Abnormal results**
      (1) Pathologic sleepiness is defined as sleep latency less than 5 minutes. A sleep latency of 5–10 minutes is considered borderline or within the "gray zone."
      (2) The finding of more than two episodes of REM during these brief naps is considered abnormal.
   2. **Indications:** An MSLT, which is required for the diagnosis of narcolepsy, may be helpful in evaluating patients who complain of EDS but do not have a sleep disorder, or who continue to complain of EDS despite adequate treatment of a previously identified sleep disorder. MSLT can also be used to confirm the symptoms of EDS in a patient with a complicated presentation. An MSLT is not usually included in the initial evaluation of snoring, OSA, RSL, or PLMS.
C. **Cardiorespiratory sleep study.** In the majority of cases, attended overnight polysomnography is required to make a diagnosis of OSA, the overlap syndrome, and upper-airway resistance syndrome. In some cases with very high pretest clinical suspicion for OSA and in areas without easy access to attended polysomnography, a cardiorespiratory sleep study [i.e., pulse oximetry, electrocardiogram (ECG), airway flow, and respiratory effort] may be an acceptable alternative. This should only be done with the understanding that these limited studies are not as sensitive, and repeat testing with polysomnography will be required to appropriately rule out sleep-disordered breathing and to evaluate for other intrinsic sleep disorders. It is important that all studies be "attended" by a technician for sake of quality and the ability to intervene if necessary.
D. **Overnight oximetry.** While the presence of cyclic oxygen desaturation during overnight pulse oximetry may suggest the possibility of OSA, the sensitivity is not high enough to rule out apnea (because severe OSA may occur without significant oxygen desaturation). The clinical consequences of OSA and sleep-disordered breathing are not strictly related to oxygen desaturation. Sleep disruption related to fragmentation, arousals, and respiratory event-related arousals all contribute to the clinical manifestations in a manner independent of oxygenation status.

SUGGESTED READING

Chesson A, Ferber R, et al: An American Sleep Disorders Associated Review. The indications for polysomnography and related procedures. *Sleep* 20(6):423–487, 1997.

54

Evaluation of Cerebrospinal Fluid

Majaz Moonis, Michael Mitchell, and Howard Sachs

I. **Overview.** Lumbar puncture (LP) is most useful in detecting abnormalities of intracranial pressure, meningeal inflammation, subarachnoid hemorrhage, and neoplasm.

   A. **Specimen collection.** LP is usually performed with the patient lying in the lateral decubitus position. Fluid is withdrawn usually from the L3–L4 intervertebral space, although the L4–L5 space is also suitable. The opening pressure should be measured as an initial step.

   B. **Contraindications.** LP is contraindicated in the presence of papilledema and focal neurologic signs, without prior neuroimaging (fulminant bacterial meningitis is an exception). Bleeding disorders are a relative contraindication.

II. **General Laboratory Considerations**

   A. **Amount of fluid.** Submit the maximum amount of cerebrospinal fluid (CSF) that can safely be taken from the patient. Fluid is concentrated by centrifugation for smear preparation and media inoculation.

   B. **Transport of fluid.** If transport of CSF to the laboratory will be delayed, incubate at 35°C–37°C. CSF should never be refrigerated, as this may kill *Neisseria meningitidis.*

III. **Diagnostic Considerations**

   A. **Initial evaluation.** In all cases, the initial evaluation of CSF sampling would include a cell count with differential, glucose and protein determination, Gram's stain and culture for bacteria and fungi, and cytologic evaluation. Specialized studies would follow based upon clinical suspicions.

   1. **Cell analysis**

      a. **CSF is normally acellular,** although a red blood cell (RBC) count or white blood cell (WBC) count of 0–3 mm³ may be considered normal.

      b. **WBC analysis**

         (1) A WBC count > 1000 mm³ is generally seen in bacterial meningitis. Counts of 5–1000 mm³ may be seen in early or partially treated bacterial meningitis, viral meningitis, and encephalitis.

         (2) The cell differential is useful as well. If $> 50\%$ of the cells are polymorphonuclear leukocytes, bacterial infection is likely. If $< 10\%$ of the cells are polymorphonuclear leukocytes, nonbacterial causes are suggested.

         (3) Using a ratio of ~1 WBC/mm³ for every 700 RBC/mm³ is useful in distinguishing the presence of WBCs from a traumatic tap and other causes.

    c. RBC analysis: When interpreting red cells in CSF, it is important to distinguish between a traumatic tap and pathologic bleeding (as seen in subarachnoid hemorrhage).

       (1) A traumatic tap will note a differential cell count between tubes 1 and 4.

       (2) Xanthochromia suggests that blood has been present in the CSF greater than 2 hours. It is characterized by a pink or yellowish discoloration of the supernatant on a centrifuged specimen (i.e., hemoglobin degradation products).

2. Chemistry analysis

    a. Glucose: The CSF glucose is normally maintained at a level lower than present in blood plasma (approximately 50%–60% less). Markedly decreased glucose may be seen in bacterial meningitis, as well as in tuberculous and some fungal causes. Other entities that are associated with decreased levels of glucose (i.e., a ratio of CSF:serum < 0.4) include subarachnoid hemorrhage, malignancy, sarcoid, syphilis, certain viruses, and hypoglycemia.

    b. Protein is elevated in virtually all types of meningitis. Many other processes can elevate the CSF protein (e.g., tumor, stroke, demyelinating disease).

3. Microbiologic studies. It is noteworthy that patients with partially treated meningitis have persistent abnormalities of chemistry and hematology tests of CSF. False-negative cultures may be the only impediment to diagnosis.

    a. A **Gram's stain** may be positive in 75%–80% of cases with untreated bacterial meningitis. It is useful in selecting initial antibiotic therapy.

    b. Bacterial antigen detection rarely provides information over and above that yielded by Gram's stain and culture. Consider antigen testing if the patient has been treated with antibiotics prior to culture, and in those patients where the initial cultures are negative after 24-hr incubation.

    c. Culture may be positive in 70%–85% of cases with bacterial meningitis.

    d. Venereal Disease Research Laboratory (VDRL): The VDRL test should be obtained on serum and CSF in all cases of aseptic meningitis.

B. Specialized studies

1. Oligoclonal bands should be obtained in cases of suspected multiple sclerosis (~97% sensitive). They reflect intrathecal inflammation, which is more common in chronic than in acute diseases, as it takes 7–10 days for plasma cells to secrete immunoglobulin G (IgG) molecules. It is important to note that other inflammatory conditions (e.g., subacute sclerosing panencephalitis, neurosyphilis, adrenoleukodystrophy) may also be associated with oligoclonal bands.

2. Cytology is especially useful in cases of suspected carcinomatosis or gliomatosis. In these instances, cytology may be positive in as many as 70% of cases.

3. Ziehl-Neelsen stain is useful for acid-fast bacilli (AFB) [although it is rarely positive even in confirmed cases]. Polymerase chain reaction (PCR) is much more sensitive and specific and should always be done when available.

4. **India ink smear** may be positive in as many as 50%–75% of cases of cryptococcal meningitis. Yeasts are identified by their budding, sharply demarcated capsules; doubly refractile cell wall; and refractile cytoplasmic inclusions. If a high index of suspicion exists, a latex agglutination test is useful. A titer of 1:8 or greater is present in more than 90% of cases (see also Chapter 48, GENERAL ASPECTS, II A 3).

5. **Herpes simplex virus (HSV)** should be suspected in appropriate clinical settings. CSF shows mild to moderate pleocytosis, with either normal or elevated protein.

   a. **PCR** can detect HSV DNA in the CSF (sensitivity of 95%).

   b. The **CSF:serum quotient** for the antibody titer can be used to detect the intrathecal synthesis of antibody against HSV.

   c. **Viral isolation** has not been a useful diagnostic procedure, as positive results are obtained in less than 5% of cases.

6. **Neuroborreliosis** is usually characterized by pleocytosis, elevated protein, or both. There is evidence of localized antibody production (i.e., the ratio of CSF:serum antibody > 1.0).

SUGGESTED READING

Thompson EJ: Cerebrospinal fluid. *J Neurol Neurosurg Psychiatry* 59(4):349–357, 1995.

Otolaryngology

55

Hoarseness
Daniel Y. Kim

I. Etiology. Overall, the most common cause of hoarseness is voice abuse, which can lead to irritation, inflammation, edema, nodules, polyps, keratosis, and leukoplakia. Acute viral laryngitis is the most common of the infectious causes (Table 55–1).

A. Vocal cord paralysis. Hoarseness can be caused by any factor that interferes with proper closure of the vocal cords. The causes of vocal cord paralysis are varied and numerous, ranging from idiopathic causes, to infectious causes, to trauma, to neurologic processes, to neoplastic involvement.

1. Too wide an opening of the vocal cords causes a weak and hoarse voice.
2. Too strong a glottic closure produces high pressure and results in a spastic or hyperkinetic voice.

B. Dysfunction of the laryngeal muscles. There are seven paired and one unpaired intrinsic muscles of the larynx. Dysfunction of any of these muscles can lead to dysphonia and hoarseness.

II. Clinical Evaluation of Hoarseness (Figure 55–1)

A. History

1. **Mode of onset:** Sudden onset is usually more consistent with an irritative, inflammatory, or traumatic cause.
2. **Pain** is worrisome and should always arouse suspicion of malignancy. Unexplained unilateral ear pain can be an indication of laryngeal or pharyngeal carcinoma.
3. **Alteration of vocal quality:** An alteration of vocal quality is often the first symptom associated with carcinoma. Thus, hoarseness that persists beyond 2 weeks requires visualization of the larynx.
4. Assess for **additional symptoms**, including:

   a. Associated dyspnea and dysphagia
   b. Cigarette and alcohol use
   c. Allergies or exposures (e.g., environmental, food, chemical, toxins)
   d. Infectious symptoms

TABLE 55–1. Differential Diagnosis of Hoarseness

Mechanical and Inflammatory Causes

Voice abuse or overuse

Edema: bacterial, viral, allergic, traumatic

Smoking

Nodules or polyps

Postnasal drip

Breathing through the mouth: causes dryness and irritation of laryngeal membranes

Leukoplakia: thick whitish layer of hyperkeratotic epithelial cells

Keratosis: abnormality of growth or maturation of the epithelium

Trauma: physical, surgical, cough

Laryngeal ulcer: the most common site is the vocal process of the arytenoid cartilage

Gastroesophageal reflux disease (GERD): causes irritation and inflammation of the posterior portions of the larynx; can cause ulceration

Intubation granuloma: usually seen on the vocal process of the arytenoid cartilage

Arytenoid subluxation: physical trauma, intubation

Cricoarytenoid ankylosis: intubation, trauma, rheumatoid arthritis, gout, collagen disease

Laryngeal web: on the anterior commissure, from surgery or trauma

Presbylaryngia: weakness of the laryngeal muscles as a function of aging

Foreign body: food, physical object

Infections (other than the common viral and bacterial agents):
- Tuberculosis
- Sarcoidosis
- Syphilis
- Scleroma: *Klebsiella rhinoscleromatis*
- Wegener's granulomatosis: necrotizing granulomas of upper and lower respiratory tract, pulmonary vasculitis, necrotizing glomerulonephritis
- Leprosy: *Mycobacterium leprae*
- Diphtheritic laryngitis: *Corynebacterium diphtheriae*

continued

TABLE 55–1. Differential Diagnosis of Hoarseness (*Continued*)

Mycotic infections of the larynx (*Candidiasis, Coccidioidomycosis, Histoplasmosis, Actinomycosis, Blastomycosis*)

Rheumatoid arthritis

Angioneurotic edema

Endocrine dysfunction (hypo- or hyperthyroidism, pregnancy, adrenal hypo- or hyper-functioning, acromegaly)

Neurologic Causes

Recurrent laryngeal nerve paralysis
- Malignant disease (25%): lung or neck
- Surgical trauma (20%): surgery on thyroid, parathyroid, neck, lung, mediastinum, heart, esophagus
- Idiopathic (13%): viral
- Inflammatory (13%): pulmonary tuberculosis is a major cause
- Nonsurgical trauma (11%): stretching of the nerve by enlarged left atrium, aortic aneurysm

Traumatic recurrent or superior laryngeal nerve paralysis
- Surgical: thyroid and parathyroid surgery
- Physical: blunt or sharp trauma to laryngeal nerves, cerebrovascular accident (CVA)

Neoplastic invasion of laryngeal nerves: in the neck or mediastinum

Myasthenia gravis: autoimmune disease with damage to the acetylcholine receptors in the motor end plate

Palatal myoclonus: rhythmical movements of the soft palate; believed to be a disorder of the olivocerebellar modulatory projection on the rostral brain stem

Progressive bulbar palsy: degeneration of motor neurons in the anterior horns of the spinal cord

Neoplastic Causes

Benign	Malignant
Keratosis	Squamous cell carcinoma (SCC)
Papillomatosis [human papilloma virus (HPV)]	Verrucous carcinoma
	Adenocarcinoma
Chondroma	
	Adenoid cystic carcinoma

continued

TABLE 55–1. Differential Diagnosis of Hoarseness (*Continued*)

Neoplastic Causes (*Continued*)

Benign	Malignant
Neurofibroma/schwannoma	Sarcoma
Myoma	Chondrosarcoma
Leiomyoma	Merkel cell tumor
Angiofibroma	Thyroid carcinoma
Hemangioma	Esophageal carcinoma
Chemodectoma	Metastatic carcinoma
Fibroma	
Lipoma	
Adenoma	
Granular cell myoblastoma	
Laryngocele	
Saccular cyst	
Retention cyst	
Amyloidosis	
Pleomorphic adenoma	

     e. Cough
     f. Gastroesophageal reflux disease (GERD)
     g. Trauma
     h. Prior history of neck radiation
  B. Physical examination. A complete head and neck examination should be performed with special consideration of:
     1. Quality of voice: Is it breathy, squeaky, froggy, or staccato?
     2. Stridor: Is it inspiratory or expiratory?
     3. Effort of breathing: Check for retractions and accessory muscles of respiration.

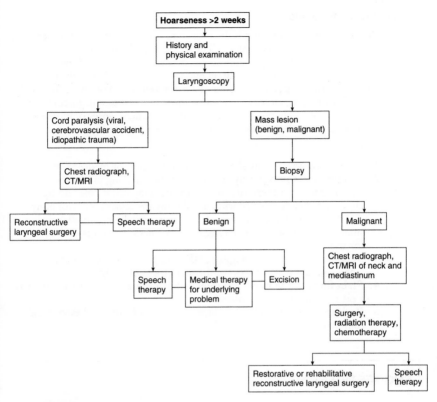

■ **FIGURE 55–1.** Algorithm for the evaluation of hoarseness. *CT* = computed tomography; *MRI* = magnetic resonance imaging.

4. **Nose:** Evaluate patency. Blocked nasal passages may result in chronic mouth breathing, causing laryngopharyngeal mucosal dryness and irritation.
5. **Oral cavity, tongue, and floor of mouth:** Check for inflammation, ulcers, and mucosal or submucosal lesions or masses.
6. **Larynx:** Evaluate appearance and mobility of vocal cords, size of airway, subglottic patency, pyriform sinuses, and postcricoid region.
7. **Neck:** Check for masses, adenopathy, infection, pain, and subcutaneous emphysema. In the trachea, look for deviation and masses. In the thyroid, check for size, consistency, mobility, and pain.
8. **Lymph nodes:** Lymphadenopathy may be present.
C. **Vocal cord paralysis.** If the evaluation of a patient with hoarseness reveals vocal cord paralysis, it is essential to rule out malignancy. Estimates suggest that neoplasm accounts for 10%–20% of cases.

III. Diagnostic Evaluation

A. **Visualization of the larynx** is the cornerstone of evaluation of hoarseness and diagnosis of its true etiology. The larynx is evaluated by using a mirror, a flexible fiberoptic endoscope, or a rigid telescope. Biopsy is dictated by findings during indirect and direct visualization of the larynx.

B. **Oral panendoscopy.** The finding of a paralyzed vocal cord mandates oral panendoscopy (i.e., laryngoscopy, bronchoscopy, and esophagoscopy) to rule out a laryngopharyngeal, esophageal, or tracheal causes of hoarseness.

C. **Purified protein derivative** should be positive in cases of tuberculosis.

D. **Imaging**

1. **Chest radiograph** may show lesions in the chest or mediastinum.

2. A **computed tomography (CT) scan** is the imaging procedure of choice, given its superiority in delineating bony detail. Specifically, the clinician is less concerned with actual bony processes than with bony extension of soft-tissue tumors. CT is extremely helpful in diagnosing submucosal lesions and mass lesions of the neck, as well as evaluating for trauma.

3. **Magnetic resonance imaging (MRI)** may be a suitable alternative when soft-tissue structures are the main focus of study.

4. **Plain films of the neck** may show radio-opaque foreign bodies, such as a piece of bone or metal object.

5. **Barium swallow** would be indicated in cases of suspected esophageal tumors or GERD.

SUGGESTED READING

Gates GA (ed): *Current Therapy in Otolaryngology: Head and Neck Surgery*, 6th ed. St Louis: Mosby, 1998.

56

Sinusitis
Daniel Ervin

I. Definition. Sinusitis is an **inflammatory condition of the paranasal sinuses.**

II. Overview

A. Pathogens. Sinusitis occurs secondary to the extension of nasal and dental infections into the pathogen-free milieu of the paranasal sinuses.

1. The most frequently recovered pathogens are *Streptococcus pneumoniae* and *Haemophilus influenzae,* accounting for more than 75% of the cultured organisms. Additional pathogens such as *Moraxella catarrhalis,* anaerobes, and *Staphylococcus aureus* are also common offenders.

2. Fungi have been increasingly recognized as playing a role in community-acquired sinusitis.

B. Complications of sinusitis

1. **Local complications:** Alteration of the nasal mucosa leads to chronic mucosal inflammation, mucocele/mucopyocele, or osteomyelitis.

2. **Orbital complications:** The eyes are bordered on three sides by sinonasal cavities, making extension of disease more prevalent. Patients may develop orbital cellulitis, dacryocystitis, or superior orbital fissure syndrome.

3. **Central nervous system (CNS) complications** are the most life threatening and include meningitis, brain abscesses, and cavernous sinus thrombosis.

III. Differential Diagnosis. Inflammatory conditions of the nasal cavity and sinuses can be grouped into three broad categories (Table 56–1).

IV. Clinical Evaluation

A. History. The major diagnostic dilemma for most physicians is to differentiate between sinus infection and allergy. Although no true clinical or pathologic classification exists for sinusitis, the following classification of symptoms can help.

1. **Sinus infection**

a. **Major factors** include facial pain or pressure, nasal obstruction or blockage, hypoosmia or anosmia, nasal discharge, and purulence.

b. **Minor factors** include headache, fever, halitosis, fatigue, dental pain, cough, ear pain or pressure, and fullness.

c. Assess for discolored nasal and postnasal drainage

2. **Allergic causes** include itchy, runny nose; paroxysmal sneezing; thin, watery, nasal discharge; nasal obstruction; head pressure; congestion; and a history of sinusitis primarily during allergy season but sometimes perennially.

TABLE 56–1. Differential Diagnosis of Sinusitis

Category	Condition
Infectious causes	Acute infection (> 4 weeks)
	Subacute infection (4–12 weeks)
	Recurrent acute infection (> 4 episodes per year)
	Chronic infection (> 12 weeks)
	Fungal infection
	Granulomatous disease
Allergic rhinosinusitis	Inhalant allergy
	Food allergy
	Chemical allergy
Nonallergic/noninfectious rhinitis	Structural abnormalities: Deviated nasal septum, obstructing masses (intranasal, paranasal, nasopharyngeal, foreign bodies)
	Rhinitis medimentosa: Multiple systemic and topical medications
	Endocrine: Pregnancy, hypothyroidism, diabetes, menstrual cycle
	Irritative: Idiopathic, vasomotor rhinitis, eosinophilic nonallergic rhinitis, mixed cellular rhinitis, nasal mastocytosis
	Other: Postlaryngectomy, tracheostomy rhinitis, recumbent rhinitis, granulomatous disease

B. Physical examination

1. **Nonspecific findings:** Many of the findings on physical examination are nonspecific. Mucosal changes such as edema and thickening, color variations, purulent discharge, posterior pharyngeal changes or drainage, and maxillofacial tenderness to palpation are all suggestive features.

2. **Structural abnormalities** often narrow the sinus ostium, which can lead to infection. The physical examination can often demonstrate areas of obstruction. Predisposing local factors include septal deviation, mucosal hypertrophy from allergic or vasomotor rhinitis, obstructive adenoids, tumors, foreign bodies, and unilateral choanal atresia.

3. **Mucopurulent discharge:** Thick, brown, tenacious nasal secretions suggest extramucosal fungal disease.

V. Diagnostic Evaluation

A. Laboratory studies

1. **Culture**

   a. **Nasal cultures** are often not helpful because the nasal cavity has a number of common bacterial flora.

    b. **Sinus cultures** are sometimes beneficial in chronic infections or for refractory states.

    c. **Special bacterial and fungal smears and cultures** should be obtained as indicated by the history.

2. **Fungal infections:** Both opportunistic and nonopportunistic infections are often confirmed by culture, biopsy, and examination of nasal secretions. Allergic aspergillus sinusitis is substantiated by a positive immunoglobulin G (IgG)-mediated skin test or by antigen-specific serum IgE elevations. Mucormycosis is a very aggressive infection confirmed on biopsy by demonstrating nonseptate, branching hyphae.

3. **Granulomatous diseases** (e.g., tuberculosis, sarcoid, syphilis, Wegener's granulomatosis) can be confirmed after extrinsic medical workup by purified protein derivative, fluorescent treponemal antibody, absorbed test (FTA-ABS), and antineutrophilic cytoplasmic antibody (ANCA). The diagnosis requires heightened clinical suspicion.

4. **Allergy evaluation**

    a. **Inhalant allergy diagnosis:** Using either skin testing or in vitro techniques, the patient is tested for the eight most common antigens found in the geographic area.

    b. **Food allergy diagnosis:** Either provocative neutralization tests or individual deliberate feeding tests may be performed.

    c. **Chemical allergy diagnosis:** Patients should be tested via provocative neutralization.

B. **Imaging studies**

1. **Transillumination** is controversial in its usefulness. It is generally considered insensitive, and positive findings do not necessarily indicate sinusitis.

2. **Nasal endoscopy** is recommended to supplement the clinical evaluation of chronic or recurrent disease.

3. **Plain films:** The diagnostic value of plain films is controversial. Serial plain films document episodes of acute sinusitis. Selective films, rather than the traditional four-view sinus series, may be useful.

4. **Computed tomography (CT) scanning** has become the imaging study of choice for sinus disease. It allows for excellent assessment of soft tissue and bony changes and also helps evaluate extension of disease beyond the sinonasal cavity. Its use is indicated in refractory cases and cases with diagnostic uncertainty or suspicion of malignancy (persistent unilateral symptoms). CT is also used to assess for obstructing lesions.

5. **Magnetic resonance imaging (MRI)** has some role in evaluation. It is best for complications of inflammatory disease, differentiating tumors, fungal sinusitis, or cribriform plate pathology.

SUGGESTED READING

Williams J, Simel D, Roberts L, et al: Clinical evaluation for sinusitis. *Ann Intern Med* 117: 705–710, 1992.

57

Otitis Media
Cliff Megerian

I. **Definition.** Otitis media (OM) is characterized by **inflammation in the middle ear.** Subcategories include acute OM, OM with effusion, recurrent OM, and chronic suppurative OM.

II. **Overview**

A. **Pathophysiology.** The pathophysiology of OM is similar in adults, children, and infants. Eustachian tube obstruction or dysfunction typically results in decreased drainage and ventilation of the middle ear, and hence the development of a relative vacuum and/or negative-pressure phenomenon. An effusion subsequently develops (from a serum transudate or secretions of middle ear mucosa) followed by contamination from upper respiratory tract pathogens including, in order of frequency, *Streptococcus pneumonia, Haemophilus influenzae,* and *Moraxella catarrhalis.*

B. **Course of OM.** Episodes will either be self-limited or proceed to suppuration and drainage via spontaneous eardrum rupture. Antibiotics are given in an attempt to diminish pain and drainage while also decreasing the complication rates of perforation, tympanosclerosis, hearing loss, and central nervous system (CNS) damage.

C. **Etiology**

1. **Causes of OM in children:** OM in children is often a consequence of an underdeveloped and immature eustachian tube that does not adequately ventilate the middle ear and hence results in obstruction and the cascade of events mentioned in II A.

2. **Causes of OM in adults:** In adults, the same scenario may occur if there is eustachian tube obstruction. Obstruction may occur in a variety of settings, such as allergies, congestion, masses of the nasopharynx, barotrauma (e.g., air flight, scuba diving), or in any situation where there can be a pressure lock within the middle ear space.

III. **Clinical Approach to OM**

A. **History**

1. **History in children:** In children, OM is heralded by the presence of pain, irritability, and ear drainage (in the setting of spontaneous eardrum perforation). Tugging or pulling at the ear is an unreliable sign of OM.

2. **Other relevant history** includes pain (acute purulent OM), hearing loss, drainage, popping or a full sensation (eustachian occlusion), headache, alcohol or tobacco abuse (nasopharyngeal carcinoma), and barotrauma.

B. **Physical examination.** The appearance of the tympanic membrane typically reveals erythema and bulging. However, it may simply be opaque with loss of the normal landmarks.

1. **Uncomplicated OM:** An ear that has recently resolved an uncomplicated course of OM may have an amber effusion. Some children who have had chronic OM will have a thick opaque effusion.
2. **Suppurative OM** is heralded by the presence of purulent drainage through the external canal. This can be confused with otitis externa if the drum is not visualized.
3. **Mastoiditis:** The presence of erythema or pain at the mastoid bone, especially over the mastoid tip, suggests mastoiditis. The presence of a fluctuant mass or a bulging retro-auricular area can be indicative of a subperiosteal abscess.
4. **Meningitis:** The finding of fever, stiff neck, and any other meningeal signs, or the presence of paralysis in the distribution of the facial nerve, should raise suspicion for meningitis and intracranial complications of OM.

C. **Therapy.** When OM is identified, therapy is recommended. Treatment often results in prompt resolution of pain within 2–3 days.

IV. Diagnostic Evaluation

A. **Tympanocentesis.** Recurrent OM or effusion that does not resolve in the presence of first- and second-line antibiotics should then be evaluated with tympanocentesis for identification of pathogens and directed antibiotic therapy.
B. **Pneumatic otoscopy** should be included in the otoscopic evaluation. This helps determine the presence of fluid or retraction of the tympanic membrane. If this test is ambiguous, then formal tympanometry will demonstrate normal compliance, retraction, fluid, or perforation.
C. **Indications for computed tomography (CT) scanning**

1. **Cholesteatoma:** The presence of a white mass behind the tympanic membrane raises suspicion for cholesteatoma.
2. **Mastoiditis:** The presence of mastoiditis warrants imaging so as to determine the extent of temporal bone involvement.
3. **Neoplasm:** When the attacks of OM recur frequently, imaging studies are desirable to rule out the presence of a neoplasm.

V. Complications

A. **Persistent infection,** despite appropriate antibiotic therapy, should be addressed by tympanocentesis so the organism may be identified. Persistent infection is quite rare. More commonly, problems result from recurrent infections or a persistent sterile effusion.
B. **Persistent effusion.** It is not uncommon for a case of resolved OM to be associated with persistent effusion for 4–6 weeks after the infection. In this case, only observation is required.
C. **Progression of OM to acute mastoiditis,** an uncommon occurrence, is a problem that needs to be considered when a patient has tenderness over the mastoid and erythema of the mastoid tip. Typically, there is an associated bulging tympanic membrane. If the infection progresses, the pinna becomes displaced outward and forward, and an abscess may develop in the subperiosteal region of the mastoid.
D. **Failure to resolve acute OM or the presence of frequent recurrences** raises suspicion for underlying systemic processes such as atopic disease,

chronic sinusitis, cystic fibrosis, hypogammaglobulinemia, and immotile cilia syndrome. Most commonly, failure to resolve OM implies resistant organisms or failure to achieve adequate drainage. In adults, nasopharyngeal carcinoma should be considered, especially when there are unilateral recurrences.

SUGGESTED READING

Gates GA (ed): *Current Therapy in Otolaryngology-Head and Neck Surgery*, 6th ed. St. Louis, MO: Mosby, 1998.

58

Otitis Externa

Cliff Megerian

I. **Definition.** Otitis externa (OE) is defined by the **presence of pain, itching, and drainage from the ear resulting from infection limited to the external auditory canal.**

II. **Overview.** Typically, the eardrum is intact. The diagnosis is suspected in the patient presenting with exquisite pain, which is exacerbated during examination with the otoscope.

A. **Etiology.** OE commonly results from water contamination to the external canal or from local heat, humidity, or trauma. The patient may not have a clear-cut history of swimming or water exposure. Nonetheless, the presence of moisture initiates the cascade of inflammation, which begins initially with erythema of the squamous epithelium followed by edema and subsequent obliteration of the lumen of the external canal.

B. **Pathogens.** Typical organisms identified include *Pseudomonas aeruginosa*, *Enterobacteriaceae* (60%), *Staphylococcus aureus* (20%), anaerobic unknown organisms (15%), and fungi (e.g., *Candida*, *Aspergillus*) [4%].

C. **Malignant OE.** Patients who are at risk for malignant or progressive necrotizing OE are those with immune deficiencies or diabetes mellitus (DM). These patients can have progression of OE to the point where granulation tissue is visualized in the external canal and chondritis sets in followed by osteomyelitis of the temporal bone and skull base. Subsequent cranial neuropathies may develop.

III. **Clinical Approach to Otitis Externa**

A. **History**

1. **Presenting features:** Patients will complain of muffling and unilateral ear pain. Drainage is often present. There may be a history of swimming or working outside in a humid environment.

2. Inquire about a history of **DM** or an **immunocompromised condition.**

3. Patients with **dermatitis** (seborrhea) or **chronic itching** are predisposed to OE.

4. Patients who complain of itching around the ear that gets worse after application of a neomycin-based regimen may have **drug sensitivity.**

B. **Physical examination**

1. **Painful auricle:** An auricle that is painful on manipulation is often present early in the course of OE. This finding can help differentiate OE from chronic suppurative otitis media (OM).

2. **Otoscopy:** An erythematous and narrowed external auditory canal is often visualized on otoscopy. The erythema may be quite mild. Drainage and exudate that obscures visualization of the tympanic membrane may be present.

3. **Tympanic membrane:** When the tympanic membrane is visualized, it is usually intact but thickened and frequently erythematous. If the tympanic membrane is perforated, ototoxic antimicrobials should be avoided (e.g., neomycin sulfate, gentamicin, tobramycin).
4. **Cellulitis:** Progression of OE to involve cellulitis of the auricle as well as the retro-auricular region is not uncommon and can masquerade as mastoiditis.
5. **Necrotizing or malignant OE:** Granulation tissue at the bony carti-laginous junction indicates the presence of necrotizing or malignant OE (see II C).

C. **Therapy.** In a patient who fails to respond to 1 to 2 courses of appropriate antimicrobial therapy, the potential for a nonbacterial infection must be suspected. Specifically, visualization of fungal elements such as hyphae is suggestive of infection by organisms such as *Aspergillus* or *Candida*. Cultures would be appropriate in this setting.

IV. Diagnostic Evaluation

A. **Cultures.** Most cases of acute OE do not necessitate immediate culture. Instead, empiric therapy directed against *S. aureus* and *P. aeruginosa* is indicated. If drainage and pain fail to resolve with topical and/or oral anti-biotics, a culture is warranted to rule out resistant organisms or fungal causes. A culture should be considered in patients at high risk for compli-cations (i.e., those who are immunocompromised or have DM).
B. **Computed tomography (CT).** Extension of the inflammation medially to involve the eardrum, the presence of a retro-auricular edema, or evidence of mastoid involvement warrants CT to rule out concomitant OM and mastoiditis.
C. **Technicium-99 and gallium scans.** The presence of granulation tissue or an unresponsive case of OE in high-risk patients warrants the use of a technicium-99 scan to detect bony involvement or osteomyelitis. Gallium scanning may be used to monitor response to treatment of osteomyelitis in the temporal bone.

SUGGESTED READING

Gates GA (ed): *Current Therapy in Otolaryngology-Head and Neck Surgery*, 6th ed. St. Louis, MO: Mosby, 1998.

59

Hearing Loss
Cliff Megerian

I. **Definition.** Hearing loss is the **subjective complaint of decreased hearing ability in either one or both ears.**

II. **Overview.** Hearing loss is typically classified as conductive or sensorineural (i.e., nerve related). The majority of cases of progressive sensorineural hearing loss are due to genetic traits, usually autosomal recessive traits. Unilateral hearing loss that is found to be sensorineural should raise a red flag for potential retrocochlear problems, such as acoustic neuroma, meningioma, or other cerebellar pontine angle lesions.

III. **Differential Diagnosis** (Table 59-1)

A. **Conductive hearing loss in children** that is not identified at or around the time of birth and is sudden in onset typically represents an infectious process, such as otitis media (OM) or serous effusion.

B. **Adult conductive hearing loss**

1. **Physical examination** is indispensable in evaluating hearing loss in adults. Findings may include occlusion of the external canal by wax, infection, or a foreign body; otosclerosis; tympanic membrane perforation; and middle ear masses such as cholesteatoma.

2. **Acquired conductive hearing loss:** The most common cause of acquired conductive hearing loss in adults is otosclerosis. Otosclerosis is characterized by the gradual onset of unilateral hearing loss. The diagnosis is supported by the findings of a normal, intact eardrum and a Weber test that lateralizes to the affected ear.

3. **Unilateral serous effusion:** A prolonged history of unilateral serous effusion raises suspicion for nasopharyngeal carcinoma or eustachian tube obstruction.

C. **Adult sensorineural hearing loss.** Hearing loss that is not remedied through addressing external or middle ear concerns is typically shown by audiogram studies to be sensorineural.

1. **Etiology:** Common causes in adults are noise-induced hearing loss, presbycusis, genetic hearing loss, Ménière's disease, and acoustic neuroma.

2. **Viral cochleitis:** Sudden sensorineural hearing loss in adults that is accompanied by the findings of a normal-appearing ear, no effusion, and the complaint of unilateral tinnitus and near-complete hearing loss often suggests the presence of viral cochleitis. Immediate treatment with steroids has a higher incidence of resolution than expectant management. Audiometry can confirm the suspicion.

3. **Acoustic neuroma:** The complaint of sudden unilateral hearing loss can also represent an undetected acoustic neuroma, which is the cause

TABLE 59–1. Differential Diagnosis of Hearing Loss

Conductive hearing loss	Sensorineural hearing loss
External auditory canal occlusion (e.g., from wax)	Congenital
	Hereditary
Otitis externa (OE)	Ototoxicity
Foreign body	
	Noise-induced
Tympanic membrane perforation	Presbycusis
Serous effusion or otitis media (OM)	
	Metabolic
Chronic OM with or without cholesteatoma	Ménière's disease
Otosclerosis	Cochlear otosclerosis
Ossicular discontinuity	Retrochochlear (acoustic tumor, meningioma, multiple sclerosis)
Middle ear tumor, neoplasm, or aural atresia with or without microtia of the auricle	Traumatic (temporal bone fracture, perilymphatic fistula)
	Viral (sudden sensorineural hearing loss)
	Bacterial (meningitis, suppurative labyrinthitis)
	Spirochete (syphilis)
	Autoimmune disorders with or without systemic vasculitis (e.g., autoimmune hearing loss, Wegner's disease, systemic lupus erythematosus)

of 5%–10% of cases of unilateral, adult-onset, sudden sensorineural hearing loss. Ménière's disease may also present this way.

IV. Clinical Evaluation (Figure 59–1)

    A. History

        1. Onset

            a. When hearing loss is of **sudden onset,** assess for pain, pressure, and fever (suggestive of an infectious cause such as OM or serous effusion).

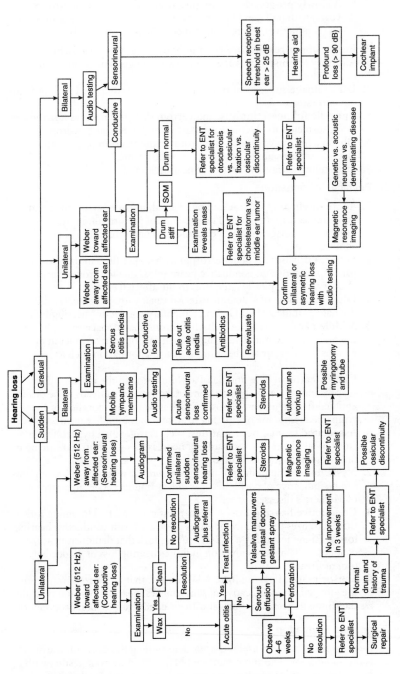

■ **FIGURE 59–1.** Algorithm for the workup of hearing loss. *ENT* = ear, nose, and throat; *SOM* = serous otitis media.

    b. A **slowly progressive onset** (i.e., over the course of months to years) with unilateral hearing loss suggests the presence of otosclerosis (conductive) versus acoustic neuroma (sensorineural).

  2. Recent **upper respiratory tract infection** suggests viral cochleitis.

  3. A history of **noise exposure** and **tinnitus** suggests noise-induced hearing loss.

  4. **Ear drainage** suggests otitis externa (OE) or chronic OM with or without cholesteatoma.

  5. **Episodic fullness, tinnitus,** and **vertigo** that accompanies hearing loss raises suspicion for Ménière's disease or endolymphatic hydrops.

  6. Obtain a history of exposure to **ototoxic medication** (e.g., aminoglycosides, furosemide, chemotherapeutic agents).

  7. Determine the **family history** of hearing loss.

B. Physical examination

  1. **Acute or chronic OM:** A finding of a red, inflamed tympanic membrane indicates acute OM. The presence of perforation in the ear with a history of drainage indicates **chronic OM** and is usually associated with conductive hearing loss.

  2. **Serous effusion:** An intact eardrum with amber fluid in the retrotympanic space indicates conductive hearing loss due to serous effusion. Weber testing typically lateralizes to the affected ear.

  3. **OE:** The finding of a stenotic external canal with white debris and drainage is indicative of OE and temporary conductive hearing loss.

  4. **Middle ear tumor:** Redness in the retrotympanic space can indicate the presence of a middle ear tumor such as glomus tympanicum or glomus jugulare, or an aberrant vascular malformation such as an aberrant carotid artery.

  5. **Cholesteatoma:** The finding of a white lesion in the retrotympanic space is indicative of cholesteatoma. Cholesteatoma needs to be differentiated from tympanosclerosis, which is white discoloration of the tympanic membrane or scarring from previous middle ear infections.

  6. **Associated cranial neuropathies,** such as trigeminal hyperesthesia or facial paralysis, can be indicative of neoplasms such as an acoustic neuroma or glomus jugulare tumor.

  7. **Nystagmus:** The finding of nystagmus with acute onset of hearing loss can be indicative of cochleitis or cochlear trauma versus an active case of Ménière's disease.

  8. **Conductive hearing loss:** A Weber test using a 512-Hz tuning fork that lateralizes to the affected ear is associated with conductive hearing loss. A Rinne test using a 512-Hz tuning fork that demonstrates air conduction < bone conduction indicates hearing loss of 25 decibels (db) or greater.

  9. **Sensorineural hearing loss:** A Weber test that lateralizes away from the affected ear is indicative of sensorineural hearing loss, and typically the Rinne test remains normal with air conduction > bone conduction.

V. Diagnostic Evaluation

  A. Audiogram. The most useful test for determining the cause of hearing loss is the audiogram. The audiogram should include pure-tone testing with bone and air conduction for both ears with appropriate masking.

B. **Tympanogram.** A tympanogram with speech discrimination testing will help diagnose hearing loss and will allow for prognosis of the majority of causes of hearing loss.

C. **Pneumatic otoscopy** that reveals vertigo with positive pressure to the tympanic membrane can be indicative of perilymphatic fistula, a traumatic disruption of the oval or round window with resulting hearing loss.

D. **Laboratory testing** is necessary in only a few instances.

1. **Latent diabetes:** A finding of recurrent OE raises suspicion for latent diabetes and warrants fasting blood glucose level testing.

2. **Immune deficiencies:** Recurrent unexplained OM accompanied by problematic sinusitis and bronchitis in children raises suspicion for immune deficiencies, most commonly immunoglobulin A (IgA) and IgG subclass deficiencies, immotile cilia syndrome, or cystic fibrosis. Appropriate testing is indicated.

3. **Immune-mediated sensorineural hearing loss:** Rapidly progressive, bilateral, unexplained sensorineural hearing loss may be indicative of immune-mediated sensorineural hearing loss and an autoimmune panel including testing for antibodies against the inner ear is indicated (68 kilodalton antibody).

4. **Otic syphilis:** The finding of sudden, unilateral sensorineural hearing loss warrants an evaluation for otic syphilis despite concurrent treatment for likely viral cochleitis.

E. **Neuroimaging.** Magnetic resonance imaging (MRI) of the internal auditory canal and cerebellar pontine angle is indicated in cases of unexplained, unilateral sensorineural hearing loss that is associated with a disparity in speech discrimination between both ears. Meningioma, acoustic neuromas, and demyelinating diseases may be discerned.

F. **Auditory brain-stem response testing** is also used in the workup of asymmetric sensorineural hearing loss, although it has decreased sensitivity in the detection of small acoustic tumors when compared to MRI scanning. It cannot be used in patients who have significant sensorineural hearing loss (i.e., > 60 dB pure-tone average); in these cases, MRI scanning must be used. The main indication for this study is in the workup of asymmetric or unilateral sensorineural hearing loss when MRI is medically contraindicated or not tolerated by a claustrophobic patient.

SUGGESTED READING

Nadol J: Medical progress: Hearing loss. *N Engl J Med* 329(15):1092–1102, 1993.

60

Solitary Neck Mass

Daniel Y. Kim

I. **Background.** For the purposes of diagnosis, it is often convenient to group neck masses into three categories: congenital, inflammatory, and neoplastic lesions (Table 60–1). Further subdivision into midline and lateral lesions will aid in the evaluation.

II. **Clinical Evaluation** (Figure 60–1)

A. **History**

1. **Mode of onset:** In general, inflammatory and traumatic lesions occur over a much shorter period of time than neoplastic lesions. A congenital lesion may be unnoticed until it becomes inflamed during or after a bout of upper respiratory tract infection.

2. **Duration of the mass:** A lesion that has been present for many years without any or only a slight change in size or character is likely benign.

3. **Consistency and character of the mass:** Fluctuant masses tend to be benign. Tender masses tend to be inflammatory. Firm or hard masses tend to be neoplastic.

4. **Mobility of the mass:** Although malignant lesions can be mobile, fixation of the mass makes them more suspicious for malignancy.

5. **Age and gender:** There is a higher incidence of malignancy in adults than in children. Certain malignancies are more common in men, especially smokers (e.g., squamous cell carcinoma of the upper aerodigestive tract manifesting as a metastatic cervical node). Thyroid tumors are more prevalent in women than in men, although a significantly higher percentage of thyroid tumors are malignant in men than in women.

6. **Social history:** There is a very strong correlation between tobacco and alcohol use and squamous cell carcinoma of the upper aerodigestive tract. Poor oral hygiene is also a risk factor.

7. **Family history:** Medullary carcinoma of the thyroid and paragangliomas has a familial tendency.

8. **History of recent trauma:** Trauma may cause edema or hematoma.

9. **History of recent infection:** Infections, such as upper respiratory infection, can cause reactive lymphadenopathy and inflammation of heretofore unnoticed thyroglossal or branchial cleft cyst. Lymphangiomas can also become acutely infected and enlarged during a bout of upper respiratory infection. Obtain a travel history to assess infectious exposures.

10. **Past medical history:** Prior history of malignancy is extremely important since a cervical mass may represent either metastasis or recurrence.

11. **Review of systems:** Evaluate for symptoms of dysphagia, dyspnea, odynophagia, weight loss, choking, aspiration, hoarseness, and regurgitation.

TABLE 60–1. Classification of Neck Masses

Classification	Description
Congenital lesions	Although most congenital lesions manifest themselves early in life, many older patients can present with congenital lesions as well. For diagnostic purposes, congenital lesions of the neck can be divided into midline and lateral masses:
	Midline cervical mass: Thyroglossal duct cyst, dermoid cyst, lymph node (delphian node) cyst, and lipoma
	Lateral cervical mass: Branchial cleft cyst and sinus, cystic hygroma; hemangioma; thyroid cyst; parotid cyst; thymus remnant; congenital muscular torticollis
Inflammatory lesions	Bacterial and viral infections often produce lateral neck masses. Diagnostic considerations include lymphadenopathy, submandibular sialadenitis, parotitis, infectious mononucleosis, cat-scratch disease, tuberculosis, sarcoidosis, HIV, toxoplasmosis, actinomycosis, brucellosis, neck abscess, localized edema, and hematoma.
Neoplastic lesions	In metastatic carcinoma to a cervical node, the primary site is in the head and neck (85%), but it can also metastasize from a site below the clavicles such as the lung, breast, gastrointestinal tract and genitourinary tract, including prostate and ovaries. Seventy percent of nasopharyngeal carcinomas will initially present as a metastatic neck mass.
	Specific malignancies to consider include lymphoma, thyroglossal carcinoma, bronchogenic carcinoma, thyroid carcinoma, salivary gland carcinoma, chondrosarcoma, rhabdomyosarcoma, fibromatoses (desmoid tumors), fibrosarcoma, myxofibrosarcoma, neurofibrosarcoma, and neuroblastoma.
	Specific benign neoplasms to consider include hemangioma, lymphangioma, fibroma, lipoma, thyroid nodule, parathyroid cyst, benign salivary gland tumors, neurogenous tumors, paragangliomas, and laryngocele.

B. Physical examination

1. **Head and neck region:** The entire head and neck region should be thoroughly evaluated by visual inspection, palpation, and indirect or endoscopic visualization of the upper aerodigestive tract.
2. **Ears, nose, and nasal membranes:** Look for signs of edema, inflammation, ulceration, mass lesions, and obstruction. Check for mobility of tympanic membranes to rule out middle ear infection or mass. A pulsatile mass behind the drum may be seen. Check for cutaneous lesions on the auricle and mastoid.
3. **Nasopharynx:** Tumors are readily visible as either a mass lesion or as

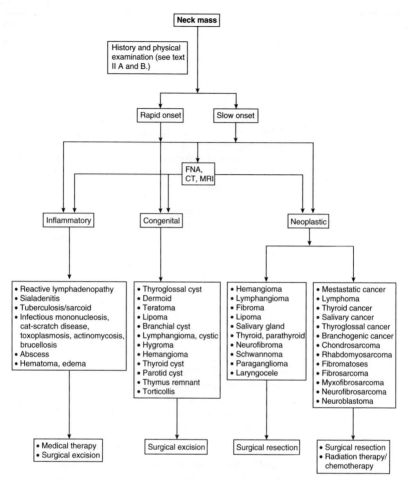

■ FIGURE 60–1. Algorithm for the workup of patients with neck mass. *CT* = computed tomography; *FNA* = fine-needle aspiration; *MRI* = magnetic resonance imaging.

ulceration. If tumors are large, they can cause choanal obstruction, eustachian tube dysfunction, or both.

4. **Oral cavity and oropharynx:** Examine and palpate the mucosa for lesions, inflammation, or ulceration. Carefully examine the tonsillar fossae, base of tongue, vallecula, epiglottis, and posterior and lateral pharyngeal wall. Manually palpate these structures if necessary, and check for symmetry of form and function.

5. **Larynx and hypopharynx** (direct/indirect laryngoscopy): Note the mobility of vocal cords, color and size of the true and false cords, size of the glottic airway, subglottis, arytenoids, laryngeal surface of epiglottis,

pyriform sinuses, and postcricoid regions. Check for pooling in the pyriform sinuses, which may be indicative of a mass lesion.

6. **Face, neck, and scalp:** Visual inspection and manual palpation of the face, neck, and scalp is important. Note the location, size, number, consistency, mobility, and tenderness of the mass. Check for signs of inflammation, compression, or deviation of adjacent structures.

7. **Complete examination:** Perform a complete examination to assess pulmonary structures, breasts, lymph nodes, and abdomen. Perform rectal and pelvic examinations to assess primary sites of tumor or infection.

III. Diagnostic Evaluation

A. **Fine-needle aspiration (FNA) biopsy** is a quick and simple way to make a fairly accurate diagnosis. It will yield information on whether the lesion is solid or cystic, absence or presence of malignant cells and, at times, even the cell type. There is no danger of seeding the tract in case of malignancy.

B. **Computed tomography (CT) and magnetic resonance imaging (MRI).** CT is the preferred study in the head and neck because of its ability to define bony and cartilaginous detail, including erosion and invasion. MRI gives greater detail and information about soft tissues. At times, both studies are indicated.

C. **Panendoscopy.** In cases of suspected malignancy, in addition to CT and MRI, the workup should include panendoscopy (i.e., direct laryngoscopy, bronchoscopy, and esophagoscopy). If a primary tumor is found on panendoscopy, there is no indication or need to biopsy the neck mass. If no primary tumor is found after an appropriately exhaustive search, an incisional or excisional biopsy is indicated to make a definitive diagnosis.

IV. Diagnosis

A. **Benign lesions.** In most instances, the history and physical examination, radiographic studies, and FNA will be sufficient to make a diagnosis of a benign lesion. If a benign lesion is diagnosed, the treatment of choice is surgical excision. In certain instances, observation may be appropriate. If FNA biopsy is inconclusive, either an excisional or incisional biopsy of the lesion may be required.

B. **Malignant lesions.** If a malignancy is suspected or noted on FNA, every effort should be made to find the primary lesion, and the urge to biopsy the mass should be suppressed. Untimely incisional or excisional biopsy will increase the chance of local recurrence.

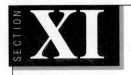

Pulmonary

61

Cough

Majid Yazdani

I. **Definition.** Cough is a **sudden explosive forcing of air through the glottis, occurring immediately on opening the previously closed glottis, and incited by mechanical or chemical irritation of the trachea or bronchi or by pressure from adjacent structures.**

II. **Overview**

    A. Cough is the **most common complaint for which patients seek medical attention** and the second most common reason for a medical examination.

    B. **Pathophysiology.** Effective cough is generally desired to enhance clearing of excess mucus and the irritants found in the airways. Mechanical irritant receptors, which are most numerous along the posterior wall of the trachea, carina, and the branching points of the large airways, represent the afferent limb of the cough reflex. The signals are carried via the vagus nerve to the central nervous system (CNS), ultimately arriving at the presumed cough center. A reflex arc is established with efferent input to the respiratory muscles and larynx initiating the cough.

    C. **Etiology**

        1. **Common causes:** The most common causes of chronic cough in the nonsmoker, not on an angiotensin-converting enzyme (ACE) inhibitor, who has a normal chest radiograph, are postnasal drip, asthma, and gastroesophageal reflux disease (GERD). These causes may occur either singly or in combination.

        2. **Postnasal drip** either singly, or in combination with other conditions, is the single most common cause of chronic cough for which patients seek medical attention.

III. **Differential Diagnosis** (Table 61–1)

IV. **Notes on the Differential Diagnosis**

    A. **Acute cough.** Although no definitive studies are available, clinical experience suggests that the most common cause of cough is postnasal drip. Acute cough in the elderly may be the manifestation of more serious underlying disease [e.g., pneumonia, pulmonary embolism, congestive

TABLE 61–1. Differential Diagnosis of Cough

Acute (< 3 weeks)	Chronic (> 3 weeks)
Viral upper respiratory infection	Postviral bronchitis
Bacterial infection	Chronic bronchitis
Pulmonary edema	Asthma
Pulmonary embolism	Postnasal drip syndrome
Aspiration pneumonitis	Drug-induced
Inhalation of irritants	Gastroesophageal reflux disease (GERD)
Foreign body	Smoker's cough
External or middle ear disease	Neoplasm
	Mitral stenosis
	Cystic fibrosis
	Aortic aneurysm
	Pacemaker wires
	Interstitial pulmonary fibrosis
	Bronchiectasis
	Abscess
	Chronic aspiration

heart failure (CHF)]. As the elderly often lack typical manifestations, diagnostic testing should be considered early in the evaluation.

B. **Postnasal drip.** There is no specific sign or symptom that is diagnostic for postnasal drip. The patient may have no symptoms other than a chronic cough. Thus, a favorable response to therapy with resolution of the symptom is crucial in establishing postnasal drip as the cause of cough.

C. **Asthma** is defined as the cause of chronic cough only with the disappearance of cough following treatment with appropriate asthma medications (see Chapter 65, Asthma).

D. **GERD.** Patients with GERD may manifest cough as their only symptom, lacking other gastrointestinal symptoms 75% of the time.

E. **Chronic bronchitis.** This is among the most common causes of cough in the community, but is a less common cause for patients seeking medical attention. Presumably, this is due to the prevalence of tobacco abuse among patients with chronic bronchitis, who appropriately identify tobacco use as the cause of their symptom.

F. **Induced by ACE inhibitors.** The time of onset can be variable, anywhere from immediate (i.e., within 1 week) to months after the initiation of the medication.

G. **Bronchogenic carcinoma.** Suspect bronchogenic carcinoma in the smoker with a change in his/her cough pattern, in patients with red flag symptoms (see V A 6), and in patients with high-risk occupational exposures (e.g., working with asbestos or uranium). The incidence of this disorder in patients being evaluated for chronic cough is less than 2%.

V. **Clinical Approach to Cough.** The history and physical examination are the mainstays in evaluating the patient with cough. This information permits a focused evaluation to be pursued.

A. **History**

1. **Postnasal drip:** Patient will present with the frequent need to "clear their throat" (they will do so often during the visit), hoarseness, something dripping into the throat, nasal congestion, nasal discharge, sinus tenderness, or discomfort. Assess for a history of prior upper respiratory infection, use of medications (e.g., decongestants, illicit drugs), occupational exposures, and environmental irritants.

2. **Cough-variant asthma:** Elicit a family history of asthma or a personal history of atopy. Identify triggers (e.g., cold, exercise, environmental), as well as the characteristic symptoms of wheezing and dyspnea.

3. **GERD:** Patients may present with heartburn, a sour taste in their mouth, or complications of chronic heartburn such as spasm (chest pain or pressure) or stricture (dysphagia). Symptoms may be positional and are worse postprandially or with recumbency.

4. **Medications:** Cough associated with ACE inhibitors is generally described as an irritating, tickling, dry cough.

5. **Other features** of the history include tobacco abuse, change in pattern of cough (especially in a smoker), productive cough, dyspnea, occupational or environmental exposures, and prior evaluation or treatments for cough.

6. Assess for **red flag symptoms,** including hemoptysis, weight loss, night sweats, fever, constitutional symptoms, and concomitant risk factors for head and neck malignancy.

B. **Physical examination.** After a thorough history, a focused physical examination may help to elucidate the underlying cause of cough.

1. **Head and neck:** Focus on sinus congestion and tenderness, signs of lymphadenopathy, tracheal position, thyroid enlargement, nodularity, and tenderness. Assess the nasal turbinates, looking for hypertrophy and polyps. The pharynx may be noted with drainage, mucopurulent secretions, or "cobblestoning" (which is suggestive of chronic postnasal drip).

2. **Pulmonary examination:** Note the presence of crackles, wheezes, or diminished breath sounds. Localized wheezing suggests bronchiectasis or an obstructing mass.

3. **Cardiac examination:** The cardiac examination should identify evidence of CHF, valvular disease, or cardiomyopathy. Assess for the presence of jugular vein distention, a third heart sound (S_3), a displaced apical impulse, or the auscultatory finding of significant valvular disease.

VI. Diagnostic Evaluation

A. **Acute cough.** In the setting of acute cough, diagnostic testing is generally undertaken when:

1. **Comorbidities are present** (e.g., underlying pulmonary disease, malignancy)
2. **A complicating diagnosis is suspected** (e.g., pneumonia, CHF, pulmonary embolism)
3. **Complicating signs or symptoms are present** (e.g., fever, hemoptysis, dyspnea)

B. **Chronic cough** (see Appendix B for Chronic Cough algorithm)

1. **Initial assessment:** The initial assessment of patients with chronic cough includes a history (focusing on the common causes and red flag symptoms), physical examination, and chest radiograph. If the diagnosis is still uncertain, a therapeutic trial consisting of treatment for postnasal drip is recommended.
2. **Laboratory investigation:** Outside of baseline evaluation or assessment of comorbid symptomatology, laboratory studies do not have a definitive role in the evaluation of chronic cough. However, chest radiography should not be overlooked in evaluating the patient presenting with chronic cough.

C. **Postnasal drip**

1. **Diagnostic evaluation**

   a. **History** is the primary method for diagnosis.
   b. **Sinus radiographs** (four-view) may be able to detect signs of chronic sinusitis, but this will not confirm that postnasal drip is the cause of chronic cough. Specifically, sinus radiographs have a positive predictive value of 81% and a negative predictive value of 95% for predicting that chronic sinusitis was responsible for the postnasal-drip–induced cough.
   c. **Sinus computed tomography (CT) scans:** Insufficient data exist about the value and utility of sinus CT scans and the predictive value in the setting of chronic cough.

2. **Treatment:** Prior to initiating an evaluation for postnasal drip in the low-risk patient, a course of empiric therapy should be undertaken. If the cough does not respond to therapeutic interventions, further evaluation is indicated. It is important to ensure that therapy is aggressive, compliance is assessed, and the trial is of adequate duration (i.e., at least 4 weeks).

D. **Cough-variant asthma** (see Chapter 65, Asthma)

1. **Diagnostic evaluation**

   a. **Reversible airflow obstruction:** The presence of reversible airflow obstruction does not guarantee this as the cause of symptoms.

    b. **Response to therapy supports the diagnosis.** The effectiveness of anti-inflammatory medications may take several weeks to manifest.

  2. **Treatment:** The clinician may attempt a therapeutic trial with beta-agonist therapy prior to pursuing formal pulmonary function tests (especially if there is a recent upper respiratory infection or abnormal peak flows). If no clinical response is noted, the diagnosis of asthma is not excluded. Further diagnostic testing is indicated.

E. GERD

  1. **Diagnostic evaluation:** The ideal candidate for evaluation of GERD-related cough has failed treatment trials for postnasal drip and asthma, has a normal chest radiograph, does not smoke, and is not on an ACE inhibitor.

    a. The most sensitive and specific evaluation is **24-hour ambulatory esophageal monitoring** (sensitivity for GERD > 90%).

    b. Other evaluations may include **esophagogastroduodenoscopy** to assess for mucosal damage as a result of reflux.

    c. **Barium swallow or radionuclide studies** may provide important clues as well, but may not be as definitive as the pH-probe.

  2. **Treatment:** The clinician may undertake a therapeutic trial (with a proton pump inhibitor) prior to diagnostic testing. It is important to note that the cough may take several months to resolve in this setting. Failure to respond to an empiric therapeutic trial does not exclude the diagnosis.

F. Induced by ACE inhibitors

  1. **Diagnostic evaluation**

    a. There are **no diagnostic tests** to evaluate for cough induced by an ACE inhibitor.

    b. The **diagnosis is confirmed** when the cough improves or disappears after stopping the drug.

  2. **Treatment:** If a patient presents with cough and is taking an ACE inhibitor, cessation of the drug is recommended. Improvement should be noted within 4 weeks.

G. Bronchiectasis. Patients with this condition have cough as a cardinal manifestation. Conversely, however, bronchiectasis is an uncommon cause of chronic cough. Chest radiographs and high-resolution CT are diagnostic.

SUGGESTED READING

Irwin R, Boulet L, Cloutier M, et al: Managing cough as a defense mechanism and as a symptom. *Chest* 114(2, supplement), 133s–181s, 1998.

Irwin R, Madison JM: The diagnosis and treatment of cough. *NEJM* 343(23):1715–1721, 2000.

62

Dyspnea
Frederick Curley

I. **Definition.** Dyspnea refers to **shortness of breath.**
II. **Overview**
   A. **Mild dyspnea is common.** Dyspnea intensity is modified by learning, experience, and emotional/behavioral state. No single neurologic pathway mediates the sensation of dyspnea. Multiple stimuli, receptors, nerves, and pathways are involved and moderated by cognitive factors.
   B. **Although hypoxemia and hypercapnia are important stimuli for dyspnea,** information regarding load, effort, and impedance from muscle afferents are probably more clinically important. For example, it is the change in muscle afferent data, not chemoreceptor data, which mediates relief of dyspnea after thoracentesis. Dyspnea in most diseases persists even when hypoxemia is corrected.

III. **Differential Diagnosis.** The differential diagnosis varies primarily with acuity and age (Table 62–1).
IV. **Notes on the Differential Diagnosis**
   A. **Common causes.** As five disease groups account for 75%–94% of the causes of chronic dyspnea, these disease groups should always be screened first. The five disease groups are cardiac, pulmonary, psychogenic, deconditioning, and gastroesophageal reflux disease (GERD).
   B. **Less common causes.** The common causes of dyspnea are frequently overdiagnosed when a less common cause of dyspnea is actually present. The cause of dyspnea should always be confirmed by diagnostic testing or by a documented response to specific therapy.
   C. **Multiple causes.** Approximately one-third of patients have multiple causes of dyspnea. This fact suggests that a sequential systematic evaluation is necessary.
   D. **Pacemakers.** The presence of a pacemaker should prompt consideration of a pacemaker syndrome; 65% of patients with VVI pacing, due to superimposition of atrioventricular contraction, develop elevation of the wedge pressure.
   E. **Hyperventilation–anxiety syndrome.** This diagnosis may be suggested by associated symptoms of panic, undue fear and anxiety, or frequent sighing. The hyperventilation provocative test asks the patient to hyperventilate by taking deep breaths, up to 30–40 breaths per minute, until dizziness occurs or 5 minutes have passed. If the patient's symptoms of dyspnea are reproduced, the test is scored as positive. Most physicians recommend excluding cardiopulmonary diagnoses before making a diagnosis of hyperventilation–anxiety syndrome.

TABLE 62–1. Differential Diagnosis of Dyspnea

Symptom	Possible diagnoses
Acute dyspnea	Anxiety–hyperventilation syndrome Cardiac: Angina, arrhythmia, pulmonary edema, pericarditis Pulmonary: Asthma, chronic obstructive pulmonary disease (COPD), pneumothorax, pulmonary embolism, noncardiogenic edema, gastroesophageal reflux disease (GERD) Trauma: Contusion, rib fracture, laryngeal-tracheobronchial injury Upper airway: Laryngospasm, epiglottitis, foreign body, pneumonia
Chronic moderate-to-severe dyspnea	Cardiac: Arrhythmia, cardiomyopathy, ischemia, pacemaker syndrome, valvular disease Pulmonary: Asthma, COPD, interstitial lung disease GERD Anxiety–hyperventilation syndrome Deconditioning Obesity
Mild dyspnea	Anxiety–hyperventilation syndrome Deconditioning Common cold Obesity Postnasal drip syndrome Pregnancy

V. A Clinical Approach to Dyspnea

A. Background

1. **Acute dyspnea:** The combination of all historical elements and physical examination findings is helpful in diagnosing the cause of acute dyspnea in 66%–97% of cases.
2. **Chronic dyspnea:** In contrast, chronic dyspnea is identified from the history and physical examination findings only 66% of the time.

B. History

1. **Vague descriptions:** Many patients have a hard time describing dyspnea; therefore, taking a thorough history may confirm that the patient is really complaining about uncomfortable breathing. Patients with dyspnea may describe their breathing as inappropriate with:

   a. **Timing:** "I cannot breathe fast enough."
   b. **Quantity:** "I cannot get a deep breath or need more air."
   c. **Effort:** "I struggle to breathe."
   d. **Quality:** "My air is bad or my chest is raw when I breathe."

2. **Intensity:** The intensity of dyspnea is usually described by how much activity the patient can perform. The physician should ask what tasks can no longer be performed due to dyspnea, which tasks require the patient to slow down or pause, and which tasks can be done continuously but with an increased sense of effort.
3. **Exclusion of conditions:** History is most helpful in ruling out common conditions or suggesting rare ones.

   a. The fact that the patient has never smoked rules out **tobacco-induced chronic obstructive pulmonary disease (COPD).** A history of smoking, on the other hand, is only 20% predictive of a diagnosis of COPD.
   b. The absence of wheezing, throat clearing, or a sensation of postnasal drip rules out **upper airway disease** with predictive values of 88%–97%.

4. **Specific questions** regarding change in weight, exercise habits, occupational exposures, asthmatic triggers, cardiac risk factors, psychiatric history, sources of stress and anxiety, or symptoms suggestive of GERD should always be asked.
5. **Lung cancer:** Sixty-five percent of patients with lung cancer have dyspnea during the course of their disease, and 15% have dyspnea as the presenting symptom.
6. **Pregnancy:** Dyspnea is extremely common in pregnancy; however, dyspnea hindering daily activities is unusual and should prompt further evaluation.

C. **Physical examination.** Due to the wide spectrum of causes of dyspnea, a full physical examination is warranted. However, solitary findings on physical examination have low predictive value in establishing a diagnosis. The utility of the physical examination is only realized in the context of the entire clinical picture.

1. **Weight** and **height** should always be measured. Dyspnea occurs in 76% of men and 93% of women 53–57 years of age with a body mass index of 30 kg/m^2.
2. The **absence of crackles** is 98% predictive in ruling out interstitial lung diseases as the cause of dyspnea.

VI. Laboratory Assessment

A. **Specific diagnosis.** Whenever the history and physical examination suggest a specific diagnosis, that diagnosis should be initially evaluated (Figures 62–1 and 62–2).

1. **Acute dyspnea:** A chest radiograph, electrocardiogram (ECG), and peak flow measurements represent the initial series of studies.

   a. If there is **stridor** or **inability to phonate,** laryngoscopy, a lateral neck radiograph or computed tomography (CT) should be performed.
   b. **Pulmonary embolism** should always be ruled out when suspected or if other tests are not diagnostic. A ventilation-perfusion scan remains the initial diagnostic procedure of choice.

2. **Chronic dyspnea:** Initial screening tests include a chest radiograph, ECG, oximetry at rest and on walking, and peak flow measurements.

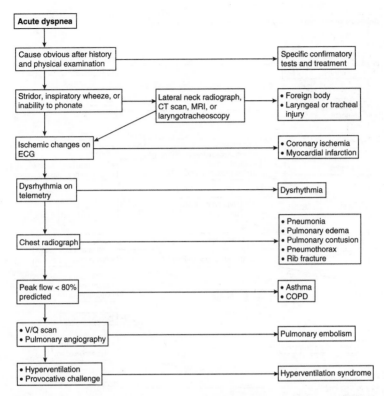

■ **FIGURE 62–1.** Algorithm for the evaluation of acute dyspnea. *COPD* = chronic obstructive pulmonary disease; *CT* = computed tomography; *ECG* = electrocardiogram; *MRI* = magnetic resonance imaging; *V/Q* = ventilation-perfusion.

*Arrows pointing down indicate normal or nondiagnostic results. Arrows pointing right indicate abnormal or diagnostic results.

Tests with high predictive value should be performed early in the evaluation and should serve as diagnostic branch points.

a. Chest radiograph [positive predictive value (PPV) 0.75; negative predictive value (NPV) 0.91]
b. Bronchoprovocation challenge (PPV 0.95; NPV 1.00)
c. Spirometry (PPV 0.32; NPV 1.00)
d. Diffusing capacity (PPV 0.79; NPV 0.95)

B. Unclear diagnosis

1. **Comprehensive gas exchange exercise testing (CPEX)** has a PPV of 0.93. Many clinicians recommend CPEX as the initial screening test when the diagnosis is unclear. CPEX is the only test that confirms the absence or diagnosis of cardiopulmonary disease. It can also confirm the presence of psychogenic (inappropriate hyperventilation) or deconditioning.

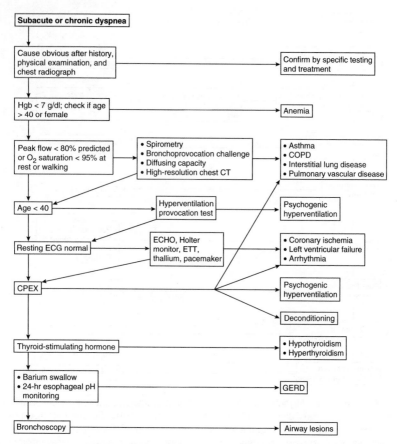

■ **FIGURE 62–2.** Algorithm for the evaluation of subacute or chronic dyspnea in adults. *COPD* = chronic obstructive pulmonary disease; *CPEX* = comprehensive gas exchange exercise testing; *CT* = computed tomography; *ECG* = electrocardiogram; *ECHO* = echocardiography; *ETT* = exercise tolerance test; *GERD* = gastroesophageal reflux disease; *Hgb* = hemoglobin.

*Arrows pointing down indicate normal or nondiagnostic results. Arrows pointing right indicate abnormal or diagnostic results.

    2. **Rhinolaryngotracheoscopy:** Patients with upper airway symptoms, such as stridor, should undergo rhinolaryngotracheoscopy.
    3. **Ambulatory esophageal pH monitoring:** GERD may be clinically silent except for the symptom of dyspnea and may require ambulatory esophageal pH monitoring to confirm the diagnosis.

63

Evaluation of Pleural Effusions
Eric Alper

I. Overview

A. **Definition.** Pleural effusion is defined as an increased amount of fluid in the pleural cavity. It is a common problem in clinical medicine.

B. **Dual challenge.** The challenge with evaluating pleural effusions is attempting to identify the underlying cause of the effusion as well as minimize fluid accumulation.

II. Pathophysiology

A. **Fluid accumulation.** The pleural space normally contains a small amount of fluid, generally less than 20 ml. Fluid accumulates in this space when the rate of fluid production exceeds the rate of removal. There are two primary mechanisms through which this occurs:

   1. **Transudate:** The pressure gradient favors secretion of fluid from capillary beds (via hydrostatic and oncotic pressure mechanisms). Fluid that accumulates in this fashion is generally referred to as transudate.

   2. **Exudate:** There is excessive capillary leak of the pleural vessels, generally as a result of inflammation of the pleura. Fluid that accumulates in this fashion is generally referred to as exudate.

B. **Additional causes.** There are additional ways by which fluid may accumulate, such as fluid in the peritoneal cavity crossing through the diaphragm or through thoracic duct injury, where rupture or obstruction may occur, leading to accumulation of lymph (chylothorax).

III. Differential Diagnosis (Table 63–1). The most common causes of pleural effusion are, in order, congestive heart failure (CHF)/fluid overload, pneumonia, and malignancy (i.e., direct infiltration of pleura).

IV. Notes on the Differential Diagnosis

A. **Tuberculous pleural effusion.** The most common site for extrapulmonary tuberculosis is the pleura. Patients with tuberculous pleural effusion may have no other signs of lung disease on chest radiography. Hallmarks of tuberculous effusions include exudative, pH usually 7.3–7.4, and low glucose (may be < 30 mg/dl). It is rare to recover acid-fast bacilli from thoracentesis.

B. **Empyema** is a pleural effusion that is grossly purulent and frequently form loculations. Empyema requires immediate surgical drainage.

C. **Parapneumonic effusion.** When a patient develops a pleural effusion associated with pneumonia, it is referred to as a parapneumonic effusion.

   1. **Types:** Simple parapneumonic effusion may resolve with resolution of the pneumonia. Complicated parapneumonic effusions have the potential to become an empyema.

TABLE 63–1. Differential Diagnosis of Pleural Effusion

Transudate	Exudate
Congestive heart failure (CHF)	Malignancy (e.g., of the lung, breast, ovary, gastric, lymphoma most common)
Cirrhosis	
	Infectious:
Nephrotic syndrome	Parapneumonic effusion
	Tuberculosis
Peritoneal dialysis	
	Pancreatitis (usually left-sided effusion)
Atelectasis	
	Esophageal rupture
Pulmonary embolism	
	Collagen vascular diseases:
Hypoalbuminemia	Systemic lupus erythematosus
	Rheumatoid arthritis
Superior vena cava obstruction	
	Drug-induced effusion
Sarcoidosis	
	Chylothorax
Myxedema	
	Hemothorax
	Postsurgical effusion
	Trauma

2. **Thoracentesis:** While somewhat controversial, it is generally recommended that all patients with parapneumonic effusions undergo thoracentesis. It is difficult to predict which parapneumonic effusions will become complicated.

    a. Free-flowing parapneumonic effusions in which the pH > 7.30, glucose > 60, and lactate dehydrogenase (LDH) < 1000 are unlikely to organize and, therefore, require surgical drainage.

    b. If the pleural pH is < 7.10, glucose < 40, and LDH > 1000, there is a higher likelihood that the effusion will require surgical debridement, and many physicians recommend early chest tube placement.

  D. Pulmonary embolism and **sarcoidosis** are the most common conditions that can present with either a transudate or exudate.

V. Clinical Approach (Figure 63–1). The history and physical examination are directed toward assessing symptoms resultant from and causative of the effusion. Given the broad range of causes, the history and examination should be comprehensive.

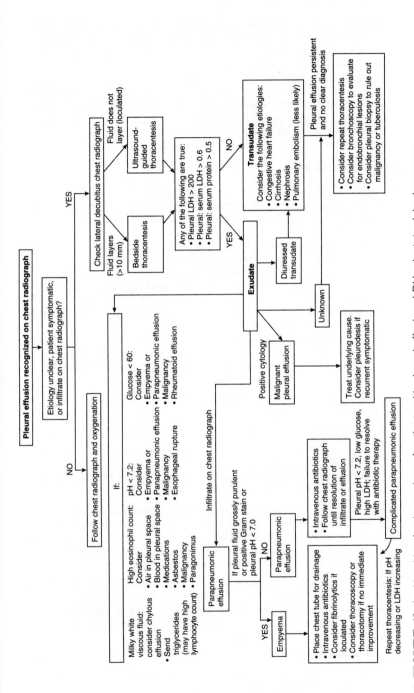

■ **FIGURE 63–1.** Algorithm for the workup of patients with pleural effusion. *LDH* = lactate dehydrogenase.

A. History. Assess for dyspnea, chest pain (pleuritic, anginal), cough, fever, sputum production, weight loss, tobacco abuse, risk factors for deep venous thrombosis, trauma, travel, medications, invasive procedures, and dermatologic and rheumatologic symptoms.

B. Physical examination. Assess for reduced breath sounds, wheezing, bronchial breath sounds, a third heart sound (S_3), displaced point of apical impulse, elevated jugular venous pressure, auscultatory evidence of significant valvular disease, peripheral swelling, ascites or stigmata of chronic liver disease, and lymphadenopathy. Perform a breast, pelvic, and rectal examination.

VI. Diagnostic Evaluation

A. Radiologic guidance

1. **Plain radiography** will contribute information toward identifying the cause of effusion, such as heart size, presence of infiltrate, nodules, or lymphadenopathy.

2. **Chest radiography:** Pleural effusion is most frequently diagnosed on chest radiography. Findings suggestive of pleural effusion include blunting of the costophrenic angle and the presence of a meniscus posteriorly on a lateral chest view. This generally occurs with approximately 150 ml of fluid. However, the chest radiograph does not reach 100% sensitivity for diagnosis of pleural effusion until there is greater than 500 ml of pleural fluid.

3. **Lateral decubitus films** are used to define whether or not a pleural effusion is loculated, and can provide an additional estimate of the volume of fluid. It is better than plain films at detecting small effusions.

B. Thoracentesis. It is generally safe to perform thoracentesis without radiologic guidance if the pleural fluid layer is > 10 mm.

1. **Indications:** Thoracentesis is indicated primarily for:

   a. **Diagnostic purposes,** when the pleural effusion cannot be easily explained by the clinical presentation

   b. **Therapeutic purposes** to relieve dyspnea, drain infection, and prevent complications

2. **Contraindications:** There are no absolute contraindications to thoracentesis, but relative contraindications include anticoagulation, bleeding diathesis, small volume of fluid ($\leq$ 10 mm by imaging study), mechanical ventilation, an uncooperative patient, tapping a postpneumonectomy space, and an overlying skin disease.

C. Pleural fluid analysis. Various studies may be performed on pleural fluid to help determine the underlying cause. There are few conditions for which there is a single pleural test that clinches the diagnosis. Initial studies are directed at determining whether the fluid is transudate or exudate.

1. **Chemistries**

   a. **Exudate versus transudate:** Fluid is considered exudative if it meets one of the following criteria:

(1) Pleural fluid: LDH ≥ 200
(2) Pleural:serum LDH ratio ≥ 0.6
(3) Pleural:serum protein ≥ 0.5

b. **New criteria:** Recent meta-analyses have shown that the following criteria are as accurate in identifying an exudate:

(1) Pleural LDH above 0.45 of upper limits of normal serum values
(2) Pleural cholesterol > 45 mg/dl
(3) Pleural protein > 2.9 g/dl

c. **LDH criteria:** If exudate is determined by LDH criteria alone, cancer and parapneumonic effusion should be strongly considered.

2. **Fluid appearance:** The appearance of pleural fluid may be informative.

a. A **milky, viscous pleural fluid** suggests chylothorax or pseudochylothorax. Triglyceride level and lymphocyte count should be obtained.
b. If the fluid is **grossly bloody,** a finding of > 100,000/mm³ red blood cells (RBCs) is suggestive of trauma, malignancy, and pulmonary embolism. If the fluid hematocrit approaches the blood hematocrit (ratio > 50%), the effusion is a hemothorax.
c. If the fluid is **grossly purulent,** it is an empyema.
d. **Straw-colored fluid** is not helpful in classifying the effusion.

3. **Cell count**

a. **RBCs** > 100,000/mm³ are frequently seen in malignancy, trauma, and pulmonary embolism.
b. **White blood cells** (WBCs): The differential of WBCs is more important than the absolute number of cells.

(1) **Neutrophils > 50%** are seen in any acute inflammatory or infectious process, such as parapneumonic effusion or empyema.
(2) **Lymphocytes > 50%** are seen in lymphoma or malignancy, tuberculosis, fungal infections, sarcoid, and postpericardiotomy syndrome.
(3) **Elevated eosinophils** are seen in patients with air or blood in the pleural space, malignancy, drugs, parasitic infection, asbestos-related conditions, and Churg-Strauss syndrome. High eosinophils contraindicate tuberculosis.

4. **Cytology studies** are positive in 66% of samples ultimately found to have malignant pleural effusions. Repeated thoracentesis will increase the yield.
5. **Culture and Gram stain:** If the Gram stain is positive for organisms, it is an empyema.
6. A **pH < 7.2** is seen in empyema, complicated parapneumonic effusion, rheumatoid disease, esophageal rupture, tuberculosis, and sometimes malignancy.
7. **Glucose < 60 mg/dl** is seen in empyema, complicated parapneumonic effusion, rheumatoid disease, malignancy, and tuberculosis.
8. **Specialized studies** on pleural fluid can be used in the appropriate clinical scenario:

a. **Amylase > 200** is seen in acute pancreatitis and esophageal rupture.

    b. Rheumatoid factor $> 1:320$ is very supportive of rheumatoid effusion.

    c. Antinuclear antibody $> 1:160$ is seen in lupus pleuritis.

    d. Carcinoembryonic antigen (CEA) > 10 indicates malignancy.

    e. Adenosine deaminase > 43 **U/l** indicates tuberculous pleuritis.

    f. Pleural biopsy (via thoracoscopy) is indicated for evaluation of exudative pleural effusion of unclear etiology. The most common indication is to evaluate for potential pleural tuberculosis, and it may improve the yield for malignancy as well.

SUGGESTED READING

Bartter T, Santorelli R, Akers S, et al: The evaluation of pleural effusion, *Chest* 106:1209–1214, 1994.

Light RW: Diagnostic principles in pleural disease. *Eur Resp J* 10:467–481, 1997.

64

Hemoptysis

Erika Cappelluti

I. **Definition. Hemoptysis** is spitting of blood from the lungs or bronchial tubes. **Pseudohemoptysis** is spitting of blood from a source other than the lower respiratory tract.

II. **Overview**

    A. Seventy percent of patients with hemoptysis will have **bronchitis, bronchogenic carcinoma,** or an **infection** (e.g., bronchiectasis, pneumonia, tuberculosis, lung abscess).

    B. **Classification of hemoptysis** is usually based on the rate of blood loss.

        1. **Mild:** Expectoration of less than 15–20 ml in 24 hrs

        2. **Moderate:** Expectoration of 20–600 ml in 24 hrs

        3. **Massive:** Expectoration of more than 600 ml of blood in 24 hrs (occurs in 3%–10% of all patients with hemoptysis)

    C. **Severity.** The amount, rate, and duration of bleeding are not reliable indicators of the severity of the underlying cause. However, the rate of bleeding does correlate with mortality.

III. **Differential Diagnosis.** Categories may overlap in their clinical presentation (Table 64–1).

IV. **Notes on the Differential Diagnosis.** On average, the cause of hemoptysis can be determined in about 90% of patients.

    A. **Essential hemoptysis.** Approximately 12% of patients will have **idiopathic** or **essential hemoptysis** (most commonly seen in men between 30–50 years of age).

    B. **Pseudohemoptysis.** It is important to rule out causes of pseudohemoptysis by completing a thorough examination of the nose and pharynx using a nasopharyngoscope. If a clear-cut source of the pseudohemoptysis cannot be determined, the spitting up of blood is assumed to be true hemoptysis.

    C. **Hematemesis** is usually dark red, not frothy, and has an acid pH. Hemoptysis is usually bright red, frothy, and has an alkaline pH.

    D. **Hemoptysis before the third decade of life** is likely due to congenital heart defects, bronchiectasis, tracheobronchitis, cystic fibrosis, pneumonia, tuberculosis, or blood dyscrasias.

    E. **Menses.** Hemoptysis that accompanies menses suggests pulmonary endometriosis.

    F. **Hematuria.** Hemoptysis that accompanies hematuria suggests Goodpasture's syndrome, Wegener's granulomatosis, or systemic lupus erythematosus.

    G. **Chronic sputum production** that precedes hemoptysis is suggestive of bronchiectasis, chronic bronchitis, or cystic fibrosis.

    H. **Sputum characteristics**

        1. **Pink frothy sputum** is the hallmark of increased pulmonary venous pressure.

TABLE 64–1. Differential Diagnosis of Hemoptysis

Category	Etiology
Pseudohemoptysis	Upper respiratory infection (of the nose or mouth) Upper gastrointestinal tract infection Malingering
Infection	Bronchitis Bronchiectasis Pneumonia Tuberculosis Lung abscess Cystic fibrosis Fungal organisms Viral pneumonitis
Neoplasm	Bronchogenic carcinoma Bronchial adenoma Metastatic cancer
Cardiovascular	Congestive heart failure (CHF) Mitral stenosis Pulmonary embolism
Systemic	Wegener's granulomatosis Goodpasture's syndrome Idiopathic pulmonary hemosiderosis Vasculitis Scleroderma
Miscellaneous	Trauma Foreign body Coagulopathy Iatrogenic
Idiopathic	

2. **Slight blood streaking** in the sputum is most common with bronchitis.
3. **Purulent bloody sputum** is most often seen in cases of bronchiectasis or lung abscess.
4. **Gritty sputum** is diagnostic of broncholithiasis.
5. **Frankly bloody sputum** without much mucus is seen in tuberculosis, pulmonary embolism, and bronchogenic carcinoma.

V. Clinical Approach to Hemoptysis

A. **Presentation.** Hemoptysis is a disconcerting symptom that will cause most people to seek medical attention. The clinician's first responsibility is to determine the rate, duration, and amount of blood loss. In the nonurgent situation, the workup may be completed in the outpatient setting. Otherwise, admission to the hospital, with consultation from a pulmonologist or surgeon, may be indicated.

B. History

1. Determine the **characteristics** of the hemoptysis in the initial evaluation. This includes determining the amount, duration, and rate of bleeding, as well as patterns of recurrence.
2. Assess for factors that **induce, exacerbate, or accompany** the hemoptysis (e.g., exercise, menses, hematuria).
3. Assess for a **previous history** of pneumonia, tuberculosis, or bronchiectasis. Determine occupational exposures (e.g., asbestos, silica), tobacco use, and travel history.
4. **Pneumonia:** If a patient with pneumonia, who is receiving appropriate therapy, has hemoptysis for more than 24 hours, consider an alternative source of bleeding such as a coagulopathy or an endobronchial lesion.
5. **Anticoagulation therapy:** A history of anticoagulation therapy may suggest an intrapulmonary bleed from excess anticoagulation, pulmonary embolism from insufficient anticoagulation, or congestive heart failure (CHF).

C. Physical examination

1. **Skin examination** may show ecchymoses or petechiae consistent with a hematologic abnormality, or telangiectasias consistent with hereditary hemorrhagic telangiectasia.
2. **Otolaryngologic examination** may reveal evidence of bleeding gums, epistaxis, oropharyngeal ulcers, or hemotympanum.
3. **Respiratory examination** may reveal tachypnea, friction rub, crackles, diminished breath sounds, or wheezes. Localized wheezing suggests bronchiectasis or an obstructing lesion.
4. **Cardiovascular examination:** Jugular venous distention (JVD) may indicate right or left heart failure. Auscultatory examination may reveal mitral stenosis, pulmonary artery stenosis, or pulmonary hypertension.

VI. Diagnostic Evaluation (Figure 64–1)

A. Initial evaluation

1. **Complete blood count** (CBC) [assessing for infection, chronic blood loss, thrombocytopenia]
2. **Coagulation studies** (to rule out a primary hematologic disorder)
3. **Urinalysis** (may suggest the presence of systemic disease)
4. **Electrocardiogram** (ECG) [useful in considering cardiovascular disorders]
5. **Chest radiograph** (20%–60% of patients will have a normal chest radiograph)
6. **Arterial blood gas** (may indicate coexisting pulmonary disease or diffuse intrapulmonary hemorrhage)

B. Flexible bronchoscopy and high-resolution computed tomography (CT) should be considered in all cases and used in a complementary fashion. If the patient is actively bleeding, bronchoscopy should be

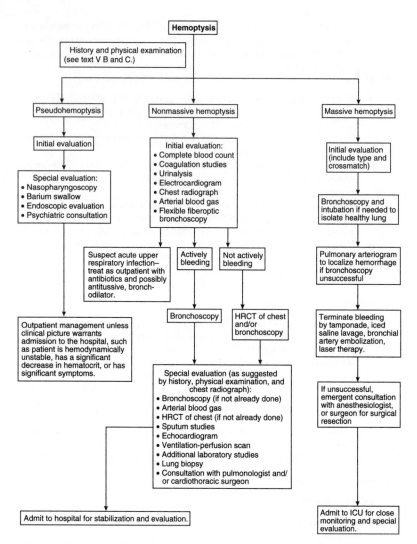

■ **FIGURE 64–1.** Algorithm for the evaluation of patients with hemoptysis. *HRCT* = high-resolution computed tomography; *ICU* = intensive care unit.

performed as soon as possible to determine the location of the hemorrhage. This also permits patient positioning and other maneuvers to limit the amount of blood that spills into normal alveoli.

C. **Additional tests.** Depending on the results of the initial evaluation and the suspected cause of hemoptysis, the following tests may be useful:

1. **Sputum studies** for acid-fast bacillus (AFB), fungi, cytology may be useful for arriving at a diagnosis.

2. **Cardiovascular causes:** Consider echocardiogram and cardiac catheterization.
3. **Thromboembolic disease suspected:** Consider ventilation-perfusion scan, spiral CT, and angiography.
4. **Interstitial or parenchymal disease suspected:** Consider a rheumatologic assessment [antinuclear antibody, rheumatoid factor (RF), complement levels, antineutrophilic cytoplasmic antibody, antiglomerular basement membrane antibody], lung biopsy, or both.

SUGGESTED READING

Boyars MC: Hemoptysis: Current strategies for diagnosis and therapy. *J Resp Dis* 17:959–974, 1996.

Hirshberg B, Biran I, et al: Hemoptysis: Etiology, evaluation, and outcome in a tertiary referral hospital. *Chest* 112(2):440–444, 1997.

Lenner R, Almenoff PL, Lesser M: Workup and management of hemoptysis. *Intern Med* 19(11):27–32, 1998.

65

Diagnostic Approach to Pulmonary Disorders
Michael McCormick and Oren P. Schaefer

Asthma
Michael McCormick

I. **Definition.** Asthma is a **chronic inflammatory condition of the airways** that is characterized by airway inflammation, airway hyperresponsiveness, and reversible airway obstruction.

II. **When to Suspect Asthma**

A. **History**

1. Patients with asthma have **episodic wheezing** often with **dyspnea, cough, sputum production,** and **chest tightness.**
2. **Nocturnal** or **early morning symptoms** are common.
3. In some cases, patients with asthma do not present with wheezing. Cough or dyspnea may be the only presenting symptom.

B. **Physical examination**

1. **Chronic asthma** is characterized by polyphonic expiratory wheezing heard on chest auscultation.
2. **Acute severe asthma:** Patients with acute severe asthma are tachypneic and may be in respiratory distress. Use of accessory muscles of inspiration and hyperinflation of the chest can be seen on inspection. Wheezing is frequently heard but does not correlate with the degree of airflow obstruction.

III. **How to Confirm the Diagnosis**

A. **Pulmonary function tests**

1. **Spirometry:** In a nonsmoker with the appropriate clinical history, asthma may be diagnosed with spirometry. A positive finding demonstrates airflow obstruction, as shown by a decrease in the ratio of forced expiratory volume in 1 second to forced vital capacity (FEV_1:FVC), that is at least partially reversible with bronchodilation.
2. **Bronchoprovocation testing** is used to diagnose asthma in patients who do not have reversible airway obstruction on spirometry. The presence of hyperresponsiveness in the correct clinical context is strongly supportive of asthma. The sensitivity of bronchoprovocation testing is close to 100%. The specificity is approximately 80%. False-positive results can be seen in chronic obstructive pulmonary disease (COPD), congestive heart failure (CHF), and allergic rhinitis.

B. **Imaging.** Shortness of breath, cough, and wheezing can be seen in several clinical entities. If the diagnosis of asthma is not certain, particularly when a patient is presenting to a physician for the first time, a chest radiograph can help to exclude CHF, pneumonia, bronchiectasis, and interstitial lung disease.

C. Ancillary tests

1. **Allergen skin testing for inhalants** (e.g., tree, grass and weed pollens, mold and mold spores, dust mite allergens, animal dander) can aid in establishing triggers for the patient's asthma.
2. **Peripheral blood eosinophilia** is frequently seen in patients with allergic asthma.

SUGGESTED READING

Boushey HA Jr, Corry DB, and Fahy JV: Asthma. In Murray JF, Nadel JA (eds): *Textbook of Respiratory Medicine*, 3rd ed. Philadelphia: W.B. Saunders Company, 2000, pp 1247–1289.

Chronic Obstructive Pulmonary Disease

Michael McCormick

I. Definitions

A. COPD is defined as a disease state that is characterized by the presence of airflow obstruction due to chronic bronchitis or emphysema. The airflow obstruction is generally progressive.

B. Chronic bronchitis is characterized by a chronic productive cough that lasts for at least 3 months in each of 2 successive years. Other causes of chronic cough must be excluded before diagnosing chronic bronchitis.

C. Emphysema is defined as abnormal permanent enlargement of the airspaces distal to the terminal bronchioles, accompanied by destruction of their walls and without obvious fibrosis. While there are patients who have pure chronic bronchitis or pure emphysema, the majority of COPD patients have both.

D. α_1-protease inhibitor deficiency should be suspected in the following patients:

1. Patients with early-onset COPD (i.e., patients younger than 50 years of age)
2. Patients with chronic bronchitis and airflow obstruction who have never smoked
3. Patients with bronchiectasis without clear etiology
4. Patients with basilar emphysema on chest radiography
5. Patients with difficult-to-control asthma

II. When to Suspect COPD

A. History

1. **Smoking:** A significant smoking history is required for the development of clinical symptoms related to COPD. In fact, only 15%

of smokers actually develop clinically significant COPD. Patients do not usually present until the fifth decade.

2. **Symptoms** include chronic cough, sputum production, wheezing, and dyspnea.

3. **Clinical course:** The clinical course of COPD is punctuated by acute exacerbations that include increased cough and sputum volume, purulent sputum, wheezing, and worsening dyspnea.

4. **Hemoptysis** is common and more likely to occur during an acute exacerbation.

5. **Sputum production** initially occurs only upon arising but will progress to occur throughout the day.

6. **Dyspnea,** which usually begins years after the development of a productive cough, is often insidious.

7. **Hypoxemia**

   a. **Oxygen desaturation:** Patients with COPD will frequently develop oxygen desaturation with exercise well before they become hypoxemic at rest.

   b. **Chronic hypoxemia,** often seen in the late stages of COPD, leads to cor pulmonale with resultant right heart failure and peripheral edema.

B. **Physical examination.** In mild cases of COPD, the physical examination is usually normal. As the condition worsens, hyperinflation of the chest with an increased anteroposterior diameter and low-lying diaphragms is characteristically seen.

1. **Breath sounds** are diminished and **wheezing** is heard on exhalation with a prolonged expiratory phase.

2. **Exhalation** may be through pursed lips with forceful contraction of the abdominal musculature in more severe cases.

3. **Positions:** Patients may assume characteristic positioning to improve diaphragmatic function, such as by leaning forward and resting on the arms.

III. How to Confirm the Diagnosis

A. Pulmonary function tests

1. **Airflow obstruction,** as evidenced by a reduced FEV_1:FVC ratio, is necessary for diagnosis. A value less than 70 usually indicates airflow obstruction. The severity of the obstruction is obtained from the FEV_1 rather than the FEV_1:FVC ratio. A possible grading system follows:

   a. Mild obstruction: % predicted $FEV_1 < 100$ and > 70
   b. Moderate obstruction: % predicted $FEV_1 < 70$ and > 60
   c. Moderately severe obstruction: % predicted $FEV_1 < 60$ and > 50
   d. Severe obstruction: % predicted $FEV_1 < 50$

2. **Lung volumes,** although not necessary to establish the diagnosis, show an increase in total lung capacity, most of which is due to an increase in residual volume.

3. **Diffusing capacity** is reduced in proportion to the severity of disease.

4. **COPD versus asthma:** COPD can be difficult to distinguish from asthma when reversibility of airflow obstruction is seen with broncho-

dilators or bronchial hyperresponsiveness is demonstrated with a positive methacholine challenge.

B. **Imaging.** The chest radiograph may be normal in mild cases of COPD, but it can be helpful in excluding other diseases. Findings that are characteristic of more severe emphysema include hyperlucency of the parenchyma; low, flat diaphragms; and a large retrosternal air space.

C. **Ancillary tests.** An arterial blood gas is indicated in the evaluation of COPD when the patient is hypoxemic and there is a question about pCO_2 and acid-base status. All patients admitted to the hospital with COPD exacerbation should have an arterial blood gas. Arterial blood gas analysis initially shows hypoxemia without hypercarbia. Hypercarbia becomes more common as the FEV_1 falls below 1 liter and should be suspected in asymptomatic patients with a serum bicarbonate level > 30 mg/dl.

1. **Erythrocytosis** without leukocytosis and thrombocytosis can be seen in patients with chronic hypoxemia.
2. **An α_1-protease inhibitor level** should be drawn when α_1-protease inhibitor deficiency is suspected (see I D).

SUGGESTED READING

Madison JM, Irwin RS: Chronic obstructive pulmonary disease. *Lancet* 352:467–473, 1998.

Pneumonia

Oren P. Schaefer

I. Differential Diagnosis

A. **Community-acquired pneumonia (CAP)** is pneumonia in an immunocompetent host that develops outside the hospital or nursing home setting.

1. **No etiologic pathogen:** Rigorous prospective studies on CAP fail to demonstrate the etiologic pathogen in almost one-half of all cases.
2. *Streptococcus pneumoniae:* Among the multitude of organisms shown to be responsible for causing CAP, *S. pneumoniae* is the leading cause, accounting for 20%–60% of all cases.
3. **Additional microorganisms**

   (a) Other, less frequent microorganisms causing CAP are *Haemophilus influenzae* and *Moraxella catarrhalis*. These cases occur particularly in patients with COPD.
   (b) *Chlamydia pneumoniae* and *Mycoplasma pneumoniae* are common in younger individuals and together may account for 25% of cases of CAP.
   (c) Legionella species have been reported in 2%–6% of cases.
   (d) Anaerobes should be considered in patients with a predisposition to

aspiration such as a history of altered consciousness or dysphagia. Anaerobes are the most common pathogen isolated from pulmonary abscesses and are common in empyema as well.

   (e) *Staphylococcus aureus* and Gram-negative bacilli are much less common causes of CAP.

   (1) *S. aureus* predominantly affects the elderly and is also seen more frequently in association with influenza pandemics.
   (2) Gram-negative bacilli are associated with underlying alcohol abuse, or the nursing home patient.

   (f) Viruses, such as influenza, parainfluenza, adenovirus, and respiratory syncytial virus, account for 2%–15% of cases.

B. Hospital-acquired pneumonia (HAP) is defined as pneumonia occurring ≥ 48 hours after hospital admission. The most frequently associated bacterial pathogens are enteric Gram-negative rods and *S. aureus.*

C. Tuberculosis generally presents with classic symptoms and radiographic patterns, but atypical presentations mimicking pneumonia are commonly reported in elderly, debilitated, or HIV-infected patients.

D. Endemic fungal infections, such as histoplasmosis, coccidioidomycosis, and blastomycosis, should be considered in appropriate geographic regions (or in patients who have traveled to these regions).

E. Noninfectious conditions, such as CHF, pulmonary thromboembolism, atelectasis, immune-related lung disease, drug-related lung disease, or malignancy, may mimic pneumonia.

II. When to Suspect Pneumonia

A. History. A history of cough, sputum production, dyspnea, chest pain (commonly pleuritic), fever, chills, sweats, fatigue, malaise, mental status changes, and gastrointestinal symptoms should be noted. The medical history should also include travel and animal contacts.

B. Physical examination. Fever, tachycardia, tachypnea, crackles, rhonchi, and signs of pulmonary consolidation may be found.

III. Diagnostic Evaluation

A. Chest radiography. A chest radiograph can be used to exclude other diseases such as CHF or pneumothorax. Patients who have multilobar infiltrates or pleural effusions are at higher risk for a complicated course.

B. Laboratory investigations. The laboratory evaluation of a patient with CAP needs to be a focused attempt to obtain, if possible, a definitive microbiologic diagnosis, as well as to gather information that will aid the physician in deciding whether admission to the hospital is necessary. Treatment should never be delayed while attempting to obtain microbiologic specimens.

   1. Sputum evaluation remains perhaps the most controversial in the evaluation and management of patients with CAP and HAP.

   a. CAP: Approximately 30% of patients presenting with CAP will not have a productive cough. Approximately 25% of patients presenting with CAP have already been taking an antibiotic, thus significantly reducing both the sensitivity and specificity of the sputum Gram stain and culture.

    b. HAP: The role of a routine Gram stain of sputum in the evaluation of HAP is even less clear. In cases where sputum is obtained, the sample should be produced from a deep cough and be grossly purulent.

    c. Induced sputum samples can be obtained in cases where the patient cannot spontaneously produce sputum. Induced sputum samples are required from patients who are suspected to have an opportunistic infection (e.g., *Pneumocystis carinii* pneumonia), tuberculosis, or fungal infection. Sputum should be immediately transported to the laboratory for rapid processing.

    d. Though routine sputum culture has a lower sensitivity and specificity than Gram stain, it may take on more importance in the identification of resistant microorganisms.

2. **Blood cultures** are recommended for all patients; two sets should be obtained prior to antibiotic therapy. The overall yield of blood cultures is low (8%–11%), though it may be higher in those patients with pneumococcal pneumonia. A positive blood culture provides a definitive diagnosis and portends a more complicated course.

3. **Arterial blood gas** should be performed on patients who are hypoxemic (by pulse oximetry) and should be considered in patients with underlying cardiopulmonary disorders such as CHF or COPD.

4. **Invasive studies** such as bronchoscopy with quantitative microbiologic cultures can be considered in patients with HAP. Bronchoalveolar lavage and lung biopsy may be necessary in immunocompromised patients, especially if *P. carinii* pneumonia is suspected.

SUGGESTED READING

Neiderman MS, Bass JB, Campbell GD: Guidelines for the initial management of adults with community-acquired pneumonia: Diagnosis, assessment of severity, and initial antimicrobial therapy. *Am Rev Respir Dis* 148:1418–1426, 1993.

Bronchogenic Carcinoma

Michael McCormick

I. Overview

    A. Lung cancer is the most common cause of death from malignancy in the United States.

    B. Cell types

        1. **Non-small-cell carcinoma:** For purposes of staging and treatment, the first three cell types can be grouped together as non-small-cell carcinoma:

            a. Squamous cell carcinoma

            b. Large cell carcinoma

            c. Adenocarcinoma (most common type of lung cancer in nonsmokers)

2. **Small cell carcinoma:** Because of the propensity for early widespread dissemination, small cell carcinoma is separated from the other three cell types.

II. When to Suspect Bronchogenic Carcinoma

A. **Signs and symptoms** of bronchogenic carcinoma can result from local growth of tumor, intrathoracic and extrathoracic metastases, and paraneoplastic syndromes. Only 10% of patients are asymptomatic at the time of diagnosis.

B. **Central endobronchial tumor growth** can cause cough, hemoptysis, wheezing, and postobstructive pneumonia, and it is more likely to lead to an early presentation.

C. **Peripheral growth** can lead to pleural or chest wall invasion with resultant dyspnea, cough, and chest pain. Involvement of the recurrent laryngeal nerve can cause vocal cord paralysis and hoarseness.

D. **Pancoast syndrome.** Bronchogenic carcinoma arising in the lung apex at the superior thoracic inlet frequently causes a constellation of characteristic signs and symptoms referred to as Pancoast syndrome. Local extension of the tumor into the brachial plexus, parietal pleura, vertebral bodies, and first three ribs leads to pain in the shoulder, radicular pain along the distribution of the ulnar nerve without muscle wasting, and Horner's syndrome (ptosis, miosis, and anhidrosis). The tumor is usually a non-small-cell carcinoma.

III. Diagnostic Evaluation

A. **Purpose of diagnostic studies**

1. **To make a pathologic diagnosis of malignancy** (can be established with either cytological or surgical biopsy specimens)
2. **To stage the extent of disease**
3. **To evaluate the patient as a candidate for lobectomy or pneumonectomy**

B. **Sputum cytology.** In patients with central lesions, the sensitivity of sputum cytology is approximately 65%, while the specificity is 99%. The sensitivity is much lower with peripheral lesions.

C. **Bronchoscopy** remains a major tool for both diagnosis and local staging.

1. **Diagnosis** can be made from cytologic examination of specimens, bronchial brushings, bronchial washings, and transbronchial needle aspirations. Biopsy specimens can be obtained from both endobronchial lesions as well as peripheral lesions not visible with bronchoscopy. If the lesion is visible bronchoscopically, the diagnostic yield is greater than 90%. A pathologic diagnosis can also be made at the time of mediastinoscopy or at the time of surgical resection of the tumor.
2. **Local staging:** In addition to making a diagnosis, a transbronchial needle aspiration of mediastinal nodes allows local staging. Bronchoscopy can also exclude synchronous but unsuspected lesions.

D. **Cytologic diagnosis** can be made via transthoracic needle aspiration usually done under computed tomography (CT) guidance. While the diagnostic yield is high, the procedure is rarely able to prevent a thoracotomy, since only a definitive negative diagnosis (unlikely with cytology) will accomplish this. Pleural fluid cytology is positive in more than 50% of patients with lung cancer and pleural effusion. A second pleural fluid sampling increases the diagnostic yield.

E. **Thoracoscopy** can confirm pleural involvement in greater than 95% of patients with pleural extension of tumor.

F. **Imaging**

1. **Chest CT** is the primary modality used. In addition to localizing the primary tumor and determining its relationship to nearby structures, chest CT allows an excellent view of the pulmonary hilum, mediastinal nodes, as well as the liver and adrenal glands. CT evaluation of mediastinal adenopathy is mandatory in all patients with bronchogenic carcinoma. Due to the low specificity of lung cancer in enlarged lymph nodes, all nodes with a short-axis diameter of more than 1 cm need to be evaluated pathologically for accurate staging.

2. **Magnetic resonance imaging (MRI)** is useful when chest wall invasion is an issue. MRI has become a routine part of the staging regimen for patients with superior sulcus tumors.

3. **CT scan of the brain** is necessary in patients with neurologic symptoms as well as in patients with signs or symptoms suggestive of widely metastatic disease.

4. **Radionuclide scans** are done to evaluate bony metastases.

IV. **Staging.** Once a diagnosis of lung cancer is confirmed, staging of the cancer is done to group patients into anatomic subsets, which assists in predicting prognosis and determining therapeutic options.

V. **Solitary Pulmonary Nodule.** A solitary pulmonary nodule can be defined as a well-circumscribed spherical lesion completely surrounded by aerated lung and not associated with atelectasis or adenopathy. The size is normally less than 3 cm, but different size criteria have been used.

A. **Etiology.** More than 50% of solitary pulmonary nodules are due to granulomatous disease, and approximately 35% are due to malignancy, usually bronchogenic carcinoma.

B. **Malignancy risk**

1. In nonsmokers younger than 35 years, the risk of malignancy is less than 1%, and consequently, these lesions can usually be followed with serial radiologic studies.

2. In patients older than 35 years or with a smoking history, unless the lesion has been radiographically stable for 2 years or shows a distinctive benign pattern of calcification on chest CT, a **thorascopic biopsy** will likely be needed.

SUGGESTED READING

Adjei AA, Marks RS, Bonner JA: Current guidelines for management of small cell lung cancer. *Mayo Clin Proc* 74:809–816, 1999.

Jett J, Feins R, Kvale P, et al: Pretreatment evaluations of non-small-cell lung cancer. *Am J Respir Crit Care Med* 156:320–332, 1997.

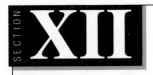

Renal/Genitourinary

66

Dysuria
David Hatem

I. **Definition.** Dysuria is defined as **difficulty or pain in urination** and occurs when fluid (urine or discharge) passes over an inflamed urethra.

II. **Differential Diagnosis of Dysuria** (Table 66–1)

A. **Local causes.** Urinary tract infections, deep-seated infections (e.g., of the prostate or kidney), vaginal and pelvic infections, and inflammation account for the majority of cases of dysuria. **Acute cystitis** is the most common bacterial infection in women.

B. **Systemic illness** involving the joints and selected mucocutaneous surfaces (Reiter's syndrome) and **local effects of systemic treatment** (e.g., radiation therapy for prostate cancer, certain chemotherapeutic agents) can also lead to dysuria.

C. **Nongonococcal urethritis** is typically caused by *Chlamydia trachomatis*, *Ureaplasma urealyticum*, and *Trichomonas vaginalis*. This condition is usually seen in women.

D. **Pyelonephritis** should be suspected as a cause of dysuria when symptoms last longer than 1 week, or in the following clinical scenarios:

1. The patient has diabetes mellitus (DM)
2. The patient is in an immunocompromised state
3. The patient is pregnant
4. There is a known anatomic anomaly of the urinary tract
5. The patient has vesicoureteral reflux or a ureteral obstruction
6. Symptoms relapse within 3 days of completing cystitis treatment
7. There is a history of pyelonephritis within the past year

E. **Atrophic vaginitis** in women can lead to dysuria with or without urinary tract infection.

III. **Clinical Approach**

A. **History.** There are no specific characteristics of dysuria per se that are useful in distinguishing the various causes. The diagnosis is derived through assessment of associated features that accompany dysuria.

1. **Urinary tract infections:** Patients with simple urinary tract infection complain of acute or subacute onset of dysuria, urinary frequency, and

TABLE 66–1. Differential Diagnosis of Dysuria

Local infections/inflammation

Urinary tract infection: Most commonly caused by *Escherichia coli, Proteus, Klebsiella,* and *Staphylococcus saprophyticus*

Urethritis: Commonly caused by *Neisseria gonorrhoeae, Chlamydia trachomatis, Ureaplasma urealyticum,* and herpes simplex virus

Pelvic inflammatory disease: Most common causes *include N. gonorrhoeae* and *C. trachomatis.*

Vulvovaginitis: Commonly caused by *Candida albicans, Trichomonas vaginalis,* and *Gardnerella vaginalis*

Atrophic vaginitis

Interstitial cystitis

Acute urethral syndrome

Deep-seated infection

Prostatitis: *E. coli* and *Klebsiella* are common causes

Pyelonephritis: Same pathogens as urinary tract infection

Systemic illness

Reiter's syndrome

Miscellaneous

Local radiation therapy

Prostatodynia: Symptoms and signs of prostatitis but no prostatic inflammation [normal white blood cells (WBCs) and urine culture]

Idiopathic

---

occasionally hematuria. Fever is uncommon in uncomplicated cases of urinary tract infection.

2. **Pyelonephritis:** A simple urinary tract infection can usually be distinguished from pyelonephritis by symptoms. The presence of flank pain, nausea, vomiting, fever, and signs of sepsis usually point to pyelonephritis. The presentation of pyelonephritis can also be subtle, sometimes with only cystitis-like syndrome and mild flank pain.

3. **Prostate involvement:** In men, hematuria, hematospermia, or blood-

tinged discharge often suggests involvement of the prostate in the inflammatory process.

4. **Sexually transmitted disease (STD):** If an STD is suspected, especially with complaints of uretheral discharge, a sexual history should be obtained.

   a. **Characteristics of the discharge** can range from thick and purulent (gonococcal urethritis) to mucoid, scant, or even absent (nongonococcal urethritis).

   b. **Onset of the discharge** can provide a clue: gonococcal urethritis presents with a 2- to 4-day history, while the presentation in nongonococcal urethritis is more indolent.

5. **Vaginitis:** Women with dysuria may complain of vaginitis-type symptoms, such as discharge, itching, external irritation, or dyspareunia. Discharge can vary from homogeneous white or gray (*Gardnerella*), to thick and curd-like (*Candida*), to malodorous and yellow-green (*Trichomonas*) [see Chapter 34, VAGINITIS].

6. **Acute urethral syndrome:** The history does not provide any specific distinguishing characteristics of acute urethral syndrome in women. This diagnosis is chiefly determined by eliminating alternative causes.

7. **Reiter's syndrome:** Systemic symptoms can include polyarthritis (large joints of the lower extremities most commonly), dermatitis (keratoderma blenorrhagicum), conjunctivitis, uveitis, and oral ulcers, which are all clues to Reiter's syndrome. Reiter's syndrome is associated with ~1% of cases of nongonococcal urethritis and 2% of enteric infections.

B. Physical examination

1. Assess for **fever, tachycardia, and blood pressure changes,** which can accompany a deep-seated infection or sepsis.

2. Assess for **costovertebral tenderness** (defined by the angle at which the lower ribs articulate with the vertebral facets), which is suggestive of pyelonephritis.

3. Assess for **masses, fullness,** or **tenderness in the abdomen.** The bladder should be percussed (dull percussion with urinary retention) and palpated for tenderness.

4. **Male genitalia**

   a. Check for **external lesions** (e.g., warts or ulcers), **urethral discharge** (milk the urethra from the proximal to distal), and **epididymal tenderness.** The presence of painful penile ulcers or warts suggests herpes or human papilloma virus (HPV).

   b. Examine the **prostate** to determine the presence of tenderness and bogginess (soft, mushy quality compared with the usual firm consistency), which is suggestive of prostatitis. An enlarged prostate gland suggests bladder outlet obstruction, which predisposes the patient to urinary tract infection.

   c. A distinctive feature of Reiter's syndrome is **circinate balanitis** (i.e., erythema and ulceration on the glans penis).

5. Perform a **pelvic examination** looking for vaginal erythema, urethral or vaginal discharge, cervical erosions, cervical discharge, or motion

tenderness. Bimanual examination should be performed, looking for adnexal fullness, masses, or tenderness.

6. Palpate the anterior vaginal wall on each side of the urethra to check for **tenderness of the paraurethral glands.** This examination is considered by some physicians to be consistent with acute urethral syndrome; however, the sensitivity and specificity of the examination is not known.

7. Assess for **systemic features** including signs of gonococcemia and typical features of Reiter's syndrome.

   a. In **gonorrhea,** joints and periarticular structures involve a migratory tenosynovitis, diffuse arthralgia, or purulent arthritis usually involving one joint, most commonly the knees, ankles, or wrists.

   b. The joint manifestation of **Reiter's syndrome** includes asymmetric arthritis in the large joints of the lower extremities, painful or painless involvement of the sacroiliacs, and involvement of the ligaments and tendons of the feet.

   c. Gonococcal arthritis usually presents with a relatively small but painful effusion, whereas Reiter's joint involvement usually has a large volume effusion relative to the pain.

IV. Diagnostic Evaluation (Figure 66–1)

A. Urinary tract infection

1. **Urine dipstick test** should be the initial test if urinary tract infection is suspected.

   a. **Pyuria** is the most sensitive indicator of infection, and the leukocyte esterase test on dipstick is 75%–95% sensitive in detecting pyuria due to infection.

   b. **Urine nitrite** on dipstick is a specific indicator of urinary tract infection (90% specific), but sensitivity is only 30%. Most urinary pathogens can convert nitrate to nitrite. Two exceptions are *Staphylococcus saprophyticus* and *Enterococcus.* Sensitivity of urinary nitrite can be increased to 60% if a first morning voided specimen is used.

2. **Urinalysis** demonstrating pyuria [> 2–5 white blood cells (WBCs) per high-power field in the spun sediment] and the absence of squamous epithelial cells (suggesting a contaminated specimen) is suggestive of urinary tract infection. The absence of pyuria suggests a vaginal cause of dysuria in women.

3. **Urine culture**

   a. **Indications**

      (1) Symptoms present for more than 1 week
      (2) Suspected upper tract disease
      (3) Cystitis suspected by symptoms, but urine dipstick test is negative for pyuria and nitrites

   b. **Criterion for infection:** If a urine culture is obtained, the criterion for infection in a patient with acute dysuria is a colony count of $> 10^2$ organisms per ml as opposed to the less sensitive criteria of 10^5 used previously.

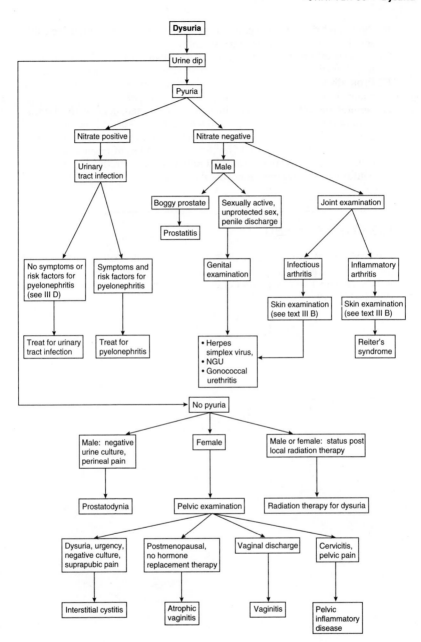

FIGURE 66–1. Algorithm for the evaluation of dysuria. *NGU* = nongonoccal urethritis.

B. **Pyelonephritis.** If risk factors for pyelonephritis are present, urine culture should be obtained to guide treatment.
C. **Acute urethral syndrome.** Pyuria in a woman without evidence of urinary tract infection or an STD is consistent with acute urethral syndrome.
D. **Prostatitis.** If prostatitis is suspected, urine culture shows greater colony counts when obtained following prostatic massage.
E. **Genital infection.** If a genital infection is suspected, begin with a Gram stain of the urethral discharge to distinguish gonococcal from non-gonococcal urethritis. Four or more polymorphonuclear neutrophils per high-power field and mixed Gram-positive and Gram-negative extra-cellular organisms are indicative of nongonococcal urethritis. This is confirmed by a negative gonococcal culture.

SUGGESTED READING

Dewan PA, Wilson TM: Idiopathic urethritis in the adolescent male. *Eur Urol* 30:494–497, 1996.
Freeman SB: Common genitourinary infections. *J Obstet Gynecol Neonatal Nurse* 24:735–742, 1995.
Stamm WE, Hooton TM: Management of urinary tract infections in adults. *N Engl J Med* 329:1328–1334, 1993.

67

Hematuria
Michael Wollin and David Clive

I. **Definition.** Hematuria is the **excretion of abnormal amounts of red blood cells (RBCs) in the urine.**

II. **Overview**

   A. **Hematuria may be a warning sign of an underlying nephrologic or urologic pathological process.** Thus, any degree of hematuria needs to be evaluated.

   1. Urinary tract bleeding that occurs while a patient is taking **anticoagulant therapy** should not automatically be attributed to that therapy. A pathological etiology is found in approximately 40% of these patients.

   2. As many as 60% of patients with hematuria will have no identified cause following evaluation.

   B. **Bleeding may be either gross (visible with the eye) or microscopic (viewed only under a microscope).** The chance of identifying significant pathology increases with the degree and duration of hematuria. Yet the severity of the pathology does not correlate with the degree of bleeding.

   C. **Gross hematuria needs to be differentiated from colored urine.**

   1. The most common causes of colored urine are myoglobinuria and hemoglobinuria, both of which can discolor urine dark brown or red.

   2. As little as 1 ml of blood/L can cause urine to become discolored. The duration of bleeding determines the urine color. For example, fresh blood is bright red, while older blood is dark burgundy or brown.

III. **Differential Diagnosis** (Table 67–1)

IV. **Notes on the Differential Diagnosis**

   A. Hematuria must be differentiated from **hematospermia** in men, **menstrual bleeding** in women, and **blood staining the urethral meatus.**

   B. Bleeding can be either **glomerular** (nephrologic) or **epithelial** (urologic).

   1. **Glomerular bleeding** is frequently associated with significant proteinuria (> 2–$3 +$ on dipstick), red cell casts, hypertension, edema, or a dysmorphic appearance of RBCs.

   2. **Epithelial bleeding** presents with eumorphic (round) RBCs in sediment.

   a. **Infection** is the most common cause of gross hematuria in young women.

   b. **Benign prostatic obstruction** is a rare cause of hematuria by itself. The incidence increases with prostate size. Bleeding often occurs after Valsalva maneuvers.

   c. **Endometriosis:** Implants may occur in as many as 20% of women with endometriosis. Implants can occur within the bladder or ureter (causing bleeding) or extrinsic to the ureter (causing obstruction).

TABLE 67–1. Differential Diagnosis of Hematuria

Nephrologic bleeding	Epithelial bleeding
IgA nephropathy (Berger's disease)	Infection
Familial nephritis (Alport's syndrome)	Interstitial cystitis
Goodpasture's syndrome	Intraurethral condyloma
Systemic lupus erythematosus	Obstruction
Poststreptococcal glomerulonephritis	Stones
Henoch-Schonlein purpura	Benign prostatic obstruction
Sickle cell disease or trait	Endometriosis
Acute interstitial nephritis	Cancer
Hypertension	Trauma
Thrombotic microangiopathy	Foreign bodies
	Papillary necrosis
	Renal vein thrombosis
	Renal infarction
	Arteriovenous fistula
	Renal embolus/thrombus
	Sickle cell disease
	Exercise-induced hematuria
	Polycystic kidney disease
	Drug-induced hematuria
	Occupational exposure

IgA = immunoglobulin A.

d. Tumors: Almost all patients with tumors of the renal pelvis, ureters, or bladder will have some degree of hematuria at some time in the course of their disease. Bladder cancer is the most common cause of gross hematuria in patients older than 50 years of age.

(1) **Tobacco use** is associated with an increased incidence of uro-epithelial tumors. One-third of patients with bladder cancer are cigarette smokers.

(2) **Occupational exposures** are noted in 25%–33% of cases of bladder cancer (e.g., leather workers, painters, apparel manufacturers).

(3) The **"classic triad"** for renal cell cancer (hematuria, flank pain, palpable mass) occurs in less than 10% of patients and is indicative of more advanced disease.

e. Papillary necrosis needs to be considered in patients with sickle cell disease, analgesic abuse, and diabetes.

f. Renal vein thrombosis typically presents with nephrotic syndrome, flank pain, azotemia, and hematuria. It is usually unilateral in location, with nephromegaly noted on radiographic studies.

V. Clinical Approach to Hematuria (Figure 67–1)

A. History

1. Distinguish between **gross** or **microscopic bleeding.**
2. Determine the **pattern of bleeding:**

a. **Initial hematuria** suggests anterior urethral bleeding.

b. **Total hematuria** suggests bleeding from the upper tracts (e.g., kidneys, ureters).

c. **Terminal hematuria** suggests bleeding from the bladder or prostate.

d. **Blood staining the meatus** suggests meatal stenosis or urethral stricture.

e. **Cyclical bleeding** suggests endometriosis.

f. **Persistent bleeding** has an increased likelihood of malignancy.

3. **Painful bleeding** usually indicates stones, while **painless bleeding** is more common with malignancies.
4. **Associated irritative voiding symptoms** suggest a lower tract inflammatory process.
5. The **family history** should focus on malignancy, stones, medical renal disease, or sickle cell disease.
6. Inquire about trauma, tobacco use, infectious symptoms, and history of sexually transmitted disease (STD), all of which can lead to urethral strictures.
7. **Medical illnesses** (e.g., diabetes, papillary necrosis, glomerulo-nephropathy, hypertension, coagulopathy) and **medication use** (e.g., cyclophosphamide, anticoagulants) should be ascertained.

B. Physical examination

1. **Abdominal examination:** An abdominal or flank mass may indicate renal tumor or hydronephrosis.

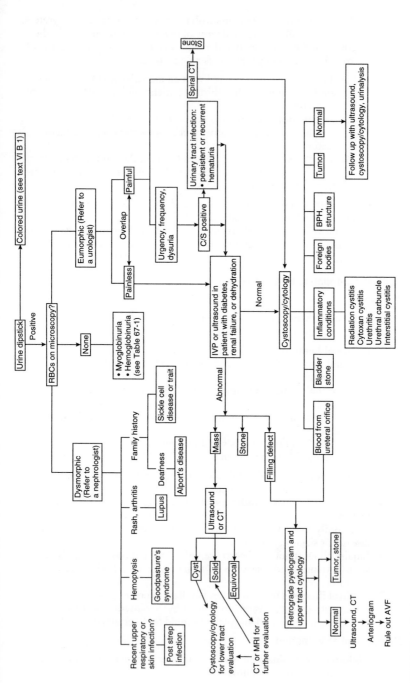

■ **FIGURE 67-1.** Algorithm for the evaluation of hematuria. *AVF* = arteriovenous fistula; *CT* = computed tomography; *IVP* = intravenous pyelography; *MRI* = magnetic resonance imaging; *RBCs* = red blood cells.

2. A **palpable bladder** may indicate retention secondary to benign prostatic hyperplasia (BPH) or prostate cancer.
3. **Pelvic examination:** Assess for urethral abnormalities in women, such as urethral caruncle or diverticulum.
4. **Genital examination:** Assess for varicocele, which may be due to a renal mass compressing the gonadal vein or vena cava.
5. **Digital rectal examination** is useful in the detection of prostate disease (e.g., BPH, prostate cancer) and in the setting of significant pelvic trauma.

VI. **Diagnostic Evaluation.** A diagnostic evaluation is appropriate for all adults, with the possible exception of women younger than 40 years of age.

A. **Initial workup.** The workup should begin with an effort to characterize the hematuria as either urologic or renal in origin.

1. **Urinalysis** can confirm the presence of RBCs in the urine.
2. **Sequential urinalyses** may be used to confirm the diagnosis because hematuria may be a transient phenomenon secondary to a nonpathologic phenomenon.

B. **Laboratory studies**

1. **Urine dipstick test:** A positive urine dipstick should always be corroborated with a microscopic assessment. The dipstick can detect as few as 5 RBCs/ml; however, as many as 50 or more RBCs/ml are required for an abnormal finding (the equivalent of 3 RBCs/high power field). Dipsticks have a sensitivity of 91%–100% and a specificity of 65%–99% for detecting microscopic hematuria. The positive predictive value for urologic malignancy is estimated to be 6%–8%.
2. **Microscopic assessment** permits the identification of RBCs versus pigments. It is also useful in distinguishing between dysmorphic and eumorphic cells. Other findings derived from microscopic assessment include white blood cells (WBCs) [inflammation/infection], red or white cell casts (medical renal disease), and crystals (stone disease).
3. **Urine culture** should be obtained if white cells or bacteria are present.
4. **Other laboratory studies** include complete blood count (CBC), blood urea nitrogen, creatinine, and coagulation studies.
5. **Urine cytology** is useful in the assessment of bladder cancer. The specificity is estimated to be approximately 95%, whereas the sensitivity is approximately 49%. This study is more sensitive when used in the evaluation of patients with high-grade tumors.

C. **Imaging**

1. **Plain films** of the kidney, ureter, and bladder can detect calcium stones, occasionally cysteine stones, and foreign bodies. Uric acid stones are radiolucent, and therefore, cannot be detected with plain films.
2. **Ultrasound** has replaced intravenous pyelography (IVP) as the initial study because it can detect smaller stones than IVP can detect. Ultrasound is the test of choice to differentiate cysts from solid lesions. It is useful in detecting hydronephrosis, renal vein thrombosis, anterior renal lesions, and small cortical lesions. Ultrasound is not useful in evaluating the lower urinary tract.
3. **IVP** is used in the radiographic analysis of the upper urinary tract. It is

most useful in detecting tumors of the renal parenchyma, renal collecting system, and ureters. IVP may be used in detecting imaging stones or papillary necrosis. It is important to note that IVP may miss as many as 10% of small cortical tumors; therefore, if these tumors are suspected, ultrasound should be obtained.

4. **Computed tomography (CT) scan** is used to evaluate renal masses because it provides better definition than ultrasound and IVP. CT enables the staging of urinary tract malignancies. It is the procedure of choice if renal injury is suspected.

5. **Spiral CT scan of the kidney, ureter, and bladder** is the procedure of choice for the detection of urinary tract calculi in patients with ureteral colic. It can detect stones at the ureterovesical junction. Diagnostic accuracy is greater than 95% (false positives may be due to phleboliths). This procedure can also detect pathology (e.g., appendicitis, diverticulitis, abdominal aortic aneurysm) in the patient presenting with pain of uncertain origin.

6. **Magnetic resonance imaging (MRI)** is an adjuvant procedure in the evaluation of equivocal renal masses. It provides superior visualization of vessels (renal embolus/thrombus, renal vein thrombosis, caval thrombus with advanced renal cancer) when compared with ultrasound and CT.

7. **Cystoscopy** is the best test to evaluate the urethra and bladder mucosa. It is mandatory in all patients with epithelial hematuria. Cystoscopy is indicated if hematuria persists after a urinary tract infection has been treated. Bladder biopsy can be performed if suspicious areas are noted. Cystoscopy done at the time of bleeding can detect the site of bleeding and lateralize bleeding from the upper tract.

8. **Retrograde pyelogram** is useful when the collecting system is not completely defined by noninvasive radiographic studies. Urine can be obtained from ureteral catheters and evaluated for cytology or infection. It is the procedure of choice if ureteral injury is suspected.

SUGGESTED READING

Lowe FC, Brendler CB: Evaluation of the urologic patient. In Walsh P, Retik A, Stamey T, et al (eds): *Campbell's Urology*, 6th ed. Philadelphia: WB Saunders, 1992, pp 307–331.

Schaeffer AJ, Del Greco F: Other renal diseases of urologic significance: Hematuria. In Walsh P, Retik A, Stamey T, et al (eds): *Campbell's Urology*, 6th ed. Philadelphia: WB Saunders, 1992, pp 2065–2072.

68

Polyuria
Wendy Lawler Mitchell

I. **Definition.** Polyuria is arbitrarily defined as **urine volume > 3 L/day.**
II. **Overview**

  A. **True polyuria.** The clinician must discern true polyuria (large excreted volumes of urine in a 24-hour period) from other similar urinary complaints:

    1. **Urinary frequency:** The frequent voiding of small volumes of urine
    2. **Nocturia:** The excretion of > 500 ml of urine at night
    3. **Urgency:** A strong desire to void (from overactive detrusor function or due to vesicourethral hypersensitivity), with a sensation of impending micturition
    4. **Urinary incontinence:** An inability to prevent the discharge of urinary excretion

  B. **Polydipsia.** Polyuria is often associated with polydipsia (excessive thirst). Either symptom may be the cause or the result of the other.
  C. **Water intake.** Under normal physiologic conditions, the chief determinant of urine volume is the intake of water. Water-loaded subjects can excrete as much as 18–20 L of water per day. The intact hypothalamic-pituitary-renal axis is effective at regulating water excretion to a level appropriate for intake.
  D. **Complications of polyuria** include hypovolemia due to excessive water losses, rapid changes in serum sodium concentration leading to neurologic manifestations, and dilation of the bladder, ureters, and kidneys.

III. **Differential Diagnosis.** Different classifications include excessive input versus output, "appropriate" diuresis versus "inappropriate" diuresis, or the site of renal abnormality. Table 69–1 classifies polyuria in terms of solute versus water diuresis.

  A. **Primary polydipsia.** As long as water intake does not exceed renal excretion capacity, patients will not develop water intoxication or hyponatremia.
  B. **Central diabetes insipidus (CDI)** is caused by an abnormality of the hypothalamic–hypophyseal tract.

    1. In **complete CDI,** antidiuretic hormone (ADH) levels are undetectable, and polyuria is severe.
    2. In **partial CDI,** ADH levels are subnormal but detectable, and polyuria is less extreme.

  C. **Nephrogenic diabetes insipidus (NDI)** denotes end-organ failure (i.e., the inability of the kidneys to respond normally to available ADH). Most forms of parenchymal renal disease can lead to impairment of urinary concentration.

TABLE 68–1. Differential Diagnosis of Polyuria

Water Diuresis	Solute Diuresis
Primary polydipsia (taking in too much water)	**Solute diuresis** (or nonelectrolyte diuresis): due to excessive filtration of a poorly resorbed solute
• Psychogenic polydipsia	• Glucosuria (diabetic ketoacidosis, hyperglycemic hyperosmolar nonketotic coma, intravenous infusions)
• Hypothalamic disease (infiltration or infarction affecting thirst center)	
• Drugs (e.g., thioridazine, chlorpromazine, anticholinergic agents) causing dry mouth, which leads to increased thirst	• Urea diuresis (high-protein tube feedings, relief of obstruction, acute tubular necrosis recovery)
	• Mannitol or glycerol infusion
Inability of kidneys to conserve water	• Radiographic contrast media
• **CDI** (vasopressin sensitive): pituitary ablation, tumor, cyst, compression by aneurysm, Sheehan's syndrome, empty sella, Guillain-Barré syndrome, trauma, infiltrative disease	• Chronic renal failure
	Natriuretic syndromes (or electrolyte diuresis): due to excessive chronic sodium loss
• **NDI** (vasopressin insensitive): acquired tubulointerstitial renal disease (e.g., hypercalcemia or hypokalemic nephropathy, pyelonephritis, analgesic nephropathy, multiple myeloma, obstructive uropathy, sarcoidosis, amyloidosis, Sjögren's syndrome, sickle cell anemia, renal transplant); drugs or toxins (e.g., lithium, ethanol, amphotericin); congenital causes (e.g., hereditary NDI, polycystic or medullary cystic disease)	• Salt-wasting nephropathy
	• Diuretic agents
	• Excessive salt ingestion
	• Intravenous saline
	• Addison's disease or aldosterone deficiency

CDI = central diabetes insipidus; NDI = nephrogenic diabetes insipidus.

    D. Osmotic diuresis is a form of polyuria in which large amounts of filtered, nonreabsorbable solute gain entry to the renal tubules. As a result, osmotic diuresis can lead to ionic imbalance, hypovolemia, and dehydration. The most common clinical example of osmotic diuresis is glycosuric diuresis seen in diabetic hyperglycemia.

IV. Clinical Approach

    A. History

        1. **Chief complaint:** The clinician should note the onset and duration of the problem, estimate of voiding volumes, number of voids per day and per night, volume of fluid consumption, and alleviating and aggravating factors.

        2. **Associated symptoms** include polydipsia, urgency, frequency, nocturia, and incontinence.

3. **Medications and habits**

   a. Use of lithium (can cause NDI), diuretics, intravenous solutions, and drugs that can cause dry mouth (leading to excessive water intake)

   b. Caffeine and alcohol intake (diuretic effect)

   c. Salt and protein intake

   d. Ethanol abuse

4. **Additional considerations**

   a. The clinician should identify any history of head trauma (suggests CDI) or the diagnosis of bladder outlet obstruction (postobstructive diuresis or prostatism).

   b. The clinician should also assess for psychiatric illness (suggestive of psychogenic polydipsia), malignancy (hypercalcemia can lead to NDI or renal sodium wasting), diabetes mellitus (DM), Addison's disease, and renal failure.

5. **Family history** of DM, malignancy, and NDI should be noted.

6. **Water diuresis:** When a patient has water diuresis, the clinician needs to distinguish between primary polydipsia, CDI, and NDI.

B. **Physical examination**

   1. Evaluate the **volume status** of the patient (i.e., blood pressure, pulse, mucous membranes, skin turgor, urine output).

   2. Evaluate for **target organ involvement** (e.g., retinopathy, neuropathy) associated with DM.

   3. Evaluate for **malignancy** (e.g., lymphadenopathy, cachexia, palpable masses).

   4. **Kidney examination:** Assess for enlargement.

   5. **Neurologic examination:** Rule out focal findings consistent with a mass lesion or encephalopathy.

   6. **Genitourinary examination:** Check for penile, testicular, scrotal, prostate, and vulvar/adnexal masses.

V. **Diagnostic Evaluation**

A. **Obtain serum and urine samples** before patient receives any intravenous fluids, as fluid solutions will alter results.

B. **Laboratory studies**

   1. **General tests:** As indicated by the history, obtain serum sodium, potassium, chloride, bicarbonate, blood urea nitrogen, creatinine, glucose, calcium, albumin, osmolality, blood count, total protein, cortisol level, aldosterone level, cosyntropin stimulation test (if suspicious of adrenal deficiency).

      a. **Serum sodium indicates the state of water balance.**

         (1) A high level of serum sodium is consistent with CDI and NDI. Hypernatremia stimulates thirst in these patients.

         (2) A low level of serum sodium may be seen in patients with severe, compulsive water drinking.

         (3) The serum sodium in osmotic diuretic states may be difficult to interpret since the presence of the unmeasured osmole in the plasma leads to translocation of intracellular water into the

plasma, diluting the measured level of sodium. Thus, a patient with severe water deficit due to diabetic hyperglycemia may present with a normal serum sodium concentration.

b. Hypercalcemia and hypokalemia interfere with ADH activity on the collecting tubule, and can cause NDI.

2. Urine tests

a. Glycosuria: A urine dipstick test identifies the presence of glycosuria and the specific gravity.

b. 24-hour urine specimen: In the evaluation of polyuria, it is necessary to collect a 24-hour urine specimen.

(1) Polyuria needs to be confirmed by the 24-hour urine total volume (must be > 3 L).

(2) A 24-hour specimen helps to avoid errors attributable to variations in circadian rhythms.

(3) Quantification of the various urine components permit calculation of the solute excretion rates, and thus, lead to the cause of the polyuria.

(4) A 24-hour urine specimen should be sent for the following studies: volume, electrolytes, pH, osmolality, creatinine, urea, glucose, ketones, mannitol, glycerol, and specific gravity.

c. Urine osmolality is low in primary polydipsia (reflecting the kidneys' appropriate "dumping" of water) and both CDI and NDI (reflecting the disabling of the ADH-dependent process on urinary concentration). Urine osmolality in osmotic diuresis is generally close to that of plasma, since the presence of the osmoles in the urine is the force driving the diuresis.

3. Specific tests of ADH function

a. Water deprivation test: The water deprivation test is used to differentiate between CDI and NDI in a patient likely to have one or the other.

(1) Water is withheld from the patient until he or she develops frank hypernatremia (serum Na > 145) or mild hypovolemic hyperosmolarity (serum osmolarity > 295). Urine osmolality is then recorded at hourly intervals until stable on two successive readings. This measurement represents the patient's maximal baseline osmolality and, under these conditions, should be > 800 mOsm/kg. A value less than 200 suggests severe NDI or CDI; a value between 200 and 800 may reflect partial NDI or CDI.

(2) Intravenous 1-deamino-8-D-arginine vasopressin (DDAVP) or aqueous vasopressin (5 U) is then administered. Two more hourly urine osmolalities are recorded in order to determine response to exogenous hormone. Patients with CDI should have a marked increase in Uosm following administration of hormone; patients with NDI have little or no response. Response in patients with partial CDI is difficult to predict.

b. Plasma vasopressin levels should be low in patients with CDI and high in patients with NDI (due to absence of feedback inhibition).

The water deprivation test is usually adequate for distinguishing between CDI and NDI. When results are ambiguous, the plasma vasopressin assay is a useful adjunct.

C. Imaging studies have a limited place in the workup of polyuria.

SUGGESTED READING

Oster JR, Singer I, Thatte L, et al: The polyuria of solute diuresis. *Arch Intern Med* 157: 721–729, 1997.

Rippe JM, Irwin RS, Fink MP, et al: *Intensive Care Medicine*, 3rd ed. Boston: Little, Brown and Company, 1996, pp 962–964.

69

Urinary Incontinence

Stephen B. Young, Allison Howard, and Howard Sachs

Female Urinary Incontinence

Stephen B. Young and Allison Howard

I. **Definition.** Urinary incontinence is a condition in which **involuntary loss of urine is a social or hygienic problem that is objectively demonstrable.**

II. **Overview**

A. Urinary continence, in the absence of detrusor activity, results from an interplay of factors that maintain intraurethral pressure:

1. The internal urethral sphincter
2. The extrinsic urethral sphincter
3. Anatomic support of the urethrovesical junction
4. Intact neurologic pathways

B. **Hypoestrogenism.** Structures of the internal urethral sphincter are estrogen dependent. Estrogen receptors have been demonstrated in the trigone and bladder as well.

1. Postmenopausal hypoestrogenism leads to atrophy of the urethral mucosa, decreased vascular and collagen integrity, and decreased sensitivity of urethral smooth muscle to α-adrenergic stimulation.
2. Hypoestrogenism is further associated with atrophic vaginitis, irritative urethral symptoms, such as dysuria and recurrent urinary tract infections, and genuine stress incontinence (GSI), which is defined as the simultaneous, involuntary loss of urine that occurs when intravesical pressure exceeds maximum urethral pressure in the absence of detrusor activity.

C. **Pregnancy.** Women may incur pudendal and perineal nerve stretch injury and pelvic-floor relaxation associated with childbearing, which is then followed by age-related collagen deficiency. Relaxation may be occult until the hypoestrogenic milieu and years of the chronic cumulative effect of weight bearing, gravity, and physical exertion permit blatant pelvic organ prolapse.

D. **GSI** is the most common cause of urinary leakage in the perimenopausal age group. Eighty-five percent of GSI occurs because the urethrovesical junction has moved out of the intra-abdominal pressure domain. Fifteen percent of women with GSI have damage to the intrinsic sphincter mechanism [i.e., intrinsic sphincter deficiency (ISD)]. Stress incontinence is often, but not purely, associated with symptoms of urine loss with coughing, sneezing, laughing, exercise, lifting, or coitus. The diagnosis is based on the objective loss of urine during physical exertion when other causes of urine loss have been excluded.

E. **Detrusor instability (DI)** is the presence of involuntary, uninhibitable detrusor activity that occurs during bladder filling with or without provocation. Commonly referred to as an unstable or overactive bladder, DI refers to idiopathic, overactive, or uninhibitable detrusor function in the absence of known neurologic abnormality. Overactivity due to neurologic pathology is termed detrusor hyperreflexia.

III. **Differential Diagnosis of Female Urinary Incontinence** (Table 69–1) and Figure 69–1)

IV. **Clinical Approach**

A. **History**

1. **Presenting complaint:** Focus on the amount and type of urinary leakage, associated activities or sensations, and the onset and duration of incontinence. GSI loss occurs in variable amounts and is usually suppressible.

2. **Urge incontinence symptoms** are described as a strong desire to urinate, followed by a sudden, irrepressible, and often large volume of urine loss or dribbling on the way to the bathroom. Urge symptoms usually coexist with complaints of frequency, nocturia greater than or equal to three occurrences, enuresis, supine incontinence, excessive caffeine intake, or a family history of unstable bladder. The onset of DI is associated with increasing age.

3. The **obstetrical/gynecologic history** (especially delivery details) and present **coital activity** are important elements of the history. Other pertinent history includes past surgical procedures for gynecologic or urinary disorders, pelvic irradiation, hormonal status, and medication use.

4. A self-administered **patient questionnaire** as well as a **voiding diary** will facilitate the clinical assessment.

5. It is important to note that **history alone is rarely sufficient in the differential diagnosis of urinary incontinence.** The reliability of stress symptoms in predicting the clinical diagnosis of GSI reveals a positive predictive value (PPV) ranging from 64%–90%. On the other hand, 53%–71% of women with pure DI reported the same history as those with pure GSI.

B. **Physical examination.** The physical examination includes assessment of the neurologic integrity of the urethra and bladder and a complete pelvic examination.

1. **S2-S4 neurologic screening test:** The S2-S4 neurologic screening test demonstrates that the sensorimotor reflex arc of the urethra and bladder are intact. Sensation to pinprick and light touch is tested over dermatomes of the inner thigh, vulvar, and perianal areas. The motor component is tested by anal and clitoral reflexes.

2. **Pelvic examination**

a. If hypoestrogenic atrophy is present vaginally, the urethra and trigone will appear the same.

(1) A scarred, fixed anterior wall may be seen in women who have had prior surgery.

(2) Tenderness or swelling may be indicative of fistula or diverticulum.

TABLE 69–1. Differential Diagnosis of Female Urinary Incontinence

Genuine stress incontinence (GSI)

Detrusor instability

GSI with detrusor instability

Sensory urgency

Detrusor hyperreflexia

Urethral instability

Urethral syndrome

Urinary tract infection

Overflow (denervation, school teacher's bladder)

Functional (ambulatory/toileting impairment)

Psychogenic

Central nervous system (CNS) dysfunction (cerebral atherosclerosis)

Detrusor sphincter dyssynergia (voiding with an uncoordinated sphincter)

Urethral diverticula

Urogenital fistulae

Congenital anomaly (ectopic ureter, bladder exstrophy, epispadias)

Pharmacologic malfunction

Polyuric syndrome (diabetes insipidus)

---

      b. **Pelvic organ relaxation:** Using a Sims retractor, any cystocele, rectocele, or uterine/vaginal prolapse is evaluated for degree of descent on Valsalva. The presence of an exteriorizing prolapse indicates the need for a complete urodynamic evaluation, as "kinking" of the urethra by the descending organ may mask incontinence symptoms and hide the severe incontinence of ISD.

      c. **Levator tone.** Assess levator tone by placing one finger against each vaginal sidewall and asking the patient to contract her vaginal muscles as if stopping the flow of urine. An erect rectovaginal Valsalva examination further determines the presence and extent of rectocele or enterocele. Sphincter tone and presence of a fecal impaction or rectal mass is also determined.

Incontinence

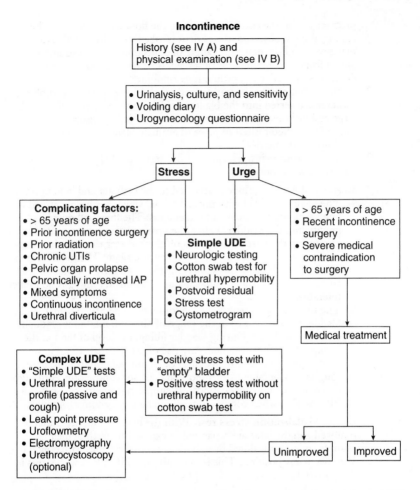

■ **FIGURE 69–1.** Algorithm for the evaluation of female urinary incontinence. *UDE* = urodiagnostic evaluation; *UTIs* = urinary tract infections; *IAP* = intra-abdominal pressure.

V. Diagnostic Evaluation

A. **Urinalysis and culture.** An initial urinalysis and culture is mandatory to rule out infective irritation as the cause of symptoms.

B. **Simple urodynamic evaluation** involves the cotton-swab test for urethral mobility, catheterization for postvoid residual, simple cystometrics, and direct-visualization stress test.

1. **Cotton-swab test:** The cotton-swab test is performed after the urethra is prepared with povidone-iodine (Betadine) and anesthetized with 2% lidocaine jelly. A sterile cotton swab is introduced into the bladder and retracted until a slight resistance is felt, indicating the position of the tip at the urethrovesical junction. The examiner aligns a goniometer or

protractor with the cotton swab, using the floor as a reference. The resting angle is observed, the patient is asked to perform Valsalva maneuver, and the maximum angle of deflection (i.e., the straining angle) from the horizontal is observed. An angle greater than 30 degrees is indicative of urethral hypermobility.

2. **Catheterization for postvoid residual:** A 12–14 French red rubber catheter is inserted into the bladder to determine postvoid residual. A large residual (i.e., > 100 ml) may indicate a voiding disorder (retention). The catheter is left in place to evaluate bladder storage function by simple cystometrics.

3. **Simple cystometrics:** The goal of this test is to elicit any abnormal detrusor contractions.

   a. A 60-ml Asepto syringe is attached to the catheter and held upright. The bladder is filled with normal saline, which has been warmed to body temperature, in 50-ml increments. The fluid will flow by gravity into the bladder. When the syringe is almost empty and prior to pouring the next 50 ml, pinch off the catheter to avoid the introduction of air into the system, then release again. The measurements are "eyeballed" as the patient is enlisted to identify her first desire to void, feeling of bladder fullness, and when further filling is no longer tolerable.

   b. The next measurement is the **cystometric capacity.** Normal bladder capacity is within the range of 300–500 ml, but it gradually decreases with age. During bladder filling, the level of fluid in the syringe is carefully watched. Any rise of greater than 15 ml in the fluid column, in the absence of a rise in intra-abdominal pressure, is roughly attributable to an abnormal detrusor contraction. Although this is a crude diagnostic modality, simple cystometry has shown a PPV of 85% when compared to multichannel cystometrography.

4. **Direct-visualization stress test.** With the bladder full, the catheter is removed and the labia are separated to expose the urethral meatus. A positive stress test is noted by a fluid spurt simultaneous with cough or Valsalva in any position. This is indicative of GSI. A leak with stress in the postvoid state is suggestive of ISD.

   a. At this level of workup, the patient may be categorized as having suspected DI, primary GSI with or without urethral hypermobility, or in need of more complete evaluation.

   b. Complex urodynamics are performed in a urodynamic laboratory.

SUGGESTED READING

Bent AE: Geriatric urogynecology. In Ostergard DR, Bent AE (eds): *Urogynecology and Urodynamics: Theory and Practice.* Baltimore: Williams & Wilkins, 1991, p 522.

Summitt RL, Bent AE: Genuine stress incontinence: An overview. In Ostergard DR, Bent AE (eds): *Urogynecology and Urodynamics: Theory and Practice.* Baltimore: Williams & Wilkins, 1991, pp 394–395.

Benign Prostatic Hyperplasia

Howard Sachs

I. Overview

A. The **diagnosis of benign prostatic hyperplasia (BPH)** is made on **digital rectal examination, radiologic imaging,** or a **clinical basis,** characterized by the presence of lower urinary tract symptoms in the absence of alternative diagnoses to explain the symptoms.

1. **Lower urinary tract symptoms** are not invariably the result of BPH, although in middle-aged men, 90% will be found to have BPH as the cause of those symptoms. On the other hand, despite the almost inevitable development of histologic BPH with age, a significantly lower proportion of patients exhibit symptoms.

2. **Bladder outlet obstruction** in BPH manifests urodynamically by diminished urinary flow, increased postvoid residual urine volume, and uninhibited bladder (detrusor) contractions.

B. **Clinical course**

1. **Symptom progression:** The severity of symptoms at baseline correlates with the likelihood of progression.

2. **Stabilization** or **improvement** occurs in 50%–60% of patients.

3. A **complicated course** may be characterized by:

   a. Obstructive uropathy/renal failure (1%–2%)
   b. Urinary tract infection (< 5%)
   c. Urinary retention (1%–2% per year)
   d. Urolithiasis (2%)

II. Clinical Approach (Figure 69–2)

A. **History**

1. **Presenting complaint:** Use a standardized instrument such as the International Prostate Symptom Score (IPSS) to evaluate symptoms, assess symptom severity, monitor progression, and assess symptom impact upon the patient. The questionnaire elicits and quantifies information about incomplete bladder emptying, urinary frequency, urgency, intermittency, straining, and nocturia. The IPSS should not be used as the sole means of diagnosing BPH because symptoms are not specific.

2. **Relevant symptoms:** Although the majority of men with voiding symptoms have BPH, other conditions are present in approximately 10% of patients with lower urinary tract symptoms. Specific inquiry should focus on malignancy (prostate and bladder), infection (prostatitis, cystitis), neurologic dysfunction (neurodegenerative disease, autonomic dysfunction, spinal cord disease), diabetes, congestive heart failure (CHF), medication use, fluid consumption, caffeine and alcohol use, symptoms of urolithiasis, and prior pelvic surgery.

3. **Complications of BPH:** Assess for increased postvoid residual urinary volume, urinary retention (sense of incomplete bladder emptying or

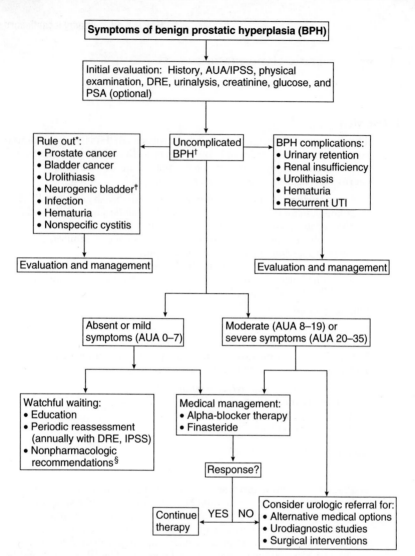

■ FIGURE 69–2. Algorithm for the evaluation of benign prostatic hyperplasia (BPH). *AUA* = American Urologic Association questionnaire; *DRE* = digital rectal examination; *IPSS* = International Prostate Symptom Score; *PSA* = prostate-specific antigen; *UTI* = urinary tract infection.

*Other conditions can present with symptoms similar to BPH.

†After the initial evaluation, it is reasonable to employ a "treat first" strategy and defer more detailed evaluation to treatment failures or patients presenting with BPH-related complications.

‡Neurogenic bladder should be suspected under certain clinical circumstances (neurodegenerative disorders, spinal cord disease, or bladder dysfunction). Cystometrogram studies can usually confirm the diagnosis.

§Nonpharmacologic methods include avoiding caffeine, alcohol, over-the-counter medications, culprit medications, and evening fluid consumption. Education should include information on the natural history of BPH and complicating diagnoses.

▲

distension), symptoms of infection or stone (dysuria, fever, pain, or hematuria), and obstructive uropathy and renal damage (history of azotemia or renal failure). Acute urinary retention may develop suddenly in asymptomatic patients or in patients with mild degrees of prostatism.

B. Physical examination

1. **Digital rectal examination:** The prostate gland should be palpated for size, symmetry, tenderness, nodularity, and texture. The pathogenesis of BPH arises from changes in the periurethral region (i.e., the transitional zone). However, digital rectal examination palpates the peripheral region of the gland. This explains why the gland is palpably normal in as many as 60% of cases, even in patients with advanced symptoms. Although the size of the gland correlates poorly with symptoms, the examination is useful in identifying diagnoses, such as prostate cancer and prostatitis.

2. **Abdominal examination**

   a. Assess the bladder for tenderness or distension.

   b. Assess for fluid overload states.

3. **Neurologic examination:** Focus on sacral nerve function as well as signs of autonomic dysfunction.

III. Diagnostic Evaluation

A. Urinalysis is obtained to assess for the presence of infection, hematuria, and glycosuria.

B. Serum creatinine is obtained for purposes of determining renal insufficiency, the cause of which may be obstructive uropathy. An elevated value is not synonymous with obstructive uropathy, but does warrant further evaluation.

C. Serum glucose is not a routine test in the evaluation of BPH per se. However, given the prevalence of type II diabetes and the overlapping symptoms (polyuria versus frequency, urgency, and nocturia), assessment for hyperglycemia is of clinical benefit. In addition, patients with diabetes may present with urinary dysfunction secondary to neurogenic bladder.

D. Prostate-specific antigen (PSA) is considered an optional test in the evaluation of patients with BPH. BPH does not increase the risk of prostate cancer, although the two diseases are common and may coexist. Furthermore, prostate cancer may present with lower urinary tract symptoms. The efficacy of PSA as a screening test for prostate cancer in this setting has not been established. Physician discretion is advised, especially if a watchful waiting approach is taken. Another potential role for PSA testing, in this setting, is in the assessment of prostate volume. A PSA < 1.5 ng/dl is indicative of a low-volume gland, which is less likely to respond to finasteride therapy.

E. Urinary flow rate (urinary flowmetry) measures the rate of urine flow in milliliters per second. Parameters measured include maximum flow rate (Q_{max}), time to maximum flow rate, voiding time, and average flow rate. The maximal (peak) flow rate correlates most closely with the degree of bladder outflow obstruction. Poor flow, however, can be secondary to poor detrusor contractility rather than outflow obstruction. Decreases in symptom scores are not proportional to increases in Q_{max}.

F. Pressure-flow studies may be helpful in patients whose history or examination suggest primary bladder dysfunction (as in patients with neurologic disease). They are also useful in patients for whom a distinction between prostatic obstruction and impaired detrusor contractility might affect the choice of therapy.

G. Cystometry measures the volume at which a bladder contraction occurs and its strength. Cystometry provides data on bladder capacity, sensation, compliance, and stability. The cystometrogram will be most useful in distinguishing between prostatic obstruction, uninhibited detrusor contractions, or impaired detrusor contractility. Distinction is most useful in patients with suspected neurologic diseases.

H. Urodynamic studies are used to identify those patients, usually with neurologic disease, where external sphincter dyssynergy is suspected.

SUGGESTED READING

Oesterling JE: Benign prostatic hyperplasia. *N Engl J Med* 332(2): 99–109, 1995.

70

Oliguria
David Clive

I. Definition. Oliguria is a **reduction in urine flow to less than 400 ml/day** (i.e., 20 ml/hr).

  A. Patients rarely complain of oliguria because people are less attuned to reductions in their urine output than to increases, unless the reduction is so severe as to approach a cessation of urine altogether (i.e., **anuria**).

  B. Oliguria is more apt to be recognized in a hospitalized patient, especially in the following cases:

    1. Patients with septic shock

    2. Patients with decreased cardiac output

    3. Following anesthesia

    4. Patients who are taking diuretics

    5. Following radiographic contrast agents

    6. Patients with chronic renal failure, although oliguria does not generally become fixed until after reaching the end stage

II. Overview

  A. Acute renal failure. By far the most important aspect of oliguria is as a sign of acute renal failure, as discussed in Chapter 76.

    1. Oliguria is seen in less than half of cases of acute renal failure.

    2. Oliguria is an **ominous sign** in acute renal failure. Patients with oliguria are more likely to die, to require interim dialysis, and to remain in renal failure longer than patients with acute renal failure who do not have oliguria.

  B. Anuria is even more rare than oliguria, and is not ordinarily expected in routine cases of toxic or ischemic acute renal failure. When a patient stops making urine altogether, greater consideration should be given to:

    1. Complete acute devascularization of the kidneys (e.g., aortic dissection involving both renal arteries)

    2. Complete acute obstruction of the urinary tract (i.e., involving either the bladder outlet or both ureters)

    3. Acute unilateral obstruction or devascularization in a patient who has only one functioning kidney at baseline

SUGGESTED READING

Klahr S, Miller SB: Current concepts: Acute oliguria. *N Engl J Med* 338:671–675, 1998.

71

Sodium Imbalance
David Clive

| Hyponatremia

I. Definition. Hyponatremia occurs **when the balance of extracellular water relative to sodium is disproportionately high.** Thus, even patients with generalized edema, reflecting a sodium overload state, may be hyponatremic.

II. Overview

A. The **concentration of sodium in the extracellular fluid is normally between 136–143 mEq/L.** The serum sodium concentration does not reflect total body sodium content as much as water balance.

B. **Pseudohyponatremia** occurs when a subnormal serum sodium concentration is observed as an artifact of unusually high levels of lipid or paraprotein in the blood since the actual ionic concentration of the aqueous component of plasma is normal. Once this situation is ruled out, the patient can be said to have **true hyponatremia.**

III. Forms of Hyponatremia

A. **Hyperosmolar hyponatremia** occurs when an osmotically active substance accumulates in the bloodstream, leading to movement of water from intracellular to extracellular space. This movement of water leads to dilution of the extracellular sodium. Examples include hyponatremia seen in patients with severe diabetic hyperglycemia, or patients receiving mannitol or radiocontrast agents.

B. **Hypo-osmolar hyponatremia** is the most common and most serious form of hyponatremia. Patients in this category have disordered water homeostasis. The amount of free water ultimately to be excreted depends on the appropriate regulation of antidiuretic hormone (ADH) release by the hypothalamic–pituitary axis. Volume-depleted patients have an ongoing stimulus for continued antidiuresis, even though they may be hypo-osmolar. There are several subtypes of this category, best differentiated by assessment of the patient's extracellular volume. Hypovolemic patients may have hypotension, orthostatic hypotension, and poor skin turgor. Patients with expanded extracellular volume may have frank edema.

1. **Decreased extracellular volume:** Patients are volume depleted, having lost electrolyte-rich body fluid, and have replaced these losses with electrolyte-poor fluids. Hyponatremia may occur in patients following hemorrhage, third-space losses, or fluid losses due to burns, excessive perspiration, vomiting, or diarrhea.

2. **Expanded extracellular volume:** These are patients with generalized edema (see Chapter 25). By definition, these patients are overloaded with total body sodium. They are simultaneously hyponatremic since their water retention is disproportionately greater than that of sodium.

3. **Normal extracellular volume** may be the result of an increase in total

body water with only minimal change in total body sodium. The increase in extracellular volume is small, and the patient appears normovolemic. A number of miscellaneous conditions fall under this heading.

a. **Syndrome of inappropriate ADH secretion (SIADH)** is a condition in which ADH release is either autonomous or poorly regulated. This condition may be seen in conjunction with certain neoplasms, pulmonary disease, central nervous system (CNS) disease, drug intake, or sustained unpleasant stimuli such as nausea or pain.

b. **Hypothyroidism,** particularly when severe, can cause hyponatremia.

c. **Glucocorticoid insufficiency,** like hypothyroidism, can cause reduced cardiac output and impaired water excretion.

d. **Inadequate solute intake** or excessive water intake can cause hyponatremia. If solute intake and renal function are normal, a person can drink and excrete up to 16 L of water per day. Thus, **primary polydipsia** (i.e., compulsive water drinking), as seen in some psychotic patients or athletes, is a rare cause of hyponatremia. Conversely, patients with normal fluid intake must have an extraordinarily low solute intake to become hyponatremic. In these conditions, ADH levels are usually suppressed, and urine osmolality (U_{osm}) is appropriately low.

e. **Thiazide-induced hyponatremia** and **SIADH** have the potential to provoke the most profound hyponatremia. The two disorders may be difficult to distinguish. While a low serum urea and uric acid level are seen in SIADH, the opposite generally applies with thiazide use.

IV. Diagnostic Evaluation. Serum osmolality, blood urea nitrogen, creatinine, electrolytes, total protein, lipid profile, urine sodium, and U_{osm} should be obtained in all patients with hyponatremia. Figure 71–1 provides an algorithm for evaluating patients with hyponatremia.

Hypernatremia

I. Definition. Hypernatremia (i.e., serum sodium concentration > 145 mEq/L) **represents an excess of sodium relative to water in the extracellular space.**

II. Overview (Figure 71–2). Although such an imbalance may come about as a result of sodium overload, more commonly it arises from free water depletion. Both hyperosmolarity and hypovolemia are stimuli for ADH release and thus reabsorption of water from renal tubular fluid.

III. Forms of Hypernatremia

A. **Primary sodium overload** is a relatively uncommon cause of hypernatremia. It has been reported in relation to dietary excess of sodium, most notoriously in infants receiving undiluted sodium-rich formulas. In adults, the most common cause of sodium overload is administration of parenteral sodium bicarbonate, as may occur during cardiopulmonary resuscitation. Correction of the sodium excess is readily accomplished when kidney function is normal. In critically ill patients with acute renal failure, hypernatremia of this form may be prolonged.

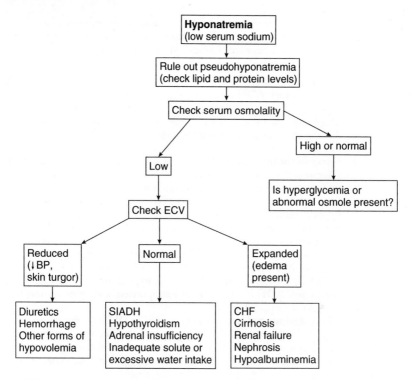

■ **FIGURE 71–1.** Algorithm for the evaluation of hyponatremia. *BP* = blood pressure; *CHF* = congestive heart failure; *ECV* = extracellular volume; *SIADH* = syndrome of inappropriate antidiuretic hormone secretion.

B. Reduced water intake. So powerful is the thirst mechanism that hypernatremia due to reduced water intake generally implies CNS dysfunction (e.g., a comatose, geriatric, or disabled patient who is unable to verbalize a desire for water), or loss of access to water. Primary hypodipsia results from damage to the thirst centers in the hypothalamus (from tumors, granulomas, vascular disease, or trauma). Even with maximal water conservation by kidneys, ongoing, unreplenished insensible water losses will eventually lead to hypernatremia.

C. Increased water losses

1. **Renal water loss:** Inability to concentrate urine normally occurs in osmotic diuresis, treatment with loop diuretics, or when ADH effect is inadequate. Renal concentrating defect is suggested when the U_{osm} of a hypernatremic patient is not well above that of the plasma osmolality (P_{osm}).

   a. If ADH is lacking, or deficient, the patient is said to have **central diabetes insipidus** (CDI) [see Chapter 68].
   b. If ADH is available, but the kidney's ability to respond to it is

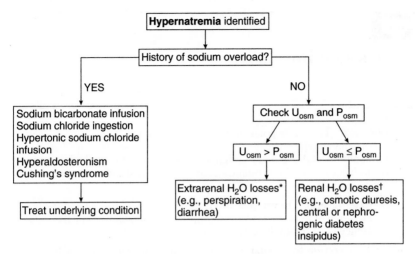

■ **FIGURE 71–2.** Algorithm for the evaluation of hypernatremia. U_{osm} = urine osmolality; P_{osm} = plasma osmolality.
*Clinical history will usually point to diagnosis prior to measuring U_{osm} and P_{osm}.
†History of polyuria will frequently enable diagnosis to be made before checking U_{osm} and P_{osm}.

    attenuated, the patient has **nephrogenic diabetes insipidus** (NDI) [see Chapter 68].

2. **Extrarenal water loss:** Hypotonic fluid may be lost through perspiration, prolonged nasogastric suction, vomiting, diarrhea, and in the setting of third space losses or through insensible routes. In these situations, a high U_{osm} is appropriate.

SUGGESTED READING

Fried LF, Palevsky PM: Hyponatremia and hypernatremia. *Med Clin North Am* 81:585–609, 1997.

72

Potassium Imbalance
David Clive

I. **Overview.** The serum potassium concentration is maintained within a very narrow physiologic range.

II. **Potassium Metabolism.** Potassium metabolism in the body fluids is under the influence of two homeostatic systems, the internal and external arms of potassium balance.

A. **External arm.** The external arm is the system by which the body's excretion of potassium is kept appropriate in relation to its intake. The kidney is central to the external arm.

1. **Secretion by tubular cells:** Secretion of potassium by tubular cells in the distal and cortical collecting tubules of the kidneys is responsible for much of the ultimate excretion of potassium. Secretion is augmented by factors that enhance the electrochemical secretory gradient, particularly metabolic alkalosis and high nephronic flow rates. Distal sodium reabsorption favors potassium excretion, such as occurs in states of increased mineralocorticoid activity.

2. **Excretion in stool:** A small amount of potassium is excreted each day in stool. This amount may increase with diarrhea.

3. **Loss via perspiration:** Potassium can also be lost via excessive perspiration. When extrarenal potassium wasting occurs, the kidneys should conserve potassium. However, if volume depletion or metabolic alkalosis is present, ongoing potassium losses may occur even in the face of established hypokalemia.

B. **Internal arm.** The internal arm of potassium balance is concerned not with maintaining the intake–excretion balance of potassium, but rather with an appropriate distribution of existing potassium content within the body. Specifically, the vast majority (> 95%) of the body's potassium is confined to the intracellular space. The concentration of potassium in intracellular fluid is about 150 mEq/L, which is much higher than the concentration of potassium in extracellular fluid (3.5–5.0 mEq/L). This disparity is critical to the electrophysiology of cardiac, skeletal, and smooth muscle myocytes.

1. β-blockers, such as propranolol, inhibit potassium uptake by cells.

2. Changes in the chemical milieu of the body can lead to transcellular fluxes of potassium independent of the Na-K exchanger.

3. Increases in the extracellular fluid osmolarity cause potassium-rich water to move from cells into extracellular fluid.

4. Alkalemia leads to movement of potassium into cells; acidemic states favor translocation of potassium into extracellular fluid.

III. **Morbidity.** The most serious morbidity of potassium imbalance relates to its adverse effects on the electrical activity of the heart. Both hyper- and hypokalemia can trigger arrhythmias, and both are associated with specific electrocardiographic abnormalities. In hyperkalemia, prolongation of the QRS complex may be seen, as well as peaking of T waves.

Hyperkalemia

I. **Definition.** Hyperkalemia is defined as **serum potassium > 5.5 mEq/L.** Spurious elevation of the serum potassium level is the most frequent cause of hyperkalemia.

II. **Pseudohyperkalemia** may occur as a preanalytical error due to released potassium from red cells, if the blood specimen is left unspun in the cold or due to intravascular hemolysis. Pseudohyperkalemia may also result from hyperleukocytosis or thrombocytosis.

III. **Diagnostic Approach** (Figure 72–1)

   A. The **source** of excess potassium should be identified.

   B. The **impediment to its excretion or metabolism** should be sought. This is best accomplished by screening for possible abnormalities in the external and internal arms of potassium balance.

SUGGESTED READING

Williams ME: Hyperkalemia. *Crit Care Med* 7:155–174, 1991.

Hypokalemia

I. **Definition.** Hypokalemia is defined as **serum potassium < 3.5 mEq/L.**

II. **Diagnostic Approach** (Figure 72–2). The approach is similar to that followed in evaluation of hyperkalemia. The electroencephalogram often demonstrates U waves, a repolarization abnormality that manifests as a prolonged positive deflection following the T wave. Prolonged conduction intervals may also be seen.

   A. **Hypokalemia due to abnormalities in the external arm of potassium balance**

   1. **Insufficient intake:** Dietary deprivation of potassium is unusual, due to the ubiquitous nature of potassium in foodstuffs. This cause of hypokalemia, therefore, is most often observed in the clinically malnourished or alcoholic patient.

   2. **Excessive excretion**

   a. **Metabolic alkalosis** not only causes shift of potassium into cells, but the resulting increase in the transtubular potassium gradient encourages secretion of potassium ions distally.

   b. **Bicarbonate excretion in the urine** (as in renal compensation for metabolic alkalosis or in the posthypercapnic state) obligates K^+ excretion.

   c. **Osmotic diuresis** causes potassium, and other ions, to be swept out into the urine.

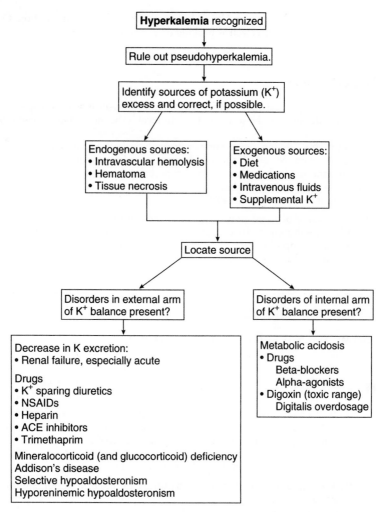

FIGURE 72–1. Diagnostic approach to hyperkalemia. *ACE* = angiotensin-converting enzyme; *NSAIDs* = nonsteroidal anti-inflammatory drugs.

d. **Mineralocorticoid excess states**

(1) Primary aldosteronism (glucocorticoid excess states can cause hypokalemia)

(2) Bartter's syndrome

(3) States of secondary mineralocorticoid excess rarely cause hypokalemia because the antikaliuretic effect of low nephronic rate offsets the tendency of aldosterone to enhance K^+ secretion.

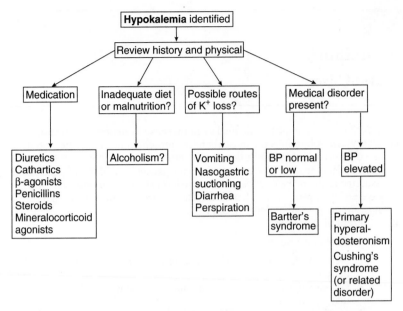

FIGURE 72–2. Diagnostic approach to hypokalemia. *BP* = blood pressure; *K⁺* = potassium.

> **e. Drugs**
>> **(1)** Diuretics (including surreptitious use)
>> **(2)** Mineralocorticoid agonists (e.g., fludrocortisone)
>> **(3)** Synthetic penicillins (especially nafcillin and carbenicillin)
>> **(4)** Cathartics
>
> **f.** Diarrhea and other states of increased enteric fluid output, pyloric stenosis, gastrointestinal suction, and drainage
> **g.** Acute monocytic and monomyelocytic leukemias
> **h.** Overindulgence of licorice, chewing certain tobaccos

B. Hypokalemia due to abnormalities in the internal arm of potassium balance

> **1. Hormonal imbalance**
>> **a.** Insulin, especially in correction phase of diabetic hyperglycemia
>> **b.** β-adrenergic excess
>
> **2. Drugs** (β-agonists, such as albuterol)
> **3. Metabolic alkalosis**

SUGGESTED READING

Gennari ME: Hyperkalemia. *Crit Care Med* 7:155–174, 1991.

73

Proteinuria
David Clive

I. **Definition.** Proteinuria is defined as an **increase in protein excretion.**

II. **Overview.** Albumin is the most abundant protein in normal urine, and it is the only protein that can be detected by urine dipstick test used in common medical laboratories. Under normal circumstances, < 200 mg of protein are excreted in the urine each day, below the level at which albumin can be detected by dipstick test. There is a certain degree of imprecision in dipstick measurement of albuminuria (see IV A).

III. **Differential Diagnosis**

  A. **Clinical conditions**

    1. **Renal disease:** Proteinuria can occur in virtually any form of renal disease.

    2. **Glomerular lesion:** When albumin excretion is > 2 g/day, a glomerular lesion is likely.

    3. **Nephrotic syndrome:** When albumin excretion is > 3 g/day, the patient is said to have a nephrotic syndrome (the terms "nephrosis" and "nephrotic range proteinuria" are also used). Patients with nephrotic syndrome often "spill" other forms of protein [e.g., peptide hormones, immunoglobulins (Ig)] besides albumin. Common complications of nephrotic syndrome include edema, hyperlipidemia, and hypercoagulability.

  B. **Types**

    1. **Tubular proteinuria** refers to excretion of protein molecules small enough to be filtered, but that, under normal circumstances, do not appear in the urine since they are readily reabsorbed from the filtrate by tubular cells. When protein is present in the urine, therefore, a tubular lesion may be present. Nephrotic syndrome may trigger secondary tubular proteinuria since the reabsorption of filtered albumin and lipid by tubular cells may damage them through overload. β_2-microglobulin is the paradigm example of a tubular protein.

    2. **Overflow proteinuria** refers to the excretion of proteins, which while filterable, are normally not found in large amounts in the urine since they are not overly abundant in plasma. In certain pathologic conditions, however, they may be overproduced and presented in abnormally large quantities to the glomerulus. Examples include the **pigment proteins** [hemoglobin (Hg) and myoglobin] and **Ig fragments.** Most familiar of these are the light chains, which are often detected in the urine in plasma cell dyscrasias and amyloidosis **(Bence Jones proteins).**

    3. **Tissue proteinuria** arises from inflammation and infection in the urinary tract causing exudation or bleeding directly into the urine. It is usually of low grade.

    4. **Glomerular proteinuria** is attributable to damage to the glomerulus.

The hallmark of glomerular proteinuria is **albuminuria;** massive albumin excretion cannot occur in the absence of significant damage to the glomerular basement membrane. In most glomerulopathies, however, nonalbumin proteins are also being lost in urine.

IV. **Diagnostic Evaluation** (Figure 73–1). Detection and quantitation of urinary protein entails the following:

   A. **Urine dipstick test.** This is actually an indirect test for albumin. The reagent is a pH indicator responding to the ability of albumin to buffer hydrogen ions in the urine. Three notes of caution include:

   1. A high urinary pH will give a false-positive result.
   2. The familiar 0 to 4+ grading system is an imprecise tool for quantifying proteinuria.
   3. Proteins (e.g., Ig and light chains) that lack albumin's buffering properties will not be detected by dipstick.

   B. **24-hour protein determinations** employ direct chemical assay of protein in urine. They are, therefore, more accurate than the dipstick test in defining proteinuria. The main concern is to make certain that a 24-hour collection is complete. For this purpose, the volume of the collection is of little use; measuring the creatinine content of the specimen is better (expect $\geq$ 12 mg/kg/day in women, $\geq$ 14 mg/kg/day in men). Many

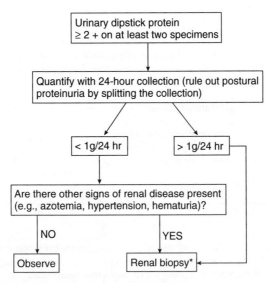

FIGURE 73–1. Diagnostic approach to proteinuria.
   *Patients with systemic disorders or taking medications known to induce secondary proteinuria may not necessitate biopsy for diagnosis. Children presenting with nephrotic range proteinuria and normal renal functions are often empirically treated with steroids based on the likelihood of diagnosis of minimal change disease. Biopsy may later be entertained if therapeutic response is inadequate.

TABLE 73–1. Drugs and Disorders That May Cause Secondary Albuminuria

Drugs	Disorders
Ampicillin	Allergic reactions
Nonsteroidal anti-inflammatory agents	Infections • Bacterial (e.g., endocarditis, *Streptococcus viridans,* leprosy, tuberculosis, syphilis)
Bismuth	• Protozoal (e.g., malaria, toxoplasmosis) • Helminthic (e.g., filariasis, schistosomiasis)
Penicillamine	• Viral (e.g., cytomegalovirus, Epstein-Barr virus, hepatitis B, HIV)
Captopril	Neoplasia (e.g., adenocarcinoma, lymphoma, Hodgkin's disease)
Probenecid	Amyloidosis
Gold salts	Collagen vascular diseases including
Tolbutamide	• Dermatomyositis
Lithium carbonate	• Sjögren's syndrome
	• Systemic lupus erythematosus
	• Rheumatoid arthritis
	• Vasculitis (e.g., cryoglobulinemia, Henoch-Schönlein purpura, polyarteritis nodosa, Takayasu's arteritis, Wegener's granulomatosis)
	Diabetes mellitus
	Goodpasture's syndrome
	Massive obesity
	Pre-eclampsia

clinicians favor the use of the urinary **protein-to-creatinine ratio**. A ratio of ≤ 0.15 mg protein/mg creatinine is normal; a ratio > 3 mg protein/mg creatinine suggests the presence of nephrotic syndrome.
C. **Urine protein electrophoresis** enhances ability to detect and quantify different urinary protein species.
D. **Microalbuminuria** refers to a tendency in the early stages of progressive glomerulopathies, particularly diabetic renal disease, to excrete small amounts of protein on a regular basis. This finding may be critical for prognostic or screening purposes, but is too subtle to define by urine

dipstick test or standard 24-hour assay methods. Albumin excretion rates of 15–30 μg/min can be detected using radioimmunoassay techniques.

V. Diagnosis of Albuminuria (see Figure 73–1). This entry will consider only the patient with glomerular proteinuria (i.e., the patient found to have albuminuria).

   A. **Confirm the presence of glomerular proteinuria.** Vigorous exercise and fever can produce transient albuminuria in normal glomeruli. The persistent presence of > 1+ protein by dipstick test should be verified on sequential samples collected on different days.

   B. **Establish excretion rate.** Using a 24-hour urine collection, the actual excretion rate of protein should be established. It is often helpful to have the patient divide the 24-hour specimen into separate daytime and nighttime collections to rule out the possibility of orthostatic proteinuria, a benign condition.

   C. **Consider the patient's medical background.** Having determined that the patient has truly pathologic proteinuria, the clinician should consider the patient's overall medical background. There are several questions to answer:

   1. **How serious is the proteinuria?** Most physicians will aggressively follow proteinuria > 1–2 g/24 hours in magnitude. Lesser amounts may be followed conservatively, unless the patient has other signs of renal dysfunction, such as hypertension, azotemia, or an active microscopic urinary sediment.

   2. Is the proteinuria **transient** [fever, exercise, congestive heart failure CHF)], **intermittent** (prolonged standing), **or persistent** (most cases of glomerular proteinuria)?

   3. Is the proteinuria likely due to **a primary or secondary renal condition?**

      a. For example, if the patient has known long-standing diabetes mellitus (DM) and a history of retinopathy, the appearance of proteinuria is overwhelmingly likely to represent diabetic nephropathy.

      b. Many medical conditions and even medications can induce proteinuria (Table 73–1).

TABLE 73–2. Primary Glomerular Diseases That Can Cause Proteinuria

Mainly Nephritic	Mainly Nephrotic
Poststreptococcal glomerulonephritis	Focal segmental glomerulosclerosis
Immunoglobulin A (IgA) nephropathy	Minimal change disease
Idiopathic crescentic glomerulonephritis	Membranous nephropathy
	Membranoproliferative glomerulonephritis

      c. In the absence of systemic diseases or medications that can evoke proteinuric states, a primary glomerulopathy must be considered (Table 73–2). Primary glomerulopathies generally require renal biopsy for precise diagnosis.

SUGGESTED READING

Orth S, Ritz E: The nephrotic syndrome. *N Engl J Med* 338:1202–1211, 1998.

74

Azotemia
David Clive

I. **Definition.** Azotemia is defined as **elevated blood levels of urea and creatinine.**

   A. Urea is a metabolic by-product of protein catabolism. Creatinine is a metabolic product of muscle and, to a lesser extent, liver cells. These nitrogenous wastes are normally formed in fairly fixed daily amounts and excreted in the urine.

   B. Azotemia results either from reduced excretion of urea and creatinine or from an increase in their production to which the kidneys are unable to respond by increasing excretion.

II. **Overview**

   A. **Azotemia versus uremia.** Azotemia is a laboratory finding and must be distinguished from uremia, the clinical syndrome comprising encephalopathy, neuropathy, anemia, bone disease, pruritus, and various other symptoms of severe renal failure. Until patients have severe enough renal failure to evoke uremic symptomatology, most patients with renal disease are asymptomatic. Azotemia is thus of paramount importance in the timely recognition of disorders of the kidney.

   B. **Chronic versus acute renal disease.** Since the significance of azotemia lies in its relation to renal failure, it is imperative to establish whether azotemia is long-standing (indicative of chronic renal disease) or of recent onset (indicative of acute renal failure). The tip-offs that renal failure is of a more chronic nature are the presence of anemia and the finding of small, scarred kidneys on imaging studies.

III. **Differential Diagnosis**

   A. **Decreased glomerular filtration rate (GFR).** For azotemia related to decreased GFR, see Chapter 76.

   B. **Elevations in blood urea nitrogen and creatinine unrelated to change in GFR**

   1. **Increased urea production** occurs when urea production increases and the kidney cannot meet increased excretory demand. Some common causes of increased urea production include:

      a. **Use of catabolic steroids** (e.g., prednisone, which increases ureagenesis)

      b. **Increase in dietary protein**

      c. **Gastrointestinal bleeding,** which, as red cells are catabolized, provides substrate for urea production (As a rule, patients will not develop a rise in blood urea nitrogen under these circumstances, unless they have preexisting renal insufficiency.)

2. **Excretory load of creatinine:** The excretory load of creatinine may be augmented endogenously by muscle breakdown or exogenously by meat consumption. As with urea, changes in the excretory creatinine burden should only raise serum creatinine levels in patients with reduced renal reserve.

3. **Low flow rate of filtrate** through the renal tubules augments the reabsorption of urea. This is most often seen in patients with prerenal azotemia (see Chapter 76). In this condition, the reduction in glomerular filtration causes urea and creatinine retention. However, because the tubular reabsorption of urea is enhanced, the ratio of urea to creatinine in the blood goes up.

4. **Drugs:** Some drugs, most notably cimetidine and trimethoprim, can inhibit tubular secretion of creatinine. This produces an elevation in the serum creatinine independent of a change in GFR, and without a concomitant increment in the serum urea level.

75

Acid–Base Disorders

Julia M. Gallagher

I. Background

A. **Systematic approach.** The electrolytes are essential in the evaluation of possible metabolic processes and should be drawn as close as possible to an arterial blood gas (ABG), particularly in dynamic or uncertain clinical situations. Remember, a patient may have as many as three primary acid–base disorders simultaneously, and failure to evaluate a set of electrolytes along with an ABG will result in missed diagnosis.

1. **Bicarbonate values:** The bicarbonate values from the ABG and electrolytes should be compared to ensure that data are internally consistent. The bicarbonate on the ABG is a calculated number, derived from the Henderson–Hasselbalch equation using the measured values of $PaCO_2$ and pH. The bicarbonate on the electrolytes is a true measured value. These values should be within 2 or 3 mg/dl of each other. If they are not, then there is either **lab error** or **internal inconsistency** (the latter term refers to the ABG) in one of the measurements. Alternatively, the electrolytes and ABG may have been drawn too far apart and the physiologic situation has since changed.

2. **Internal consistency:** The internal consistency of the ABG can be checked using a number of formulas, the simplest of which is:

$$[H^+] = 24 \times (PaCO_2/HCO_3^-)$$

Then, using a $[H^+]$-pH table (Figure 75–1), the calculated $[H^+]$ is used to find a corresponding pH. If the pH as measured by the ABG does not equal the pH as estimated by the formula, there is a lab error.

B. **Definitions**

1. **Anion gap (AG):** The AG represents unmeasured plasma anions and is calculated from the electrolytes as follows:

$$AG = [Na^+] - ([Cl^-] + [HCO_3^-])$$

or conceptually, the difference between the major serum cations (Na) and the major serum anions (Cl and HCO_3^-).

a. A "normal" AG ranges from 5–12 mmol/L depending on the lab.

b. Albumin, an anionic protein, accounts for the majority of the AG; therefore, significant changes in serum albumin may alter the AG. In particular, severe hypoalbuminemia decreases the AG. To "correct" the AG for hypoalbuminemia, add 3.0 to the AG for each 1.0 gm decrease in the albumin concentration below 4.0.

2. **Delta/delta:** The delta/delta is the ratio of the change from baseline of the AG over the change from baseline of the $[HCO_3^-]$. Conceptually, the delta/delta describes the relationship between the addition of an

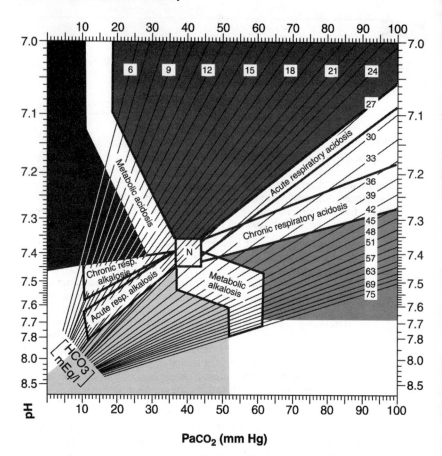

The significance bands for the various simple disorders are labeled on the map. Probable interpretations for points falling in the cross-hatched areas between are:

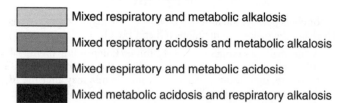

Mixed respiratory and metabolic alkalosis

Mixed respiratory acidosis and metabolic alkalosis

Mixed respiratory and metabolic acidosis

Mixed metabolic acidosis and respiratory alkalosis

■ **FIGURE 75–1.** Acid-base nomogram. (Reprinted with permission from Goldberg M: Computer-based instruction and diagnosis of acid-base disorders. JAMA 223:269, 1973.)

unmeasured "acid" to plasma (causing an increase in the AG) and the resulting decrease in plasma bicarbonate as a result of extracellular buffering. This comparison is accurate, and therefore helpful, if the patient's baseline AG is known. If there are no prior measurements of a patient's serum electrolytes, calculate the delta/delta assuming a normal AG while being mindful of possible clinical situations in which the AG is altered.

a. **Ratio ranges:** While this relationship is generally not an exact 1:1 exchange, the ratio should fall between 1 and 2 in a **simple anion-gap metabolic acidosis.**

  (1) Delta/delta ratios below 1, in which the change (increase) in AG is less than the change (decrease) in serum bicarbonate, suggest the presence of a nonanion-gap metabolic acidosis in addition to the anion-gap metabolic acidosis; in other words, the full decrease in bicarbonate is not accounted for by only the anion-gap metabolic acidosis.

  (2) Delta/delta ratios above 2, in which the change in AG is greater than the change in serum bicarbonate, suggest the presence of a metabolic alkalosis in addition to the anion-gap metabolic acidosis; in other words, the bicarbonate did not decrease as much as would have been expected based on the size of the AG, suggesting that a metabolic alkalosis is generating additional bicarbonate.

b. **Corrected bicarbonate:** For those who struggle with ratios, the delta/delta is also referred to as the "corrected bicarbonate" or the "excess anion gap." Take the increase in AG above normal (the "excess" AG) and add it to the measured serum bicarbonate from the electrolyte panel; the sum of the excess AG and the measured serum bicarbonate (the "corrected bicarbonate") should equal approximately 24 (the normal serum bicarbonate) in a simple anion-gap metabolic acidosis.

  (1) If the corrected bicarbonate is significantly less than 24, the patient should be evaluated for a coexisting nonanion-gap metabolic acidosis.

  (2) If the corrected bicarbonate is significantly greater than 24, the patient should be evaluated for a coexisting metabolic alkalosis.

3. **The plasma osmolar gap:** Under normal physiologic conditions, plasma osmolality (P_{osm}) is roughly 290 mOsm/(kg)(H_2O) and is primarily generated by serum sodium, glucose, and urea. The P_{osm} can be measured directly or calculated from serum electrolytes:

  Calculated osmolality = 2(Na) + glucose/18 + BUN/2.8

  (using conventional laboratory units of mg/dl; BUN = blood urea nitrogen)

a. **Normal osmolal gap:** The measured osmolarity should not exceed the calculated osmolarity by more than 10 mOsm/(kg)(H_2O); therefore, a normal osmolal gap is less than 10 mOsm/(kg) (H_2O).

b. **Elevated osmolal gap:** If the osmolal gap is greater than 10 mOsm/(kg)(H_2O), either the calculated serum osmolarity is falsely low (as in the case of hyperlipidemia or hyperproteinemia, both of which cause pseudohyponatremia) or the measured serum osmolarity is higher than expected due to the presence of an unmeasured, osmotically active substance in the plasma.

(1) Many ingested substances (e.g., isopropyl alcohol, ethylene glycol, ethanol, methanol) will generate an elevated osmolal gap; of these, methanol (wood alcohol) and ethylene glycol (antifreeze) also generate an anion-gap metabolic acidosis.

(2) Mannitol, radiocontrast dye, and acetone also generate an elevated osmolal gap; acetone is associated with the ingestion of isopropyl alcohol (rubbing alcohol) in the setting of a normal pH.

4. Urinary anion gap (UAG): The UAG or the urine net charge can be used to assess whether the renal system is responding appropriately to a metabolic acidosis or whether the renal system is the cause of the metabolic acidosis.

$$UAG = (\text{urine } Na^+ + \text{urine } K^+) - \text{urine } Cl^-$$

or, the major measured urinary cations minus the major urinary anion.

a. Normal response: In response to a metabolic acidosis, a normally functioning renal system is able to secrete additional acid in the form of ammonium NH_4^+, generally as NH_4Cl. While NH_4^+ is an unmeasured urinary cation, its presence in urine can be estimated by using the measurement of urine Cl^- as a proxy since ammonium (a cation) is generally secreted with chloride (an anion) to maintain electroneutrality.

b. Negative UAG: If the renal system is able to appropriately increase the secretion of ammonium in response to a metabolic acidosis, the amount of NH_4Cl in the urine increases and the UAG or net charge will be negative:

$$(\text{urine } Na^+ + \text{urine } K^+) - (\text{a larger amount of urine } Cl^-) = \\ \text{a negative number}$$

A negative UAG suggests that renal tubular dysfunction is not the cause of the metabolic acidosis.

c. Positive UAG: If, however, the renal system is not able to appropriately increase the secretion of ammonium in response to the metabolic acidosis, the amount of NH_4Cl in the urine remains unchanged or even decreases, and the UAG or net charge will be positive:

$$(\text{urine } Na^+ + \text{urine } K^+) - (\text{a smaller amount of urine } Cl^-) = \\ \text{a positive number}$$

A positive UAG suggests that there is impaired renal acid secretion and that the renal system is the cause of, or at least contributing to, the metabolic acidosis.

5. Winter's formula. In the presence of a metabolic acidosis, Winter's formula is used to determine the **expected $PaCO_2$,** assuming that the respiratory system is able to compensate appropriately.

$$\text{Expected PaCO}_2 = (1.5)(\text{serum [HCO}_3^-]) + 8 +/- 2$$

a. **Respiratory acidosis:** If the actual $PaCO_2$ is higher than the expected $PaCO_2$, then the respiratory system is not able to fully compensate for the metabolic acidosis and there is a coexisting respiratory acidosis.

b. **Respiratory alkalosis:** If the actual $PaCO_2$ is lower than the expected $PaCO_2$, then the respiratory system is "overcompensating" for the metabolic acidosis; since the body does not "overcompensate" for any acid–base disorder, there must be a coexisting respiratory alkalosis.

6. **The alveolar-arterial (A-a) gradient** measures the difference between alveolar oxygen tension and arterial oxygen tension, and is used to evaluate the causes of abnormal gas exchange. In order to be accurate, the A-a gradient must be calculated from a room air ABG, and the simplified formula is as follows:

$$\text{A-a gradient} = [150 - (PaCO_2/0.8)] - PaO_2$$

or, for those who do not like ratios, it may be written as $[150 - (1.25)(PaCO_2)] - PaO_2$.

a. **Normal A-a gradient:** The normal A-a gradient is age dependent and, in a healthy young adult, is approximately 10. Age-adjusted normal A-a gradients $= 2.5 + 0.21$ (age).

b. **Hypoxemia or hypercapnia:** The basic mechanisms involved in the generation of hypoxemia or hypercapnia generally include:

  (1) Hypoventilation
  (2) Ventilation-perfusion ($\dot{V}/\dot{Q}$) mismatching
  (3) Right-to-left shunts
  (4) Diffusion impairment

c. **Extrapulmonary causes of respiratory failure:** Calculation of the A-a gradient is useful in that it generally remains normal only in the setting of hypoventilation or extrapulmonary causes of respiratory failure.

d. **Intrapulmonary causes of respiratory failure,** such as pulmonary edema (cardiogenic or noncardiogenic), adult respiratory distress syndrome (ARDS), pulmonary emboli, pneumonia, or chronic obstructive diseases such as emphysema or asthma, will generally have an elevated A-a gradient.

II. General Approach to Acid–Base Analysis

A. **Normal values.** The normal acid–base values are as follows:

1. Serum $pH = 7.4$
2. $PaCO_2$ roughly 40 mm Hg
3. PaO_2 roughly 90 mm Hg
4. Serum HCO_3^- roughly 24 mEq/L

B. **Systematic approach.** A systematic approach to acid–base analysis generally includes the following steps:

1. **What is the pH?** Values above roughly 7.43 are consistent with alkalemia, while values below roughly 7.37 are consistent with acidemia.

2. **Is the primary acid–base disturbance a respiratory or metabolic process?** Essentially, how have the $PaCO_2$ and HCO_3^- changed relative to the pH?

   a. If the pH is < 7.4, then an increased $PaCO_2$ (respiratory acidosis) or a decreased HCO_3^- (metabolic acidosis) would be the primary disorder.

   b. If the pH is > 7.4, then a decreased $PaCO_2$ (respiratory alkalosis) or an increased HCO_3^- (metabolic alkalosis) would be the primary disorder.

3. **What is the AG?** If there is an AG, particularly if it is > 18 or 20, then a primary anion-gap metabolic acidosis exists regardless of the serum pH or bicarbonate level. Added "acids" may be in the form of organic molecules, such as lactate, ketoacids (found in patients with diabetes, starvation, and alcoholic ketosis), or intrinsic uremic anions.

4. **What is the delta/delta or the corrected bicarbonate?** In the setting of an anion-gap metabolic acidosis, this step allows for the assessment of a coexisting nonanion gap metabolic acidosis or a coexisting metabolic alkalosis.

5. **Is there a plasma osmolar gap?** In the setting of an anion-gap metabolic acidosis, the presence of an osmolar gap suggests either methanol or ethylene glycol ingestion.

6. **If there is a nonanion-gap metabolic acidosis, what is the UAP or net charge?** A negative net charge suggests a nonrenal cause of acidosis, while a positive net charge suggests renal tubular dysfunction as the cause of acidosis.

7. **In the setting of a metabolic acidosis, is there appropriate respiratory compensation?**

   a. In the presence of a metabolic acidosis, Winter's formula is used to calculate the appropriate respiratory response.

   b. If the actual $PaCO_2$ differs from the expected $PaCO_2$, then there is either a respiratory acidosis or a respiratory alkalosis in addition to the metabolic acidosis.

8. **What is the A-a gradient?** In the setting of either respiratory acidosis or alkalosis, a normal A-a gradient strongly suggests that the cause of the respiratory disorder is extrapulmonary.

9. If there is a **primary respiratory disorder,** is the disorder acute, chronic, or acute-on-chronic?

III. Differential Diagnoses

A. Metabolic acidosis (Figure 75–2)

1. **Anion-gap metabolic acidosis:** The acronym MUDPILES is frequently referred to in the differential diagnosis of an anion-gap metabolic acidosis. Causes include:

   a. **M = methanol** (found in antifreeze) or **toluene** (glue sniffing)

      (1) Consider in the setting of ingestion or when the history is not obtainable in a patient with an anion-gap acidosis.

      (2) Check for a plasma osmolal gap.

      (3) Check fundoscopic examination for optic nerve edema.

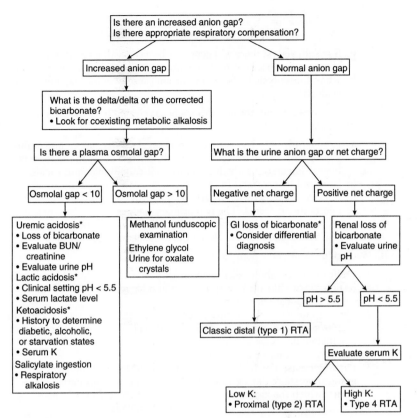

■ **FIGURE 75–2.** Algorithm for the workup of metabolic acidosis. *BUN* = blood urea nitrogen; *GI* = gastrointestinal; *RTA* = renal tubular acidosis.
  *This is one of the most common causes of metabolic acidosis.

    b. **U = uremia** or chronic renal failure; early renal failure may have a nonanion-gap metabolic acidosis.

    c. **D = diabetic ketoacidosis;** other forms to consider include alcoholic ketosis and starvation.

    d. **P = paraldehyde,** an anesthetic agent, is generally not used anymore.

    e. **L = lactate**

        (1) Lactate is probably the most common cause of an anion-gap metabolic acidosis.

        (2) The history generally includes hypoperfusion in the setting of sepsis or cardiogenic shock.

    f. **E = ethylene glycol**

        (1) Consider in the setting of ingestion or when the history is not obtainable in a patient with an anion-gap acidosis.

(2) Check for a plasma osmolal gap.

(3) Check urine for oxalate crystals.

g. **S = salicylates;** there will generally be a coexisting respiratory alkalosis due to salicylate stimulation of the central respiratory center.

h. **Rhabdomyolysis** is also an important cause of anion-gap metabolic acidosis.

2. **Nonanion-gap metabolic acidosis** (also referred to as hyperchloremic metabolic acidosis)

a. **Acid administration** is a frequently overlooked cause of nonanion-gap acidosis in the intensive care unit. It is generally in the form of hyperalimentation, which contains HCl-containing amino acids.

b. **Loss of bicarbonate:** In these cases, chloride (an anion) is retained in place of the depleted bicarbonate in order to maintain the electro-neutrality of plasma. The two primary sources of bicarbonate loss are via the gastrointestinal tract (i.e., diarrhea) and the renal system (i.e., renal failure). Calculating the urine net charge may be helpful.

B. **Metabolic alkalosis** (Figure 75–3)

1. **Definition:** Metabolic alkalosis is usually defined as either chloride responsive or chloride unresponsive, and it frequently occurs as part of a mixed acid–base disorder.

2. **Development:** Under normal circumstances, the renal system is able to excrete significant amounts of bicarbonate. Therefore, the development of a metabolic alkalosis requires some barrier to the normal ability of the kidney to excrete bicarbonate.

3. **Pathogenesis:** The pathogenesis of metabolic alkalosis involves a **generative stage** during which acid is lost and a **maintenance stage** during which the kidney cannot excrete the increased bicarbonate. Barriers to increased bicarbonate excretion include:

a. **Volume loss leading to low glomerular filtration rate** (GFR) [the increased filtered load of bicarbonate leads to increased proximal reabsorption]

b. **Chloride depletion** (the negatively charged bicarbonate is reabsorbed in place of chloride)

c. **Potassium depletion**

d. **An excess of mineralcorticoids**

4. **Additional tests:** The measurement of urine electrolytes, in particular chloride and potassium, attention to blood pressure, and measurement of plasma renin when a diagnosis is still in doubt help to narrow the differential.

5. **Chloride responsive disorders:** The clinical setting is usually characterized by some degree of volume contraction with secondary hyperreninemic-hyperaldosteronism, normal to slightly lowered blood pressure, and low serum potassium.

a. **Common causes** include:

(1) Diuretic use

(2) Loss of HCL-rich gastric fluid, generally through vomiting or nasogastric suctioning

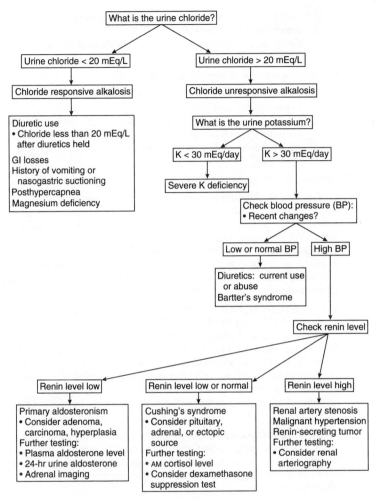

FIGURE 75–3. Algorithm for the workup of metabolic alkalosis. *GI* = gastrointestinal.

  b. **Less common causes** include posthypercapnea, magnesium deficiency, Bartter's syndrome, and high-dose intravenous penicillin (penicillin is a nonreabsorbable anion).

6. **Chloride unresponsive disorders:** The clinical setting for chloride unresponsive disorders is usually characterized by some degree of volume expansion or overload, elevated blood pressure, and low serum potassium. The increase in renin and aldosterone, or in aldosterone alone, is the primary finding.

  a. **Hyperreninemic-hyperaldosterone states**

  (1) Renal artery stenosis or renovascular hypertension
  (2) Accelerated hypertension
  (3) Renin-secreting tumors in the juxtaglomerular apparatus
  (although less common)

  b. Hyporeninemic-hyperaldosterone states

  (1) Primary aldosteronism from an adrenal adenoma, carcinoma, or
  hyperplasia
  (2) Cushing's syndrome from a primary pituitary lesion, adrenal
  adenoma, or ectopic source
  (3) Adrenal enzyme defects or licorice ingestion (although less
  common)

C. Respiratory acidosis (Figure 75–4)

1. **Definition:** Respiratory acidosis is defined by an elevation in $PaCO_2$
   (hypercapnia) and a decreased pH.
2. **Etiology:** Respiratory acidosis is generally caused by hypoventilation or
   severe V/Q mismatching.
3. **Extrapulmonary or pulmonary causes:** Calculation of the A-a
   gradient generally differentiates between these two mechanisms.
4. **Formulas** can be used to assess whether the process is acute, chronic,
   or acute-on-chronic. The simplest formula is:

   a. **Acute process:** HCO_3^- increases 1 mEq/L for every 10 mm Hg
      rise in $PaCO_2$; this small immediate increase in bicarbonate is the
      result of cellular buffering mechanisms.
   b. **Chronic process:** HCO_3^- increases 4 mEq/L for every 10 mm Hg
      rise in $PaCO_2$; this increase in bicarbonate is the result of renal
      buffering mechanisms and takes place over a period of 3–5 days.
   c. **Acute-on-chronic process:** The increase in HCO_3^- falls
      somewhere in the range of 1–4 mEq/L for every 10 mm Hg rise in
      $PaCO_2$.

5. **Coexisting metabolic alkalosis:** In response to respiratory acidosis, the renal system is generally not able to increase the bicarbonate concentration above 38; therefore, bicarbonate concentrations
   above this level suggest the presence of a coexisting metabolic
   alkalosis.

D. Respiratory alkalosis (Figure 75–5)

1. **Definition:** Respiratory alkalosis is defined by a decrease in $PaCO_2$
   (hypocapnea) and an increase in pH.
2. **Etiology:** Respiratory alkalosis is generally caused by some stimulus to
   the respiratory center resulting in increased minute ventilation either
   through an increased tidal volume or an increased respiratory rate.
3. **Extrapulmonary or pulmonary causes:** Calculation of the A-a
   gradient generally differentiates between these two mechanisms.
4. **Formulas** can be used to assess whether the process is acute, chronic,
   or acute-on-chronic. The simplest formula is:

   a. **Acute process:** HCO_3^- decreases 2 mEq/L for every 10 mm Hg
      fall in $PaCO_2$.
   b. **Chronic process:** HCO_3^- decreases 5 mEq/L for every 10 mm Hg
      fall in $PaCO_2$.

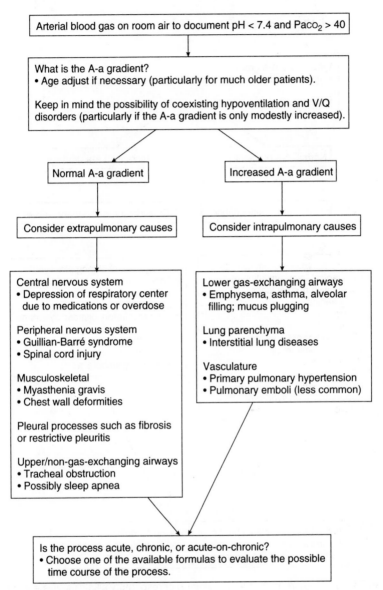

Arterial blood gas on room air to document pH < 7.4 and $Paco_2$ > 40

↓

What is the A-a gradient?
• Age adjust if necessary (particularly for much older patients).

Keep in mind the possibility of coexisting hypoventilation and V/Q disorders (particularly if the A-a gradient is only modestly increased).

| Normal A-a gradient | Increased A-a gradient |

Consider extrapulmonary causes

Central nervous system
• Depression of respiratory center due to medications or overdose

Peripheral nervous system
• Guillian-Barré syndrome
• Spinal cord injury

Musculoskeletal
• Myasthenia gravis
• Chest wall deformities

Pleural processes such as fibrosis or restrictive pleuritis

Upper/non-gas-exchanging airways
• Tracheal obstruction
• Possibly sleep apnea

Consider intrapulmonary causes

Lower gas-exchanging airways
• Emphysema, asthma, alveolar filling; mucus plugging

Lung parenchyma
• Interstitial lung diseases

Vasculature
• Primary pulmonary hypertension
• Pulmonary emboli (less common)

Is the process acute, chronic, or acute-on-chronic?
• Choose one of the available formulas to evaluate the possible time course of the process.

■ **FIGURE 75–4.** Algorithm for the workup of respiratory acidosis. *A-a* = alveolar-arterial; *V/Q* = ventilation-perfusion.

    c. Acute-on-chronic process: The decrease in HCO_3^- falls somewhere in the range of 2–5 for every 10 mm Hg fall in $PaCO_2$.

  5. Respiratory alkalosis is a common acid–base disorder in the intensive care unit. Common causes include:

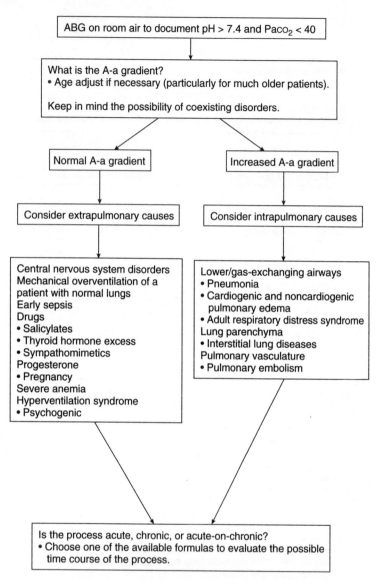

■ **FIGURE 75–5.** Algorithm for the workup of respiratory alkalosis. *A-a* = alveolar-arterial; *ABG* = arterial blood gas.

a. **Iatrogenic overventilation** with tidal volumes greater than 5–8 cc/kg or inappropriately high respiratory rates
b. **Early sepsis** in which various cytokines increase the respiratory drive

    c. Intrapulmonary processes, such as pneumonia, pulmonary edema, and ARDS

IV. Special Considerations

    A. Using only an ABG to assess a patient's acid–base status will not give an accurate picture.

    B. Do not assume that a "roughly normal" ABG and set of electrolytes exclude significant acid–base disorders, particularly if the pH is normal.

SUGGESTED READING

Adrogue HJ, Madias NE: Management of life-threatening acid-base disorders. *N Engl J Med* 338:26–34, 451–458, 1998.

76

Diagnostic Approach to Renal Disorders
Julia M. Gallagher, David Clive, and Eric Iida

Acute Renal Failure
Julia M. Gallagher

I. **Definition.** Acute renal failure is defined by **the rapid decline in glomerular filtration rate** (GFR) [as reflected by a rising creatinine], **and the retention of nitrogenous waste** (as reflected by a rising blood urea nitrogen).

II. **Overview**

A. **Etiology**

1. Three causes of acute renal failure account for the vast majority of cases:

a. Prerenal causes
b. Ischemia
c. Nephrotoxins

2. Acute renal failure in hospitalized patients is frequently multifactorial.

B. **Mortality.** The overall mortality rate for acute renal failure can reach 50% and has not changed significantly in the past 30 years.

C. **Prognosis.** Oliguria (i.e., urine output < 400 ml/day) and a rise in creatinine levels (i.e., an increase > 3 mg/dL) are associated with a poorer prognosis for recovery than patients with nonoliguric acute renal failure.

D. **Complications.** Infection is the most serious complication of acute renal failure and occurs in 50%–90% of patients. It accounts for approximately 75% of the deaths associated with acute renal failure.

III. **A Clinical Approach to Acute Renal Failure.** The physician should assume that all patients have an acute and **potentially reversible** cause of renal failure. Overlooking such diagnoses results in delays in instituting appropriate treatment and further losses in renal function (Figure 76–1).

A. **History**

1. **Predisposing conditions:** Acute renal failure may develop in patients with a history of chronic renal insufficiency or diseases that predispose them to renal microvascular disease (i.e., diabetes, hypertension, peripheral vascular disease). Such patients are already **maximally compensated** and may exhibit significant increases in blood urea nitrogen and creatinine as a result of very subtle renal insults.

2. **Recent history:** It is important to ask if any of the following occurred within the past 4–6 weeks:

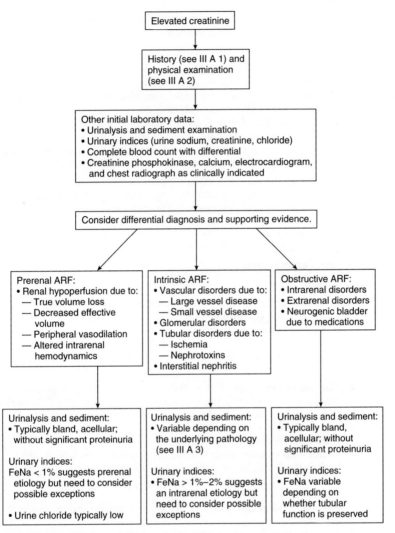

FIGURE 76–1. An algorithmic approach to acute renal failure. *ARF* = acute renal failure; *FeNa* = fractional excretion of sodium.

  a. Surgery (i.e., potential ligation of ureters) or vascular catheterization
  b. Episodes of hypotension
  c. Exposure to radiocontrast agents or antibiotics (i.e., aminoglycosides)
  d. New medications, including over-the-counter and herbal medications
  e. Symptoms that may be consistent with renal failure (e.g., nausea,

vomiting, edema, dyspnea, palpitations, change in mental status, changes in urine output or color)

3. **Prerenal state:** Obtain historical clues suggesting a prerenal state:

   a. Complaints of thirst?
   b. History of orthostatic changes?
   c. History of decreased oral intake, vomiting, diarrhea, or polyuria?
   d. Diuretic use? When was it started? Any recent dose changes?
   e. History of high fevers (increased insensible losses)?
   f. Medication use, including over-the-counter and herbal medications [e.g., aspirin-based products, nonsteroidal anti-inflammatory drugs (NSAIDs), angiotensin-converting enzyme (ACE) inhibitors]?

4. **Pain:** Does the patient complain of persistent flank pain (possible pyelonephritis, papillary necrosis, renal artery or vein occlusion, hydronephrosis with distention of the renal capsule) or a colicky pain radiating to the groin (partial ureteric obstruction)?

5. **Other symptoms:** Does the patient complain of fever, arthralgias, or a pruritic rash (possible allergic reaction)?

B. Physical examination

1. **Volume status**

   a. Where are the patient's blood pressure and pulse in relation to his or her **historical average**?
   b. Is the patient orthostatic?
   c. Does the patient have poor sternal skin turgor, dry mucous membranes, or a decrease in axillary sweat (the latter being the most sensitive finding)?

2. **Cardiac examination:** Is there a third heart sound (S_3) suggestive of heart failure or a fourth heart sound (S_4) suggestive of a "stiff" ventricle and possibly ischemia? Is the rate regular and appropriate for the blood pressure?

3. **Pulmonary examination:** Are there crackles?

4. **Abdominal examination:** Is there any evidence of ascites? Renal bruits? A palpable bladder? Costovertebral angle tenderness?

5. **Rectal examination:** Assess for prostatic hypertrophy and rectal masses.

6. **Pelvic examination:** Assess for evidence of cervical and endometrial cancer.

7. **Edema:** Does the patient have lower extremity or presacral edema, which may suggest heart failure, cirrhosis, or a protein-wasting disease?

8. **Mental status:** Assess for level of alertness.

C. Laboratory assessment

1. **Blood tests:** Test for blood urea nitrogen, creatinine, electrolytes (looking for complications of renal failure), and complete blood count (CBC) [looking for evidence of infection and anemia].

2. **Urinalysis**

   a. Proteinuria is usually mild in acute renal failure (< 1 gm/day)
   b. Both prerenal and postrenal/obstructive failure will typically have a "bland," acellular sediment.

    c. Acute renal failure due to acute tubular necrosis may have "muddy brown" casts and renal tubular cells; 20%–30% of the cases of acute tubular necrosis may lack the "classic" finding of "muddy brown" casts.

    d. Broad, granular casts [defined as > 3 white blood cells (WBCs) in diameter) may suggest chronic renal disease.

    e. Red blood cell (RBC) casts are generally consistent with glomerulonephritis or vasculitis.

    f. Leukocyte casts suggest an intrarenal infection.

    g. Dysmorphic RBCs suggest an upper tract lesion, while normal appearing RBCs suggest a lower tract lesion.

    h. A urine dipstick test that is positive for blood (generally reported as "occult blood") but without actual RBCs on microscopic examination suggests the presence of either myoglobin (consider rhabdomyolysis) or hemoglobin (consider intravascular hemolysis).

    i. A urine dipstick test for protein screens for the presence of albumin **only** (see Chapter 73); if a quantitative assessment of proteinuria estimates a much higher level of protein excretion, look for the presence of immunoglobulin (Ig) light chains.

    j. Characteristic crystals suggest specific diagnosis:

        (1) Football-shaped crystals suggest uric acid nephropathy.

        (2) Envelope-shaped crystals (oxalic acid) or needle-shaped crystals (hippuric acid) suggest ethylene glycol toxicity.

3. Urinary indices (urine sodium, creatinine, chloride)

    a. The **fractional excretion of sodium** (FeNa = urine/plasma Na divided by urine/plasma creatinine) is frequently used to separate prerenal failure (i.e., sodium reabsorption generally remains intact) from intrinsic renal failure (i.e., sodium reabsorption is disrupted). An FeNa < 1% suggests prerenal failure and an FeNa > 1%–2% suggests intrarenal failure. There are, however, many exceptions to this rule:

        (1) The FeNa may be > 1% in cases of prerenal disease in the setting of diuretic use, bicarbonaturia, and adrenal insufficiency.

        (2) The FeNa may be < 1% in cases of intrinsic disease in the setting of nonoliguric acute tubular necrosis early in the disease course, early obstruction, some forms of glomerulonephritis, and early in the course of contrast-induced nephrotoxicity.

    b. **Urine chloride** is generally low in prerenal failure and **not as variable as the urine Na.**

D. Additional data that may be helpful based on clinical suspicion include:

    1. Ca and creatine phosphokinase (CPK) levels

    2. Assessing differences in calculated and measured serum osmolarity

    3. An electrocardiogram (ECG)

    4. A chest radiograph

E. Renal ultrasound

    1. **Sensitivity:** For those cases in which there is a high clinical suspicion of renal obstruction, renal ultrasound has an 80%–85% sensitivity in detecting signs of obstruction.

2. **Limitations:** Situations in which ultrasound may fail to detect an obstruction include retroperitoneal fibrosis, obstruction in the presence of severe dehydration, and early obstruction prior to the development of ureter dilation or hydronephrosis. Ultrasound should be repeated if the clinical suspicion remains high.

F. **Renal biopsy** is generally reserved for those cases in which pre- and postrenal causes of failure have been excluded and there is not a well-defined ischemic or nephrotoxic insult by history.

IV. **Differential Diagnosis** (see Figure 76–1). A systematic approach to acute renal failure generally begins with an attempt to classify the cause as prerenal, renal, or postrenal.

A. **Prerenal acute renal failure**

1. **Definition:** Prerenal acute renal failure is defined as **renal hypo-perfusion** without parenchymal compromise; tubular and glomerular function remains intact.

2. **Frequency:** Prerenal acute renal failure accounts for approximately 50%–60% of the cases of acute renal failure.

3. **Differential diagnoses**

a. **Renal hypoperfusion** may be due to:

(1) True volume loss secondary to vomiting, diarrhea, decreased oral intake, diuretic use, hemorrhage, or insensible losses due to burns or fevers

(2) Decreased effective circulating volume secondary to a decrease in cardiac output, cirrhosis, or nephrotic syndrome

(3) Peripheral vasodilation leading to a drop in mean arterial pressure secondary to sepsis or medications

(4) Adrenal insufficiency

b. **Alteration in intrarenal hemodynamics:** Drugs in particular may impair autoregulation of the GFR.

(1) **NSAIDs** block prostaglandin production and impair afferent arteriolar dilation.

(2) **ACE inhibitors** block angiotensin II production and impair efferent arteriolar constriction.

B. **Renal acute renal failure.** Renal or "intrinsic" acute renal failure involves the renal parenchyma. Glomerular function, tubular function, or both are compromised.

1. **Frequency:** Renal acute renal failure accounts for approximately 35%–40% of the cases of acute renal failure.

2. **Etiologies:** While the possible causes of intrinsic renal failure are diverse, ischemia and nephrotoxins account for approximately 70% of these cases.

3. **Differential diagnoses:** The differential diagnosis of intrinsic acute renal failure is most easily organized by approaching the problem anatomically:

a. How is the kidney constructed (i.e., blood vessels, both large and small; glomeruli; an interstitium; tubules)?

b. What problems can occur at each of these sites?

4. Vascular disorders are not a frequent cause of intrinsic acute renal failure, but they should be considered in the appropriate clinical setting.

a. Large vessels

(1) **Renal artery occlusion as a result of emboli**

    (a) History of recent vascular surgery or heart catheterization

    (b) History of atrial fibrillation

    (c) History of myocardial infarction (MI) with aneurysm or mural thrombus

    (d) Thrombosis

    (e) Dissection

    (f) History of connective tissue disorders

(2) **Renal vein thrombosis:** Consider in cases of nephrotic syndrome with a history of clots at unusual sites.

b. Small vessels

(1) Vasculitis

(2) Malignant hypertension

(3) Various forms of microangiopathies [e.g., thrombotic thrombocytopenic purpura, hemolytic uremic syndrome, diffuse intravascular coagulation (DIC), and the HELLP syndrome (i.e., hemolysis, elevated liver enzymes, and low platelet count)].

5. Glomerular disorders are not a frequent cause of acute renal failure, but need to be considered if other, more frequent causes cannot be diagnosed. Some of these disorders are potentially treatable.

a. Postinfectious glomerulonephritis

b. Membranoproliferative glomerulonephritis

c. Autoimmune disorders (e.g., lupus, Wegener's granulomatosis, and Goodpasture's syndrome)

6. Tubular disorders are the **leading cause** of intrinsic renal failure and are generally the result of either ischemia or nephrotoxins. Patients at risk for either ischemic or nephrotoxic acute renal failure are generally older, are frequently inpatients, have some degree of either true or effective volume loss, some degree of chronic renal insufficiency, and have been exposed to multiple renal insults.

a. Ischemia

(1) The renal medullary interstitium, at baseline, borders on hypoxia; therefore, the straight segment of the proximal tubule and the thick ascending limb of Henle are at greatest risk during prolonged periods of hypoperfusion.

(2) If adequate blood flow is restored prior to the development of cortical necrosis, renal tubular cells are able to regenerate and renal function recovers over 1–2 weeks.

b. Nephrotoxins

(1) Radiocontrast agents (risk of acute renal failure is dose related)

(a) Nonionic or low anion dyes do not significantly reduce the risk of acute renal failure.

(b) Contrast nephropathy typically develops within 24–28 hours of exposure; the creatinine peaks within 3–5 days of exposure and generally declines toward baseline over the following 1–2 weeks.

(2) Antibiotics and chemotherapy

(a) Frequently implicated antibiotics include acyclovir, foscarnet, amphotericin, and aminoglycosides. Frequently implicated chemotherapeutic agents include cisplatin and ifosfamide.

(b) Toxicity generally becomes apparent 7–10 days into drug exposure as demonstrated by a rising creatinine, which may take several weeks to months to decline back toward baseline after the agent is withdrawn.

c. **Endogenous toxins**

(1) Hypercalcemia causes direct tubular toxicity, vasoconstriction, and interstitial nephritis.

(2) Myoglobinuria may complicate up to 30% of cases of rhabdomyolysis when the CPK exceeds 10,000.

(3) Hemoglobinuria is a rare cause of acute renal failure.

d. **Urate crystals** may cause obstruction of renal tubules following treatment of hematologic disorders (acute lysis syndrome).

e. **Myeloma light chains** damage renal tubules as a result of direct toxic actions and obstruction.

7. **Interstitial nephritis:** Consider in the appropriate clinical setting.

8. **Infections:** Consider acute pyelonephritis, subacute bacterial endocarditis, hepatitis, or Epstein-Barr virus.

9. **Infiltrative or connective tissue diseases** rarely cause renal acute renal failure.

C. **Postrenal acute renal failure** occurs in patients with sudden, persistent urine retention.

1. **Frequency:** Postrenal acute renal failure accounts for 5% of cases. The incidence is much higher in certain patient populations, such as men with prostatic disease, patients with solitary kidneys, and patients with a history of intra-abdominal or pelvic cancer.

2. **Renal obstruction:** Obstruction may occur intrarenally or extrarenally.

a. **Intrarenal obstruction** may occur at the level of the tubules secondary to crystal deposition (e.g., uric acid nephropathy, calcium oxalate nephropathy following the ingestion of ethylene glycol).

b. **Extrarenal obstruction** may occur at the level of the ureters (bilateral involvement of the ureters by retroperitoneal fibrosis or malignancy) or bladder (prostatic enlargement, stones, neurogenic bladder due to medications such as anticholinergics or α-blockers).

SUGGESTED READING

Clive DM, Cohen AJ: Acute renal failure in the intensive care unit. In Irwin RS, Cerra FB, Rippe JM (eds): *Intensive Care Medicine*, 4th ed. Philadelphia: Lippincott-Raven Publishers, 1999, pp 969–992.

Chronic Renal Failure

David Clive

I. **Definition.** The term chronic renal failure is applied to **irreversible loss of excretory function of the kidney.** For the purposes of this chapter, the term chronic renal failure may be used for reductions in GFR $\leq 25\%$ of normal. Lesser degrees of renal impairment will be referred to as **chronic renal insufficiency.** When the level of renal impairment is so severe as to necessitate renal replacement therapy for continued survival, the patient is said to have **end-stage renal disease (ESRD).**

II. **Etiology.** Numerous disease processes can cause chronic renal failure (Table 76–1).

   A. **Historical information.** To establish the cause, historical information is paramount.

   1. Is there a history of diabetes mellitus (DM)? Uncontrolled severe hypertension? Autoimmune disease?

   2. Has the patient had frequent urinary tract infections suggestive of reflux nephropathy or postrenal disease?

   B. **Laboratory data** comprise serologic markers, particularly useful in various autoimmune diseases, urinalysis, and radiographic studies looking for the presence of diseases that alter renal morphology or vascularity. An approach to utilizing these data is outlined in Table 76–2.

III. **A Clinical Approach to Chronic Renal Failure**

   A. **History.** Progressive kidney failure has few distinctive symptoms. It is the exceptional patient who notices flank pain or a change in urine output.

   B. **Diagnosis** is usually made on the basis of laboratory tests, most often a blood urea nitrogen and creatinine.

   1. **Differential diagnosis:** The differential diagnosis is between acute and chronic renal failure. Historical information may provide clues to the acute-versus-chronic question, but the clinician will want to look for telltale signs of azotemia and renal atrophy (typically determined by sonography) to be sure (see Chapter 74).

   2. **Staging** of chronic renal failure is part of the diagnostic process.

   a. **Stable or progressive:** Does the patient have stable mild renal insufficiency or progressive renal failure? If progressive, has the course been rapidly progressive, slow, or subacute?

TABLE 76–1. Causes of Chronic Renal Failure

Vascular diseases of the kidney

Hypertensive nephrosclerosis

Vasculitis

Atheroembolic disease

Renal artery disease (ischemic nephropathy)

Disorders related to hemolytic uremic syndrome

Inflammatory and immunologically mediated renal diseases

Glomerular diseases
  Primary
    Idiopathic crescentic glomerulonephritis
    Immunoglobulin A (IgA) nephropathy
    Poststreptococcal glomerulonephritis
    Membranoproliferative glomerulonephritis
    Focal segmental glomerulosclerosis
  Secondary
    Lupus nephritis
    Bacterial endocarditis
    Acute infectious glomerulonephritis
    Vasculitis-associated glomerulonephritis (e.g., Wegener's granulomatosis, poly-
    arteritis nodosa)
    Goodpasture's syndrome
    HIV-associated nephropathy

Chronic tubulointerstitial disease
  Analgesic nephropathy
  Gouty nephropathy
  Untreated obstructive uropathy
  Reflux nephropathy

Diabetic nephropathy

Bilateral renal cortical necrosis

Hereditary and congenital renal diseases
  Polycystic kidney disease
  Medullary cystic disease
  Alport's syndrome
  Congenital renal dysgenesis

TABLE 76–2. Clues to Etiology in Chronic Renal Failure

Class of Disease	Historical Information	Laboratory Information
Vascular	History of hypertension Peripheral vascular disease Hyperlipidemia History of vasculitis	ANCA (vasculitis) Arteriography (renovascular disease)
Inflammatory/ autoimmune, glomerular	History of hematuria, heavy proteinuria, known auto-immune disease (e.g., SLE)	Proteinuria Hematuria Serologic markers (complement levels, ANA, anti-GBM antibody titers as appropriate) Renal biopsy
Inflammatory/ autoimmune, tubulointerstitial	History of frequent urinary tract infections Polyuria Analgesic abuse	Chemical indicators of renal tubular dysfunction: • Urinary concentrating defect • Renal tubular acidosis • Hyperkalemia
Metabolic-diabetic nephropathy	History of diabetes, especially if retinopathy present	Proteinuria Glycosuria
Hereditary and congenital	Family history Hearing loss (Alport's syndrome)	Abnormal renal imaging (polycystic kidney disease) Specific genetic marker studies

ANA = antinuclear antibody; ANCA = antineutrophilic cytoplasmic antibody; GBM = glomerular basement membrane; SLE = systemic lupus erythematosus.

    b. **Tempo:** The tempo of the disease is best established by reviewing available past laboratory data, particularly serum creatinine levels.

       (1) **Uremia:** Does the patient appear uremic, or close to it? The presence of uremic symptoms in a patient with known chronic renal insufficiency usually signifies ESRD.

       (2) **Acute illness:** Occasionally, patients with chronic renal failure will exhibit uremic manifestations as a result of supervening acute illness. It is critical to rule out the existence of such a reversible acute overlay prior to committing the patient to dialysis or transplantation.

IV. Biochemical Abnormalities

    A. **Calcium and phosphorus imbalance.** Impaired ability to excrete phosphorus leads to positive phosphorus balance relatively early in the course of chronic renal failure. This has several consequences:

1. Hyperphosphatemia
2. Secondary hyperparathyroidism resulting both directly and indirectly from hyperphosphatemia

   a. Binding of calcium by retained phosphorus causes calcium phosphate salts to precipitate in tissues. The tendency of calcium to leave the circulation provides a continuous stimulus for parathyroid hormone (PTH) release. Phosphorus also inhibits enzymatic activation of vitamin D. The resultant functional vitamin D deficiency inhibits calcium absorption from the gut, further stimulating PTH secretion.

   b. The biologic roles of PTH in this setting are clear. The serum calcium level is maintained and tubular phosphorus excretion enhanced. However, these benefits come at a tremendous price with **parathyroid bone disease (osteitis fibrosa).** Vitamin D deficiency may contribute a component of **osteomalacia** to the metabolic bone disease of renal failure, which is sometimes called **renal osteodystrophy.**

B. **Metabolic acidosis.** There are two major components to the acidosis of chronic renal failure.

   1. **Retention of acid metabolites due to reduced GFR:** The unmeasured anion moieties of these acids widen the anion gap (AG) as they accumulate.

      a. Impaired acid handling by tubular cells
      b. Reduced bicarbonate reabsorption
      c. Reduced ammoniagenesis

   2. **Impaired distal hydrogen ion secretion:** These processes lower the serum bicarbonate level without increasing the AG, since hydrogen ion retention does not entail the retention of an unmeasured anion.

C. **Other electrolyte imbalances** common in chronic renal failure

   1. Hyponatremia
   2. Hyperkalemia

SUGGESTED READING

Rahman M, Smith MC: Chronic renal insufficiency: a diagnostic and therapeutic approach. *Arch Intern Med*, 158:1743–1752, 1998.

Glomerulopathies

Eric Iida and David Clive

I. **Definitions.** The glomerulopathies encompass a spectrum of renal diseases that principally involve the glomerulus. There are two subsets:

A. **Glomerulonephritis.** The term glomerulonephritis should be reserved for inflammatory diseases characterized by blood or inflammatory cells in the urinary sediment. Examples include lupus nephritis and poststreptococcal glomerulonephritis.

B. Nephrotic disorders. The term nephrotic disorders should be reserved for conditions such as diabetic nephropathy and focal glomerulosclerosis. The hallmark of these diseases is proteinuria and subtle or lacking cellular findings in the urine sediment. Nephrotic and nephritic syndromes are not formal diagnoses, but rather are clinical categories. Furthermore, some overlap in presentation is possible, but these terms are a useful starting point when instituting a diagnostic workup of a patient with urinary abnormalities.

II. Overview

A. Histologic features

1. **Focal versus diffuse:** Involving less than 50% of glomeruli (focal) versus greater than 50% of glomeruli (diffuse)
2. **Global versus segmental:** Involving glomeruli in their entirety (global) versus involving only a portion of glomeruli (segmental)
3. **Endocapillary versus extracapillary:** Refers to which population of resident glomerular cells is most affected. Note that infiltrating cells (e.g., polymorphonuclear cells) can also cause an increase in cell number within glomeruli.
4. **Sclerosis versus fibrosis:** Histologically comprising material similar to that in the glomerular basement membrane (sclerosis) versus material containing collagen I or III from the healing process (fibrosis)

B. Clinical features

1. **Primary versus secondary:** Primary glomerular disease occurs as an isolated disease process. Secondary glomerular diseases are glomerulopathies that occur as manifestations of systemic diseases (e.g., Wegener's granulomatosis, Goodpasture's syndrome, systemic lupus erythematosus, DM).
2. **Acute, chronic, and rapidly progressive** are terms that describe the course of specific types of glomerulonephritis.

   a. **Acute nephritic syndrome** refers to patients presenting with sudden onset of hypertension, oliguria, and nephritic urinary sediment. **Acute glomerulonephritis** progress to renal insufficiency over a period of days. **Poststreptococcal glomerulonephritis** generally behaves in this fashion, although it is usually reversible.

   b. **Chronic glomerulonephritis** is more indolent, and generally irreversible, leading to renal insufficiency over a period of months or years.

   c. **Rapidly progressive glomerulonephritis** refers to a group of glomerulonephritides with unique histologic features called crescents [i.e., collections of cells (parietal, epithelial or infiltrating) within Bowman's space]. If untreated, rapidly progressive glomerulonephritis will follow a subacute course, leading to irreversible renal failure over a period of weeks.

III. Evalution of Suspected Glomerular Disease (Figures 76–2 and 76–3). The history and physical examination are geared toward identifying underlying conditions that may result in secondary glomerulonephritis, as well as

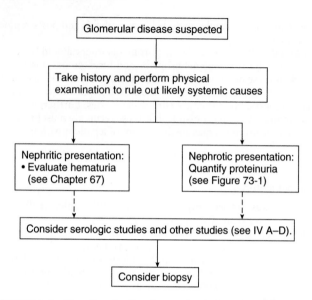

■ FIGURE 76–2. Algorithm for the diagnosis of glomerulopathies.

identifying precipitants that may result in nonglomerular causes of renal failure.

A. History

1. **Time frame:** The time frame of the development of symptoms can be useful. For instance, both IgA nephropathy and poststreptococcal glomerulonephritis often develop following pharyngitis, although typically IgA nephropathy develops within the first week following infection and poststreptococcal glomerulonephritis usually develops around day 10.

2. **Malignancies and chronic infections:** Associations with malignancies and chronic infections, such as hepatitis or endocarditis, exist for certain glomerular diseases and should be screened for when suspected.

B. Physical examination and other findings

1. **Azotemia, edema, and hypertension:** Both nephritic and nephrotic diseases can present with signs or symptoms of azotemia, edema, and hypertension.

2. **Hematuria:** Nephritic syndromes present with hematuria as a key feature (see Chapter 67). Nephrotic syndrome has a wider array of presenting symptoms, reflecting urinary losses, as well as generalized edema.

3. **Hypercoagulability** with thromboembolic events involves both arteries and veins, particularly renal vein thrombosis.

4. **Urinary losses of thyroxine, 25-hydroxyvitamin D, and transferrin** result in hypothyroidism, vitamin D deficiency, and iron-deficiency anemia, respectively.

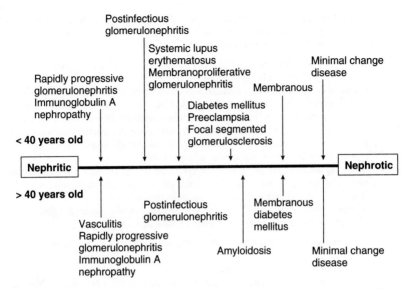

FIGURE 76–3. Algorithm of the spectrum of presentation between nephritis and nephrosis.

5. **Infections:** An increase in incidence of infections can result from losses of IgG and factors B and D of the alternate complement pathway.

IV. Laboratory Investigations

A. Urinalysis. Nephrotic syndrome by definition presents with proteinuria of at least 3 grams on a 24-hour collection and hypoalbuminemia from impaired liver production and urinary loss. **Other characteristic nephrotic features** include:

1. **Lipid droplets,** whether free, in casts, or in oval fat bodies, which can be identified by the Maltese cross shape they generate under polarized light

2. **Hyperlipidemia**

3. An **elevated erythrocyte sedimentation rate (ESR)**

   a. An ESR > 60 mm/hr is found in one-third of the cases of nephrotic syndrome; in one-fifth of cases, it is > 100 mm/hr.

   b. In the absence of other abnormalities, it is generally not considered necessary to search for an underlying malignancy based solely on an elevated ESR unless other evidence is present.

4. **Complement levels** are decreased in a number of cases of glomerulo-nephritis.

   a. C3 is depressed in most cases of poststreptococcal glomerulo-nephritis.

   b. In lupus nephritis, complement is activated via the classical pathway, leading to a preferential reduction of C4.

  c. Some nonglomerulopathic renal diseases can be associated with hypocomplementemia as well (e.g., atheroembolic disease, hemolytic-uremic syndrome).

B. Serologic studies can be useful when the cause of glomerulonephritis is not readily identifiable by the history and physical examination. A reasonable workup might include serum indirect immunofluorescence for antiglomerular basement membrane (GBM), complements, antineutrophilic cytoplasmic antibody, cryoglobulins, anti–double-stranded DNA, blood cultures, and a chest radiograph. Also consider antistreptolysin titer, antideoxyribonuclease (DNAse) and antihyaluronidase antibodies, and studies for nonglomerular causes of azotemia.

C. Imaging studies are generally not useful unless to exclude nonglomerular causes of azotemia, to assess chronicity, or occasionally to screen for a suspected complication such as renal vein thrombosis.

D. Renal biopsy is often indicated in the evaluation of glomerular diseases. Tissue can be obtained by a number of means, including:

  1. Needle biopsy under ultrasound guidance (often an outpatient procedure)
  2. An open surgical procedure
  3. Through a **transjugular approach** in patients with prohibitive bleeding risk

---

SUGGESTED READING

Schmitz PG: Glomerular and tubulointerstitial disease. In Noble J (ed): *Primary Care Medicine*, 3rd ed. Mosby, 1996, pp 1261–1274.
Orth S, Ritz E: The nephrotic syndrome. *N Engl J Med* 338:1202–1211, 1998.

Nephrolithiasis

David Clive

I. Definitions

A. Nephrolithiasis, or the formation of kidney stones, occurs when the urine becomes saturated with crystal-forming substances. Nephrolithiasis is a recurrent (or chronic) disorder in the majority of sufferers.

B. Urolithiasis is a broad term used to denote stones forming anywhere in the urinary tract (e.g., kidney stones, bladder stones).

II. Overview

A. Incidence

  1. Nephrolithiasis is common, affecting approximately 10% of Americans. Males are twice as likely as females to develop kidney stones.

2. **Bladder stones** are relatively uncommon and occur primarily in the presence of underlying bladder disease.

B. **Stone formation.** A number of different materials are responsible for stone formation. A single stone may consist of one material or a combination of different materials. Calcium-containing stones are by far the most prevalent, accounting for over 80% of all urinary calculi.

III. Causes

A. **Multifactorial etiology.** Nephrolithiasis is commonly multifactorial in origin, and several predisposing disorders may coexist in the same patient.

B. **Altered mineral metabolism.** Stones form as a result of altered mineral metabolism, which may occur as an idiopathic metabolic tendency or secondary to systemic disease.

IV. Diagnostic Evaluation

A. **History**

1. **Pain:** Patients often present with excruciating flank pain radiating toward the groin (i.e., renal colic).
2. **Renal colic** reflects transit of the stone through the ureter.
3. **Family history:** A family history of nephrolithiasis is often present.
4. **Medical history:** The medical history should aim at identifying conditions known to be associated with the formation of kidney stones (e.g., hyperparathyroidism, sarcoidosis, urinary tract infections).

B. **Laboratory investigations**

1. **Urinalysis:** On urinalysis, gross or microscopic hematuria is often present, reflecting trauma to the ureters by a stone in transit. The crystals may help to identify the stone type. Urinary excretion studies should not be done during an acute episode.
2. **Urine collections** should be taken over 24 hours to quantitate the daily excretion of calcium, uric acid, oxalate, and citrate.

   a. **Overexcretion** of stone-forming principles (e.g., oxalate, calcium) may contribute to stone formation.
   b. **Underexcretion** of citrate, an inhibitor of stone formation, may provoke recurrent nephrolithiasis.
   c. **Urine volume:** The urine volume should be recorded in order to quantify the adequacy of hydration.
   d. **Creatinine excretion** should be determined with the 24-hour urine study to ensure completeness of the collection.

3. The **metabolic workup** is done to identify the predisposing condition for stone formation.
4. **Stone analysis** requires that patients with renal colic or known to be harboring renal calculi use a strainer or basket to retrieve passed stones, which can be sent to a stone laboratory for analysis.
5. **Blood tests** should include blood urea nitrogen, creatinine, electrolytes, PTH level, calcium, and phosphorus. These tests help rule out stone-inciting conditions such as renal tubular acidosis, hyperparathyroidism, and other hypercalcemia-associated conditions.

C. **Imaging studies** help to establish the diagnosis, localize the stone, and determine whether renal obstruction is present. The size and location of the stone determine whether an acute intervention will be necessary to remove it (stones > 7 mm) or whether it can be expected to pass by itself (stones usually < 5 mm). There are several possible modalities.

1. **Abdominal plain film** (i.e., radiograph of the kidneys, ureter, and bladder) is easiest to obtain and will generally reveal radiopaque stones. Precise anatomic definition is not provided.

2. **Intravenous pyelography,** formerly the most widely used study, has fallen out of favor as the first-line imaging procedure because it requires administration of contrast, normal renal function, and it is labor intensive. However, intravenous pyelography is useful for detecting radiolucent stones (i.e., uric acid stones).

3. **Helical computed tomography (CT) is the imaging study of choice,** affording very fine resolution and anatomic detail.

4. **Renal sonography** is safe, generally readily available, and useful for ruling out renal obstruction. The level of precision of anatomic detail is less than with helical CT.

5. **Retrograde pyelography** is usually performed as part of a therapeutic urologic intervention (e.g., cystoscopic stone retrieval, ureteral stent placement).

SUGGESTED READING

Levy F, Adams-Huet B, Park CYC: Ambulatory evaluation of nephrolithiasis. *Am J Med* 98:50–59, 1995.

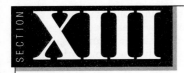

Rheumatology/Musculoskeletal

77

Arthritis
Bruce Weinstein and David Giansiracusa

I. **Definition.** Arthritis is defined by **inflammation of one or more joints** and is usually associated with pain and structural changes in the affected joints. The clinician should be aware of signs and symptoms that may be suggestive of more serious underlying pathology.

II. **Overview.** There are four basic principles when considering the clinical approach to arthritis.

   A. The **history** and **physical examination,** combined with **synovial fluid analysis** and **radiograph studies** when appropriate, are the most important components of the evaluation.

   B. **Joint symptomatology** can be caused by disorders that do not primarily involve the joint. Distinguishing articular from periarticular, soft tissue, neurologic, psychogenic, and referred symptoms is central to the initial evaluation.

   C. The clinician must **differentiate localized processes from systemic disease.**

   D. **Rheumatologic disorders,** including monarticular and polyarticular arthritis, are usually diagnosed on the basis of the complete clinical picture, and seldom on the basis of a single diagnostic test.

III. **Differential diagnosis**

   A. **Monarticular and polyarticular arthritis** can be broadly separated into structural and inflammatory disorders.

   1. **Structural disorders** are characterized by mechanical/degenerative, metabolic, or traumatic disruption of the joint. Osteoarthritis and meniscal and ligamentous injuries are common examples of mechanical/degenerative conditions.

   2. **Inflammatory arthritis** is characterized by inflammation of the synovial lining and may also involve the subsynovium or the synovial attachments to the joint capsule. These can be localized disorders, such as infection and crystal-induced disease [e.g., gout, calcium pyrophosphate disease (CPPD), hydroxyapatite), or systemic illnesses. In some of the systemic conditions, such as rheumatoid arthritis and

seronegative spondyloarthropathies, the joint manifestations are a major part of the illness, whereas in other systemic conditions, such as systemic lupus erythematosus and sarcoidosis, the arthritic aspects of the disease usually have only a comparatively minor role in the disease process.

B. Acute monarticular arthritis (Figure 77–1)

1. **Differential diagnosis:** The differential diagnosis of acute monarticular arthritis is narrow.

   a. Infectious arthritis, including causes such as staphylococcal, gono-coccal, and Gram-negative organisms (immunosuppressed patients)
   b. Crystal-induced diseases
   c. Traumatic arthritis
   d. Chronic monarticular or polyarticular arthritis with acute presentation

2. **Synovial fluid:** In addition to the history and physical examination, analysis of the synovial fluid is usually the most helpful diagnostic test (see V B).

C. Chronic monarticular arthritis (Figures 77–2 and 77–3). The differential diagnosis for chronic monarticular arthritis is broad and includes most of the disorders that cause acute monarticular and polyarticular arthritis. The initial approach consists of trying to distinguish between **inflammatory and noninflammatory conditions.**

1. **Radiographic studies** play an important role.
2. **Magnetic resonance imaging (MRI) and arthroscopy** may be helpful modalities when the diagnosis remains elusive.

D. Polyarticular arthritis (Figure 77–4)

1. **Noninflammatory causes:** The principle noninflammatory causes include osteoarthritis (primary and secondary) and avascular necrosis. Osteoarthritis can occur secondary to other disorders, including trauma, metabolic problems (e.g., hemachromatosis, hypothyroidism), and CPPD.
2. **Inflammatory causes:** Inflammatory polyarthritides include diseases that tend to affect many joints, those that involve just a few joints (pauciarticular), and those that have a special predilection to also involve the axial skeleton.

IV. Clinical Evaluation

A. History

1. Differentiate **articular from nonarticular disorders.**
2. Elicit the **acuity and tempo of symptoms** by inquiring about onset, duration, provoking and relieving factors, relationship to overuse or previous trauma, and involvement of joints in a migratory or additive fashion. Elicit a history of previous episodes.
3. Assess **symptoms of inflammation.** The presence of "gelling" or morning stiffness, in which periods of inactivity are associated with stiffness lasting longer than 30 minutes, is characteristic of inflammatory joint problems.

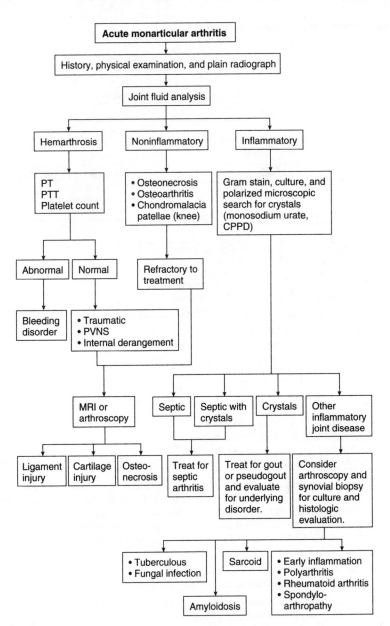

FIGURE 77-1. Algorithm for the diagnostic approach to acute monarticular arthritis. *CPD* = calcium pyrophosphate dihydrate; *MRI* = magnetic resonance imaging; *PT* = prothrombin time; *PTT* = partial thromboplastin time; *PVNS* = pigmented villonodular tenosynovitis.

(Adapted with permission from McGuire JL, Giansiracusa DF: Monoarticular arthritis. In Green HL, Glassock RJ, Kelley MA (eds): *Introduction to Clinical Medicine.* Philadelphia: Decker, 1991; and Weinstein BR, Giansiracusa DF: Primary care presentations of musculoskeletal disease. In Noble J, et al (eds): *Noble's Textbook of Primary Care Medicine,* CD-ROM Version. St. Louis: Mosby, 1996.)

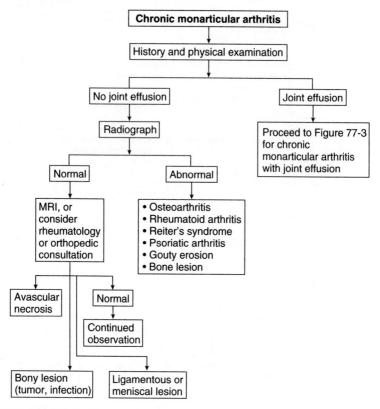

■ FIGURE 77–2. Algorithm for chronic monarticular arthritis. *MRI* = magnetic resonance imaging.

(Adapted with permission from McGuire JL, Giansiracusa DF: Monoarticular arthritis. In Green HL, Glassock RJ, Kelley MA (eds): *Introduction to Clinical Medicine,* Philadelphia: Decker, 1991; and Weinstein BR, Giansiracusa DF: Primary care presentations of musculoskeletal disease. In Noble J, et al (eds): *Noble's Textbook of Primary Care Medicine,* CD-ROM Version. St. Louis: Mosby, 1996.)

4. Assess for **systemic illnesses,** especially for constitutional symptoms. The review of systems should pay particular attention to the following:

   a. High-risk behaviors (including HIV or hepatitis risk factors)
   b. Travel to tick-inhabited regions
   c. The presence of rashes
   d. History of sexually transmitted disease (STD)
   e. Prodromal symptoms (e.g., diarrhea, viral symptoms)
   f. Ocular symptoms
   g. Xerostomia
   h. Drug use

5. **Family history:** There are genetic and familial predispositions to a number of arthritic disorders, including rheumatoid arthritis, systemic

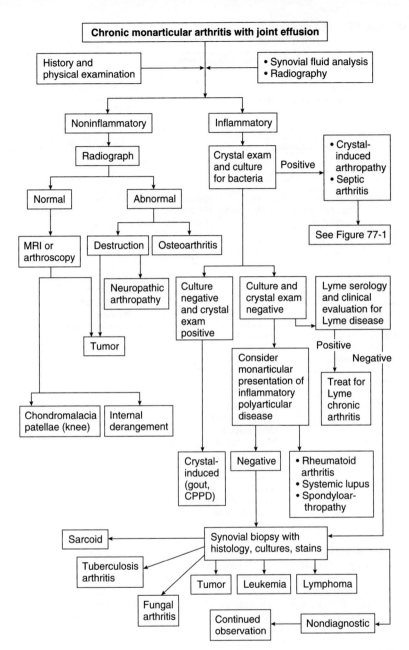

FIGURE 77–3. Algorithm for chronic monarticular arthritis with joint effusion. *CPPD* = calcium pyrophosphate dihydrate = *MRI* = magnetic resonance imaging.

(Adapted with permission from McGuire JL, Giansiracusa DF: Monoarticular arthritis. In Green HL, Glassock RJ, Kelley MA (eds): *Introduction to Clinical Medicine.* Philadelphia: Decker, 1991; and Weinstein BR, Giansiracusa DF: Primary care presentations of musculoskeletal disease. In Noble J, et al (eds): *Noble's Textbook of Primary Care Medicine,* CD-ROM Version. St. Louis: Mosby, 1996.)

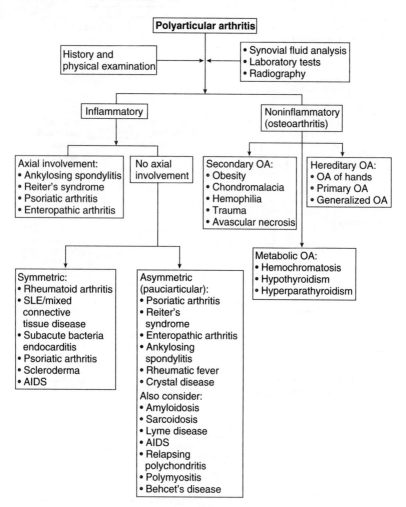

FIGURE 77–4. Differential diagnoses of polyarticular arthritis. *OA* = osteoarthritis; *SLE* = systemic lupus erythematosus.

(Adapted with permission from Doud D: Polyarticular arthritis. In Greene HL, et al (eds): *Decision Making in Medicine,* St. Louis: Mosby, 1993; and Weinstein BR, Giansiracusa DF: Primary care presentations of musculoskeletal disease. In Noble J, et al (eds): *Noble's Textbook of Primary Care Medicine,* CD-ROM Version. St. Louis: Mosby, 1996.)

lupus erythematosus, gout, osteoarthritis, and seronegative spondyloarthropathies.

B. Physical examination

  1. General principle: When examining an affected joint, the contralateral side of the patient can serve as a reference point.

2. **Nonmusculoskeletal examination:** Look for clues to systemic illness (especially dermatologic, ocular, and neurologic), and assess for lymphadenopathy.
3. **Musculoskeletal examination**
   a. **Inspection:** Assess posture, gait, and movement. Look for signs of inflammation by checking for erythema, warmth, and swelling. Joint deformity is associated with destructive changes within the joint. Active range of motion is limited with both articular and periarticular processes but is helpful in assessing function and mobility.
   b. **Palpation** of the articular and periarticular structures can usually help differentiate joint effusions, synovial thickening, bony changes, enthesitis (i.e., inflammation at sites of ligamentous and tendinous attachments to bone, a characteristic finding in seronegative spondylarthropathies), and periarticular/soft-tissue processes. Palpating areas of maximal tenderness also helps localize the problem. The presence of crepitus suggests destructive changes within the joint.
   c. **Pain with passive range of motion** characterizes articular problems, whereas in bursa and tendon disorders, pain is more prominent with **active range of motion.**
   d. **Provocative maneuvers** that stress tendons, ligaments, and the joints for stability are useful localizing techniques and can help establish a diagnosis.

V. Diagnostic Testing

A. **Laboratory testing.** In the patient where the diagnosis remains uncertain following clinical assessment, laboratory testing may be advised. These tests will have the greatest utility in patients where a systemic illness is being considered. In such instances, a complete blood count (CBC), renal functions, urinalysis, liver chemistries, and serum calcium are considered initial studies. The composite clinical picture should guide further assessment, including rheumatologic testing [erythrocyte sedimentation rate (ESR), C-reactive protein, antibody testing, rheumatoid factor (RF), serum protein electrophoresis, Lyme titer), imaging studies (MRI, plain films of sacroiliac joints, chest radiography, and nuclear imaging), and use of the microbiology laboratory.

B. **Synovial fluid analysis** constitutes the basic initial laboratory evaluation when a joint effusion is identified:

1. **Normal joint fluid** is transparent, colorless, highly viscous, and usually has < 200 white blood cells (WBCs)/mm^3, with less than 25% polymorphonuclear leukocytes.
2. In **noninflammatory disorders,** such as osteoarthritis, the fluid is yellow, clear, highly viscous, and has WBC counts between 200 and 2,000, with less than 25% polymorphonuclear leukocytes.
3. In **inflammatory arthritides,** such as rheumatoid arthritis, the fluid may be translucent or opaque, yellow in color, and have reduced viscosity. The WBC count is usually between 2,000 and 100,000, with greater than 50% polymorphonuclear leukocytes. Joints that are infected with virulent bacterial organisms may have even more inflammatory

findings, with WBC counts > 100,000, mostly polymorphonuclear leukocytes.
4. **Hemorrhagic effusions** are seen with trauma, coagulopathies, neoplasms, severe osteoarthritis, and pigmented villonodular synovitis.

SUGGESTED READING

Weinstein BR, Giansiracusa DF: Primary care presentations of musculoskeletal disease. In Noble J, et al (eds): *Noble's Textbook of Primary Care Medicine*, CD-ROM Version. St. Louis: Mosby, 1996, Chapter R.

78

Low Back Pain

Rohit Bhalla

I. Definitions and Overview

- **A. Low back pain** is defined as **pain in the lumbosacral region,** which may be associated with lower extremity symptoms. It may be acute or chronic (persisting for longer than 12 weeks). Ninety percent of patients presenting with acute low back pain will have fully recovered function and be symptom-free within 4–6 weeks.
- **B. Compression of the nerve roots or spinal cord** may occur as a result of pressure from the above structures, but most commonly occurs as a result of a herniated intervertebral disk. Approximately 95% of disk herniation in adults occurs at the L4/L5 or L5/S1 vertebral levels with compression of the L5 or S1 nerve roots.
- **C. Radiculopathy.** When compression of the nerve tissue gives rise to extremity-related symptoms in a dermatomal distribution, the process is referred to as radiculopathy (or sciatica, when the L4, L5, or S1 dermatomes are involved).
- **D. Common terms**
  1. **Spondylosis:** Degenerative changes of the vertebrae and facet joints
  2. **Spondylolysis:** Defect of the pars interarticularis, usually of a congenital nature
  3. **Spondylitis:** Inflammation of one or more of the vertebrae
  4. **Spondylolisthesis:** Anteroposterior movement of one vertebral body upon another body or the sacrum
- **E. Spinal stenosis** is narrowing of the lumbar spinal canal, with compression of the cauda equina roots, commonly as a result of progressive spondylosis and degenerative changes of ligaments and intervertebral disks.

II. Differential Diagnosis (Table 78–1)
III. Notes on the Differential Diagnosis

- **A. Disk herniation.** The absence of sciatica rules out significant disk herniation.
- **B. Vertebral compression fracture.** Patients older than 70 years of age or receiving long-term corticosteroid therapy should be considered to have a vertebral compression fracture until proven otherwise.
- **C. Cauda equina syndrome,** occurring in the presence of a large disk herniation, is characterized by urinary retention, saddle anesthesia, and radicular symptoms. Cauda equina syndrome occurs in approximately 1% of all disk herniations.
- **D. Spinal stenosis** usually occurs in middle-aged or elderly patients and gives rise to a distinctive constellation of symptoms (i.e., back pain with associated bilateral buttock pain, occasionally with associated paresthesias and paresis) termed **neurogenic claudication.** These symptoms are

TABLE 78–1. Differential Diagnosis of Low Back Pain

Musculoskeletal or disk-related sources (as many as 80%–90%)

Mechanical (majority of cases)

Herniated intervertebral disk

Herniated disk with nerve root entrapment (radiculopathy) [~ 1%]

Spinal stenosis

Vertebral compression fracture (~4%)

Spondylolisthesis (~3%)

Vertebral osteoarthritis

Scoliosis

Rheumatologic diseases (ankylosing spondylitis ~ 0.3%)

Trauma

Cauda equina syndrome (~0.0004%)

Hip osteoarthritis, fracture, avascular necrosis

Trochanteric bursitis

Neoplasm (~0.7%)

Primary malignancy, vertebral or cord elements

Metatastic (most commonly prostate, breast, or lung primary)

Multiple myeloma

Spinal infection (~0.01%)

Osteomyelitis

Intervertebral diskitis

Epidural abscess

Visceral sources

Genitourinary
    Urinary tract infection

Continued

TABLE 78–1. Differential Diagnosis of Low Back Pain (*Continued*)

Pelvic inflammatory disease
Endometriosis

Gastrointestinal
  Pancreatitis
  Duodenal ulcer

Vascular
  Cord arteriovenous malformation or fistula
  Abdominal aortic aneurysm

Psychosomatic*
  Mood, personality, and somatoform disorders
  Domestic, occupational, and financial factors
  Drug-seeking behavior
  Symptom magnification

Other
  Hernia
  Diabetic mononeuropathy
  Zoster
  Fibromyalgia

---

*Psychosomatic disorders are unlikely to be the primary cause of symptoms, but may significantly affect clinical course.

worsened by back extension, as occurs in walking or standing, and are relieved by sitting or lying with the trunk flexed.

IV. Clinical Assessment (Figure 78–1)

  A. Initial assessment. The focus of the initial assessment should be on the identification of patients with symptoms or signs suggestive of potentially serious secondary causes (i.e., red flag symptoms), which necessitate a targeted evaluation (Table 78–2).

  B. History

  1. A detailed elaboration of the **nature of pain, mechanism of onset,** and **presence or absence of associated symptoms** is imperative in narrowing the differential diagnosis.
  2. Patients should be questioned about **lower extremity pain, paresthesias or weakness,** and **bowel or bladder symptoms.**
  3. The history should further focus on eliciting those conditions noted in Tables 78–1 and 78–2.

  C. Physical examination

  1. **Routine elements** of the examination include functional observation, local examination of the lower back, pertinent neurologic examination, and testing for radiculopathy of the L4, L5, and S1 levels.
  2. **Neurologic examination:** The rationale for a neurologic assessment of

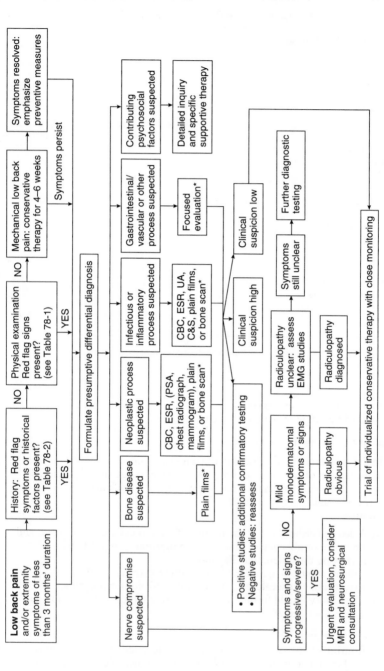

■ **FIGURE 78–1.** Algorithm for the differential diagnosis of low back pain. *CBC* = complete blood count; *C&S* = culture and sensitivity; *EMG* = electromyogram; *ESR* = erythrocyte sedimentation rate; *MRI* = magnetic resonance imaging; *PSA* = prostate-specific antigen; *UA* = urinalysis.

*Tests should be chosen based on the specific processes suspected.

TABLE 78–2. Red Flag Symptoms and Signs (and Historical Data) in the Evaluation of Low Back Pain

Red Flag Signs and Symptoms	Comorbid Conditions
Older than 50 years of age	Diabetes mellitus
Trauma	Alcoholism
Unexplained weight loss	HIV
Predominance of rest/nocturnal pain	Cancer history
Fever	Corticosteroid therapy
Bowel or bladder symptoms	Intravenous drug abuse
Progressive or severe pain, paresthesia, or weakness	
Progressive neurogenic claudication	
Symptoms persisting beyond 6 weeks	

Neurologic Findings	Nonneurologic Findings
Urinary retention	Fever
Saddle anesthesia	Weight loss
Perianal sensory loss	Abdominal tenderness or mass
Anal sphincter laxity	Severe vertebral tenderness
Polydermatomal deficit	Abnormal prostate examination
Monodermatomal or progressive motor, sensory, or reflex deficit	Abnormal pelvic examination
	Breast mass
Positive supine or seated leg raise tests	Moderate-severe kyphoscoliosis
	Conflicting supine or seated leg tests

patients with acute low back pain is to evaluate for the possibility of spinal nerve tissue impingement, most commonly as a result of a herniated intervertebral disk causing nerve root compression.

3. **Straight leg raise testing** evaluates the possibility of L5 or S1 nerve root compromise. The test is considered positive if the patient

experiences pain radiating below the knee within the first 70 degrees of motion as the examiner passively raises the patient's leg, fully extended at the knee. Clinical suspicion of (L5 or S1) nerve root compression is raised further if symptoms are intensified by foot dorsiflexion or internal limb rotation at the level where the straight leg raise test is positive.

4. **Crossed straight leg raise test** is considered positive if the examiner passively raises the uninvolved leg and pain is experienced below the knee in the contralateral resting leg. This indicates nerve root compression on the side of the contralateral (painful) leg. Although sensitivity is only 25%, the crossed straight leg raise test is among the most highly specific examination maneuvers at 90% specificity. A positive crossed straight leg raise test indicates a high likelihood of disk herniation.

5. **Ipsilateral straight leg raise test** is one of the most highly sensitive maneuvers for lumbar disk herniation at 80% sensitivity, but only 40% specificity. Hence, a negative ipsilateral straight leg raise test makes a clinically significant disk herniation very unlikely.

V. Diagnostic Assessment

A. **Laboratory studies** should be selected keeping in mind the clinical disorders that are suspected. They are rarely indicated at the initial visit. Studies may include complete blood count (CBC), erythrocyte sedimentation rate (ESR), urinalysis and culture, serum or urine protein electrophoresis, prostate-specific antigen (PSA), calcium, phosphorous, and alkaline phosphatase determinations.

B. **Electromyography.** The utility of electromyography is mainly to clarify equivocal symptoms and signs in patients with extremity symptoms prior to considering imaging studies.

C. **Imaging studies**

1. **Lumbosacral spine plain films** should be ordered when an abnormality of bone is being considered. Plain films are primarily of value in detecting fracture, malignancy, and infection (mainly vertebral osteomyelitis). Soft tissue is not visualized well by this modality. Degenerative changes and evidence of nonspecific disk disease on lumbosacral spine plain films are seen in as many as 90% of asymptomatic persons by 50 years of age. These findings are of questionable significance and are of little value in determining the precise cause of pain in symptomatic patients.

2. **Computed tomography (CT)** is mainly of value in visualizing bony tissue. When done in conjunction with intrathecally administered contrast, it is referred to as CT-myelography. CT-myelography is an excellent alternative, but given uncommon but potentially serious complications, this modality is being largely supplanted by magnetic resonance imaging (MRI).

3. **MRI** is the imaging modality of choice in visualizing nerve and soft tissue. It is highly sensitive in detecting herniated disks (approximately 90%) in patients with low back pain. MRI has the additional value of being able to evaluate other soft-tissue processes simultaneously (e.g., infection, malignancy) and is the procedure of choice in selection and guidance of surgery for lumbar disk disease. In general, MRI is rarely indicated at the initial evaluation of a patient with low back pain. It is indicated if surgery is being considered (e.g., for severe radiculopathy).

4. **Bone scan** is best utilized in detecting disorders associated with increased osteoblastic activity. It should be obtained primarily in patients in whom infectious, malignant, or inflammatory causes are being considered.

SUGGESTED READING

Bigos S, Bowyer O, Braen G, et al: Acute low back problems in adults. *Clinical Practice Guidelines, Quick Reference Guide Number 14.* Rockville, Md: U.S. Department of Health and Human Services, Public Health Service, Agency for Health Care Policy and Research, AHCPR Publ No. 95–0643, December 1994.

Deyo RA, Rainville J, Kent DL: What can history and physical examination tell us about low back pain? *JAMA* 268:760–765, 1992.

Deyo RA, Weinstein JN: Low back pain. *N Engl J Med* 344:363–370, 2001.

79

Myalgia
Nancy S. Chun

I. **Overview.** Myalgia, the subjective complaint of muscle pain, may be secondary to a localized problem (e.g., trauma, overuse) or a systemic disorder (e.g., an acute or chronic infection, a toxic or metabolic disorder). Less commonly, myalgia may reflect a primary muscle disease. Joint and bone pathology may produce complaints of muscle pain. Additionally, disease of subcutaneous tissue, fascia, tendons, and peripheral nerves may produce pain that is referred to muscle.

II. **Differential Diagnosis** (Table 79–1)

A. **Common causes** of myalgia include viral infection, trauma, fibromyalgia, the overuse syndromes, neuropathic disorders, and hypothyroidism. Rare causes of myalgia include metabolic bone diseases (e.g., osteomalacia, hyperparathyroidism) and myopathic disorders (see also page 498).

B. **Rheumatologic disorders.** Myalgia may be associated with rheumatologic disorders, including rheumatoid arthritis, systemic lupus erythematosus, polyarteritis nodosa, scleroderma, and mixed connective tissue syndrome. The systemic symptoms associated with these conditions, however, distinguish them from the clinically benign disorders.

C. **Drugs.** Many drugs may cause myalgia, but they do not generally cause weakness. Symptoms usually abate after withdrawal of the offending agent.

D. **Postviral myalgia.** Muscle pain can occur during or immediately after a viral infection.

E. **Muscle overuse syndrome**

1. **Vigorous activity and exercise** may be associated with muscle and tendon tears, which lead to muscle pain, tenderness, and swelling. The majority of patients with muscle pain related to exertion do not have any definable abnormality.

2. **Muscle damage:** Myalgia may be associated with laboratory evidence of muscle damage, including elevated serum creatine kinase (CK). If there is widespread muscle injury, myoglobinemia and myoglobinuria may occur.

F. **Fibromyalgia**

1. **Pain:** Typically, patients complain of widespread pain. Tenderness is usually symmetrical, affecting the right and left sides of the body, above and below the waist, and along the axis.

2. **Tenderness** can be found on physical examination by digital palpation of at least 11 of 18 predetermined sites, called tender points. Other than palpating tender points, the musculoskeletal and neurologic examinations are normal.

3. **Diagnosis** is based on clinical symptoms. There are no laboratory or imaging tests to confirm the diagnosis.

G. Myofascial pain syndrome is a poorly understood syndrome characterized by the presence of areas with deep tenderness. These areas are referred to as trigger points because digital palpation results in pain in a referred distribution. Regional clustering of trigger points is seen in patients with myofascial pain syndrome in contrast to the widespread distribution of pain seen in patients with fibromyalgia.

III. Clinical Evaluation. Assessment of patients with myalgia is directed at making a diagnosis of the significant disease entities noted in Table 79–1 and reassuring patients with benign disorders. A conservative approach to test ordering is directed by the history, physical examination, and serial evaluation of the patient (Figure 79–1).

A. History

1. Assess the quality, location, time of onset, and duration of **pain.** It is vital to distinguish myalgic from articular symptoms.
2. Assess for associated **weakness, fatigue, cramps,** and **functional debility.**
3. Identify **aggravating and alleviating features,** with particular attention to associations with activity.
4. Note any previous **trauma, fracture,** or **surgical procedure** in symptomatic areas.
5. A detailed **review of systems** is necessary, with a rheumatologic and endocrinologic focus.

TABLE 79–1. Classification Scheme for Myalgia with Examples of Disorders that Cause Myalgia

Classification Scheme	Examples of Disorders
Inflammatory	Viral myositis, pyomyositis, parasitic myositis, polymyositis, dermatomyositis, granulomatous myositis, interstitial myositis, localized nodular myositis, vasculitis, eosinophilic fasciitis
Toxic	Acute alcoholic myopathy, acute or subacute drug-induced myopathies, myopathies due to envenomation
Endocrine	Hypothyroidism, osteomalacia, hyperparathyroidism
Hereditary	Disorders of glycogen metabolism, carnitine palmityl transferase deficiency, myoadenylate deaminase deficiency, mitochondrial myopathy, dystrophinopathy, sodium channel myotonia, malignant hyperthermia
Other	Eaton-Lambert syndrome, fibromyalgia, polymyalgia rheumatica, postviral myalgia, muscle overuse syndromes, myasthenia gravis, neuropathy

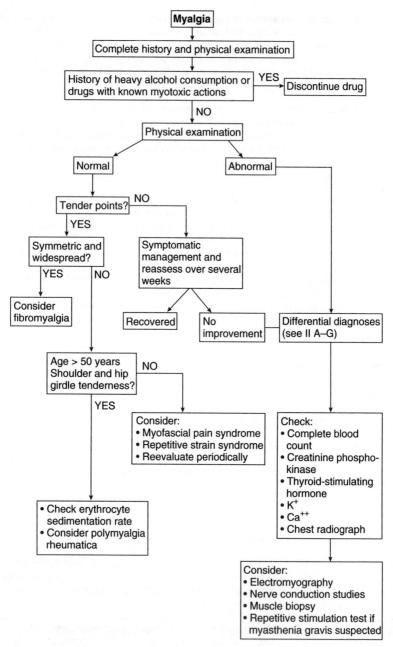

■ **FIGURE 79–1.** Algorithm for the evaluation of myalgia.

6. Obtain **additional information** by inquiring about psychosocial history, family history, complete list of medications, occupation, any previous visits to health professionals for the same complaints, use of nontraditional remedies, and any pending litigation.

B. Physical examination

1. **Musculoskeletal examination:** Focus on muscle atrophy or wasting, muscle strength, tetany, joint pain, joint effusions, range of motion, and tender/trigger points.
2. **Skin assessment:** Focus on rheumatologic manifestations.
3. A complete **neurologic examination** should be given.
4. The **thyroid gland** should be palpated for size and nodularity.

C. Laboratory evaluation.
If the history and physical examination do not provide a diagnosis or raise concerns about serious underlying disorders (see Table 79–1), symptomatic management and reassessment over several weeks is more productive than early laboratory testing.

1. **Initial assessment:** If symptoms persist, the initial evaluation should include a complete blood count (CBC) and CK level. The serum concentration of CK is the most reliable biochemical indicator of muscle disease.
2. **Other tests** should be considered, such as thyroid-stimulating hormone (TSH), potassium, and calcium levels.

D. Other diagnostic studies

1. **Electromyography (EMG)** is useful in the detection and evaluation of muscle disease. It provides information regarding the extent of the myopathic process and the pattern of muscle involvement. This test may also be useful for selecting a muscle for biopsy.
2. **Nerve conduction studies** should be considered to exclude the possibility of peripheral neuropathy as a confounding cause.
3. **Repetitive nerve stimulation** should be done if disorders of the neuromuscular junction (i.e., myasthenia gravis or Eaton-Lambert syndrome) are diagnostic considerations.
4. **Muscle biopsy** may be performed to establish a final diagnosis when myopathy is suspected on the basis of clinical abnormalities. It can help to differentiate between myopathy, denervation, and inflammatory and noninflammatory disorders.

SUGGESTED READING

American College of Rheumatology Ad Hoc Committee on Clinical Grounds. Guidelines for the initial evaluation of the adult patient with acute musculoskeletal symptoms. In *Textbook of Rheumatology*. Philadelphia: WB Saunders, 1997, pp 1880–1886.

Barth WF: Office evaluation of the patient with musculoskeletal complaints. *Am J Med* 102:3S–10S, 1997.

80

Erythrocyte Sedimentation Rate and C-Reactive Protein

Robert B. Zurier

I. **Definition.** The erythrocyte sedimentation rate (ESR) is the **distance in millimeters that erythrocytes fall during 1 hour in a sample of venous blood.** (Newer automated techniques allow the test to be performed in 30 minutes.) Normal ranges are 0–15 mm/hr in men and 0–20 mm/hr in women. The ESR is not a good screening test due to its low sensitivity.

   A. An **ESR >30 mm/hr** is suggestive of an underlying disease process. Many patients with infection, cancer, and connective tissue disease, however, will have a normal ESR (because sensitivity is < 30%).

   B. An **ESR > 100 mm/hr** indicates that the likelihood of a serious disease condition—such as malignancy, infection, or other inflammatory conditions—is > 90%.

II. **Causes**

   A. **Elevated ESR**

      1. Infections
      2. Vasculitis, including temporal arteritis
      3. Inflammatory arthritis
      4. Renal disease
      5. Anemia
      6. Malignancies and plasma cell dyscrasias
      7. Conditions associated with tissue injury, such as myocardial infarction (MI)
      8. Pregnancy
      9. Hypercholesterolemia
      10. Aging
      11. Estrogen administration

   B. **Decreased ESR**

      1. Polycythemia vera
      2. Sickle cell disease
      3. Anisocytosis, spherocytosis, acanthocytosis, and microcytosis
      4. Extreme leukocytosis
      5. Blood clotting
      6. Trichinosis and pertussis
      7. Congestive heart failure (CHF)

III. **C-Reactive Protein** (i.e., an acute-phase protein). The normal value of C-reactive protein is ≤ 2 mg/L, with a gray zone (clinically insignificant) as high as 10 mg/L. As a patient's condition improves, the ESR changes at a slow pace, whereas plasma C-reactive protein levels change rapidly. The C-reactive protein level is not affected by aging.

A. **Inflammatory disorders.** An acute-phase protein is one whose value increases or decreases by at least 25% during inflammatory disorders. Therefore, its measurement may help differentiate inflammatory from noninflammatory conditions. Among patients with values > 100 mg/L, the vast majority have bacterial infections.

B. **Rheumatoid arthritis.** Serial values are of prognostic value in rheumatoid arthritis, but not in systemic lupus erythematosus.

SUGGESTED READING

Gabay C, Kushner I: Mechanism of disease: Acute-phase proteins and other systemic responses in inflammation. *N Engl J Med* 340:448–454, 1999.

81

The Complement System
Lauren Hiestand

I. **Definition.** The complement system is a **major defense and clearance system comprised of a myriad of plasma and cellular membrane proteins that interact to augment the capacity of the immune system to eliminate foreign molecules, particles, and organisms.**

   A. **Complement plasma proteins** circulate in a nonactivated (zymogen) form and are converted to active forms in a precise sequence of intermolecular and proteolytic reactions.

   B. **Pathways of complement activations**

     1. The **classic pathway,** triggered by immune complexes
     2. The **alternative pathway,** triggered by microorganisms
     3. The **lectin pathway,** triggered by microorganisms or hypoglycosylated immunoglobulin G (IgG)

   C. **Membrane attack complex (MAC).** All three pathways lead to cleavage of C3 and terminate with the formation of the same MAC in the common pathway.

II. **Complement in Host Defense**

   A. Complement is important for **efficient bacterial killing,** influencing this process through:

     1. **Enhancement of phagocytosis** via chemotaxis mediation (C3a and C5a released during activation attract phagocytic cells to the site of infection)
     2. **Enhancement of bacterial adherence** to phagocyte membrane (C3b on the bacterial surface binds to receptors on phagocytic cells)
     3. **Direct lytic action** against some bacteria and viruses

   B. Complement is also important for the **solubilization and degradation of immune complexes.** Activation of complement on immune complexes inhibits their precipitation in tissues by:

     1. Binding to nascent complexes and preventing further growth
     2. Binding of C3b to erythrocyte complement receptor 1 (CR1) with subsequent destruction by fixed phagocytic cells in the liver or spleen

III. **Complement Deficiency and Disease.** Individuals deficient in complement components show **increased susceptibility to bacterial infection** and/or the **propensity to develop immune-complex disease.**

   A. **Genetic deficiencies of complement components** are relatively rare. Several types are especially noteworthy.

     1. **C3 deficiency** predisposes to frequent serious pyogenic infections.
     2. **Properdin, factor H, and late component deficiencies** predispose to neisserial infection.

3. **Deficiencies of early-acting components** ($C1_q$, $C1_r$, $C1_s$, C4, and C_2) strongly predispose to collagen-vascular disease, especially systemic lupus erythematosus.

4. **Deficiency of C1-INH** leads to hereditary angioneurotic edema.

5. **Deficiencies of regulatory proteins DAF, HRF, and HRF-20** predispose to hemolytic anemia.

B. **Acquired disorders of the complement system** may be due to the following:

1. **Complement activation and consumption**

   a. Posttransfusion, dialysis, apheresis syndromes, thermal injury, adult respiratory distress syndrome (ARDS)

   b. Autoantibodies to complement components

   (1) C3 and C4 nephritic factors (IgG autoantibodies to C3 convertases), which prevent binding of control proteins H or C4bp, allowing for uncontrolled C3 consumption and leading to hypocomplementemic nephritis

   (2) Autoantibody to C1-INH, leading to acquired hereditary angioneurotic edema

   (3) Anti-$C1_q$ antibody, associated with hypocomplementemic urticarial vasculitis syndrome and with proliferative glomerulonephritis in systemic lupus erythematosus

2. **Decreased synthesis** seen with malnutrition, cirrhosis, liver failure, and the newborn state

3. **Increased catabolism** seen in nephrotic syndrome and secondary to hypogammaglobulinemia

IV. Complement Testing

A. **Suspected congenital complement deficiency.** Screening for complement component deficiency is generally initiated using the **functional CH_{50} (total hemolytic complement) assay.**

1. Congenital deficiencies of C1 through C8 yield CH_{50} values approaching zero. C9 deficiency typically yields a CH_{50} value approximately 50% of normal. Abnormal CH_{50} results can be followed by immunochemical or functional assays for individual components.

2. Screening for alternative factor deficiencies can be similarly initiated with the **hemolytic (functional) AH_{50} assay** and followed up with immunochemical or functional assays of specific alternative pathway factors.

B. **Suspected complement activation.** In contrast to their role in the investigation of suspected congenital complement deficiency, hemolytic screening assays, and immunochemical measurements of native components are of limited use in the assessment of complement consumption.

1. **Hemolytic screening assays**

   a. Reduced hemolytic activity in serum (by CH_{50} or AH_{50}) might suggest complement consumption but could also reflect reduced synthesis (or increased catabolism) of any factor in the sequence.

   b. A 50% reduction in a component is required to compromise the hemolytic activity of serum, making this method relatively insensitive for detection of complement activation.

2. **Immunochemical measurements** of native complement components (usually C3, C4, or factor B) can give indirect information about activation, but have several drawbacks:

   a. **Normal concentrations vary widely.** Thus, an individual's baseline level of C3 or C4 can be reduced by 50% and still fall within the "normal" (reference) range for the assay.

   b. **Complement components act as acute-phase reactants.** Increases due to infection or inflammation may mask consumption.

   c. **Reduced concentrations may reflect inherited deficiency, decreased synthesis, or increased catabolism,** rather than consumption due to pathway activation.

   d. **Polyclonal antibodies** used in these methods detect both the native molecule and its various complement split products, potentially underestimating the extent of consumption.

3. A new generation of assays providing **direct evidence of complement activation** is expected to allow for improved monitoring of disease activity. Tests for **complement activation products** are currently available mainly through larger reference laboratories; adaptation to the hospital laboratory setting is ongoing.

   a. **Anaphylatoxins $C3_a$, $C4_a$, and $C5_a$** are extremely sensitive markers of complement consumption. Their short half-lives and tendency for false elevations due to in vitro activation limit their practical application in the clinical setting.

   b. **Biologically inert split products of C3 ($C3_{dg}$, $iC3_b$), C4 ($C4_d$), and factor B (Ba, Bb)** remain in the circulation for longer periods and are readily assayed. Split products of C4 and factor B can provide an indication of activation of the classical and alternative pathways, respectively. Ratios of fragments to parent molecules (e.g., $C4_d/C4$) can indicate activation regardless of the initial concentration of the intact component.

   c. **Functional complexes:** The **terminal** complex **$SC5_b$-9** has shown promise as a means of assessing systemic lupus erythematosus flares. Other functional complexes, such as **$C1_r$:$C1_s$:C1-INH** and **$C3_b$:Bb:P** provide evidence of activation of the early stages of the classic and alternative pathways, respectively.

SUGGESTED READING

Bing DH, Alper CA: Complement in health and disease. In Colvin RB, Bahn AK, McClusky RT (eds): *Diagnostic Immunopathology*, 2nd ed. New York: Raven Press, 1995.

Johnston RB Jr: The complement system in host defense and inflammation: the cutting of a double-edge sword. *Pediatr Infect Dis J* 1993; 12(11):933–941.

Rabson A: Complement, In Rose NR, Hamilton RG, Detrick B (eds) *Manual of Clinical Laboratory Immunology*, 6th ed. Washington DC: American Society for Microbiology, 2001.

Sullivan KE: Complement deficiency and autoimmunity. *Curr Opin Pediatr*, 1998: 10(6): 600–606.

Antinuclear Antibodies

Robert B. Zurier

I. **Definition.** Antinuclear antibodies are **autoantibodies directed against components of the cell nucleus.** They bind to single-stranded DNA, double-stranded DNA, or both. The antinuclear antibodies should be used only when there is a high clinical suspicion of disease.

II. **Causes for Elevated Antinuclear Antibodies** (Table 82–1)

A. **Systemic lupus erythematosus.** Elevated antinuclear antibodies are found in more than 95% of patients with systemic lupus erythematosus. However, the specificity of the test is low. The predictive value of antinuclear antibody testing is related mainly to the estimated likelihood of systemic lupus erythematosus before testing. A positive antinuclear antibody test has high predictive value for systemic lupus erythematosus when the diagnosis is unclear but the patient exhibits two or three features of lupus.

B. **Rheumatologic diseases**

1. Systemic sclerosis (60%–90% of patients will show elevations)
2. Sjögren's syndrome (75% of patients)
3. Polymyositis/dermatomyositis (25% of patients)
4. Rheumatoid arthritis (15%–35% of patients)

C. **Normal, healthy patients** (i.e., false-positive results)

1. Pregnancy
2. Elderly
3. Certain drugs (e.g., drug-induced lupus)
4. Family history of rheumatic disease

D. **Nonrheumatologic diseases**

1. Infections (e.g., mononucleosis, endocarditis)
2. Pulmonary fibrosis
3. Gastrointestinal diseases
4. Endocrine disease (e.g., thyroiditis, Grave's disease)
5. Neoplastic disease
6. Skin disease
7. Autoimmune hepatitis

III. **When to Order Antinuclear Antibodies** (see also Chapter 83, page 497)

A. **Supporting a diagnosis.** Antinuclear antibodies should be obtained to support the diagnosis in a patient presenting with a multisystem disease that strongly suggests systemic lupus erythematosus, systemic sclerosis, or Sjögren's syndrome. A positive test leads to testing for more specific antibodies to confirm the suspected underlying disease.

B. **Ruling out a diagnosis.** A negative test is fairly reliable in ruling out systemic lupus erythematosus, even when a patient has one or two features of lupus and no obvious alternate diagnosis.

TABLE 82–1. Interpretation of Antinuclear Antibody Test Results

Present Likelihood of Systemic Lupus Erythematosus	Antinuclear Antibody Titer	Decision
Low	≤ 80	Ignore
	≥ 160	Observe; seek alternative reason
Moderate	≤ 80	Observe; seek alternative reason
	≥ 160	Observe; seek alternative reason
High	Negative	Observe; seek alternative reason
	Positive (any titer)	Further testing: anti-<u>Sm</u>, anti–double-stranded DNA

Between 60% and 80% of patients with systemic lupus erythematosus lack antibodies to double-stranded DNA when tested by a sensitive assay. When a patient with systemic lupus erythematosus is tested at regular intervals, rising titers of anti–double-stranded DNA suggest risk of acceleration of disease.

SUGGESTED READING

Penny SL, Craft J: Antinuclear Antibodies. In Ruddy S, Harris ED, Sledge CB (eds): Kelley's Textbook of Rheumatology, 6th ed. Philadephia: WB Saunders, 2001, 161–174.

Diagnostic Approach to Common Rheumatologic Problems

Leslie R. Harrold

Gout

I. Definition. Gout is a **disease caused by the deposition of monosodium urate crystals in the tissues of and around the joint.**

II. Clinical History

    A. Location. Fifty percent of patients experience their first attack in the metatarsophalangeal joint of the great toe. Other peripheral joints, including the joints of the midfoot, ankles, knees, fingers, wrists, and elbows may be involved in a monarticular fashion. Approximately 10%–15% of patients present with acute polyarticular gout.

    B. Timing. Attacks often occur at night and may be associated with inflammation of the surrounding tendons, bursae, and skin. Even if untreated, an acute gout attack is self-limited (generally lasting 3–7 days).

    C. Frequency. Attacks may become more frequent and more prolonged, resulting in chronic, persistent gout with increasing accumulation of urate deposits (tophi).

III. Laboratory and Imaging Studies. The definitive diagnosis of gout depends on the demonstration of intracellular monosodium urate crystals in the synovial fluid in a patient with an appropriate clinical history.

    A. Laboratory studies

        1. Synovial fluid requires crystal identification by polarized light. Gout is characterized by needle-shaped monosodium urate crystals within polymorphonuclear leukocytes.

        2. Synovial white blood cell (WBC) counts are usually $\geq 2000/mm^3$.

        3. Uric acid

            a. Note that only 25% of persons with hyperuricemia develop gout.

            b. All patients with gout have hyperuricemia at some point in their diagnosis.

            c. During an acute attack, the uric acid level may be normal.

    B. Imaging. In chronic tophaceous gout, radiographic findings include cortical erosions with sharply defined sclerotic margins, cortical erosions with an overhanging margin, and round or oval cysts generally with sclerotic margins in medullary bone near joints. Unlike rheumatoid arthritis, there is preservation of joint space, absence of periarticular demineralization, and eccentric soft-tissue swelling.

SUGGESTED READING

Emmerson BT: The management of gout. *N Engl J Med* 334:445–451, 1996.
Simkin PA: Gout and hyeruricemia. *Curr Opin Rheumatol* 9:268–273, 1997.

Infectious Causes of Arthritis

I. **Nongonococcal Bacterial Septic Arthritis** (see also Chapter 35)

A. **History.** There is usually an acute onset of joint pain, warmth, tenderness, and restricted motion as a result of joint effusion.

B. **Physical examination.** Most affected patients present with a single joint involved, but 20% of patients present with polyarticular involvement. Joints commonly involved include the knee (50%), hip (13%), shoulder (9%), wrist (8%), ankle (8%), elbow (7%), and the small joints of the hands or feet (5%).

C. **How to confirm the diagnosis**

1. **Radiographic findings** early in the course of the disease may only demonstrate evidence of soft-tissue swelling and synovial effusions. After 10–14 days of bacterial infection, destructive changes including joint space narrowing, erosions, and foci of subchondral osteomyelitis become evident.

2. **Laboratory studies**

   a. Laboratory studies reveal **serum leukocytosis** in only one-third of affected patients.

   b. **Organisms**

      (1) **Gram-positive organisms** are identified as the cause of nongonococcal arthritis by Gram stain in 50%–70% of cases and by synovial culture in 65%–85% of cases.

      (2) **Gram-negative bacilli** cause 10%–15% of infections, and < 5% are caused by mixed aerobic and anaerobic infections.

   c. **A low titer positive antinuclear antibodies test** can be present secondary to nonspecific immune stimulation.

II. **Gonococcal Bacterial Septic Arthritis** (see also Chapter 35)

A. **History.** Disseminated gonococcal infection may present with symptoms of urethritis, cervicitis, proctitis, or pharyngitis; the majority of patients (80%) have no local symptoms. The condition should be suspected when a high-risk individual presents with persistent mono- or oligoarticular arthritis, usually affecting the small joints of the hands, wrists, elbows, knees, and ankles.

B. **How to confirm the diagnosis**

1. **Radiographic changes** associated with gonococcal bacterial septic arthritis are the same as for nongonococcal bacterial septic arthritis.

2. **Laboratory studies.** *Neisseria gonorrhoeae* is a fastidious organism, and

cultures from joints are often negative. Therefore, culturing synovial fluid; blood; the cervix, urethra, rectum, and pharynx; and skin lesions is recommended to increase the yield. Since a substantial proportion of patients have negative cultures, patients with clinical suspicion should be treated for the condition regardless of the culture results. Nonspecific markers of infection, such as leukocytosis, an elevated erythrocyte sedimentation rate (ESR), and an elevated C-reactive protein are commonly seen.

III. Lyme Arthritis

A. **When to suspect.** A diagnosis of Lyme arthritis is suspected when patients at risk for a tick bite present with chronic monarthritis or oligoarticular arthritis affecting large joints of the lower extremity. Musculoskeletal symptoms early in the illness consist of migratory pain in the joints, tendons, bursae, muscle, or bone. The pain is usually not accompanied by joint swelling. Months later, 60% of untreated patients develop frank arthritis with brief intermittent attacks of monarticular or oligoarticular arthritis affecting the large joints, especially the knees.

B. **How to confirm the diagnosis**

1. **Radiographs** of the involved joints may show effusions. In chronic Lyme arthritis, erosions may be seen.

2. **Laboratory tests**

   a. **Serologic tests** [e.g., enzyme immunoassay (EIA), immunofluorescent antibody (IFA)] may be used to support a clinical diagnosis of Lyme disease. Tests may be negative before the second month of illness. Patients treated earlier may never develop specific antibodies. False-positive results occur due to infection with other spirochetes or systemic inflammatory conditions.

   b. **Western blot assay:** Equivocal or positive serologic tests should be confirmed by a Western blot assay. Positive titers may remain detectable for many years.

   c. **Low titers:** Early in the course of illness, laboratory tests may demonstrate low titers of rheumatoid factor (RF), antinuclear antibodies, or anticardiolipin antibodies.

   d. **Synovial WBC counts** range from 500–110,000 cells/mm^3 (average is 25,000 cells/mm^3). The antibodies to *Borrelia burgdorferi* should be positive on enzyme-linked immunosorbent assay (ELISA) after the first several weeks of infection. The test is subject to false-negative results and more commonly, false-positive results for which a Western blot assay is used.

SUGGESTED READING

Kalish R: Lyme disease. *Rheum Dis Clin North Am* 23:239–258, 1997.
Pioro MH, Mandell BF: Septic arthritis. *Rheum Dis Clin North Am* 23:239–258, 1997.

| **Systemic Rheumatic Diseases**

I. Rheumatoid Arthritis

A. Definition. Rheumatoid arthritis is a **polyarticular chronic systemic disease of unknown origin** that produces neovascularization and persistent and progressive inflammation of the synovium in peripheral joints.

B. When to suspect rheumatoid arthritis

1. **History.** Patients usually present with malaise, fatigue, and morning stiffness lasting more than 1 hour. The majority of patients complain of symmetric pain and swelling in the hands, particularly the wrists, metacarpophalangeal joints, and proximal interphalangeal joints.

2. **Physical examination.** Symmetrical synovitis will involve the peripheral joints, particularly the hands (wrists, metacarpophalangeal joints, and proximal interphalangeal joints). Synovitis also occurs in the elbows, knees, shoulders, and feet (ankle joints, talonavicular joints, and metatarsophalangeal joints). Rheumatoid nodules, when present, are specific for rheumatoid arthritis.

C. How to confirm the diagnosis

1. **Laboratory studies.** A positive RF is present in 75%–80% of patients with rheumatoid arthritis. Anemia of chronic disease may be present as well as thrombocytosis. The sedimentation rate may be elevated and usually correlates with disease activity. Elevated liver enzymes may be associated with active disease. An antinuclear antibody test is positive in as many as 68% of patient with rheumatoid arthritis. Synovial fluid from affected joints should be inflammatory with a WBC count > 2000/mm^3.

2. **Radiographic findings.** Early in the disease course, radiographs of the extremities may show periarticular osteopenia. Bony erosions on radiograph may take several months to a year of disease activity before appearing. Chest radiographs can show pleural effusions, pulmonary nodules, or interstitial fibrosis.

II. Systemic Lupus Erythematosus

A. Definition. Systemic lupus erythematosus is an **inflammatory multisystem disease of unknown origin,** which is characterized by the production of antibodies to the cell nucleus in association with a diverse array of clinical manifestations. It is five times more likely in women than in men.

B. When to suspect systemic lupus erythematosus

1. **History**

   a. Patients usually present with constitutional symptoms, including malaise, fatigue, fever, and anorexia with weight loss.

   b. Common complaints include alopecia, photosensitivity, rashes, arthralgias, and Raynaud's phenomenon.

   c. The patient's medical history may include episodes of unexplained blood dyscrasias, seizures, neurologic deficits, pleuritis, pleural effusions (often asymptomatic), pulmonary fibrosis, pulmonary hypertension, pericarditis, pericardial effusions (usually asymptomatic), nonbacterial valvular vegetation, and thromboembolism (from associated antiphospholipid antibody syndrome).

2. **Physical examination.** Skin examination may reveal raised, erythematous, hyperkeratotic lesions in sun-exposed areas (such as in the malar distribution or dorsal surfaces of proximal phalanges). Discoid lesions (i.e., raised, erythematous lesions with hyperkeratosis, follicular plugging progressing to scarring with a peripheral erythematous ring that migrates outward) may also be present.

C. Serologic findings

1. **A high titer positive antinuclear antibody test** occurs in > 95% of patients with systemic lupus erythematosus. Positive anti–double-stranded DNA antibodies, which are specific to systemic lupus erythematosus, occur in 40%–60% of patients and are associated with glomerulonephritis and vasculitis.

2. **Positive anti-Smith antibodies,** which are also specific to systemic lupus erythematosus, occur in 10%–30% of patients and are associated with renal or central nervous system (CNS) manifestations.

3. **Positive anti-Ro antibodies** occur in 20%–60% of patients and are associated with cutaneous manifestations, thrombocytopenia, Sjögren's syndrome, congenital heart block, neonatal lupus, and antinuclear antibody-negative lupus.

4. **Positive anti-La antibodies** occur in 15%–40% of patients and are associated with Sjögren's syndrome, cutaneous manifestations, congenital heart block, and neonatal lupus.

5. **Anemia,** either from hemolytic anemia (40% of patients) or anemia of chronic disease (57%–78% of patients), is common. **Leukopenia** occurs in 50%–66% of patients and rarely results in infection.

6. **Thrombocytopenia** occurs in 20%–40% of patients. The presence of the lupus anticoagulant may prolong the partial thromboplastin time (PTT), depending on the sensitivity of reagents used.

7. Positive tests for **antiphospholipid antibodies** can occur in those patients with associated antiphospholipid antibody syndrome (i.e., a syndrome with recurrent spontaneous abortions, thrombocytopenia, and arterial and venous thrombosis). A false-positive serologic test for syphilis can occur due to the presence of antiphospholipid antibodies.

8. An **elevated ESR** can occur either from disease activity or superimposed infection. Complements (C3, C4, and CH50) may be depressed during disease flares.

9. A **urinalysis** may reveal proteinuria, red blood cells (RBCs), and RBC casts in those patients with renal involvement.

III. Systemic Sclerosis (Scleroderma)

A. **Limited form.** The limited form of systemic sclerosis includes the CREST syndrome (CREST = calcinosis, Raynaud's phenomenon, esophageal dysmotility, sclerodactyly, telangiectasias). Initially, patients present with nonpitting, symmetric swelling of both the hands and fingers. Skin changes then evolve into tightening and thickening of the skin over the distal limbs without truncal involvement. There is atrophic bound-down skin with tapering of the fingers, loss of skin appendages, and hyper- and hypopigmentation.

B. **Diffuse form.** The diffuse form of systemic sclerosis results in nonpitting, symmetric bilateral swelling of the hands and fingers that evolves into tightening and thickening of the skin over the distal and proximal limbs with or without truncal involvement. There is atrophic bound-down skin with tapering of the fingers, loss of skin appendages, and hyper- and hypopigmentation.

1. **Raynaud's phenomenon** occurs in 95% of patients with the diffuse form of systemic sclerosis.
2. **Gastrointestinal symptoms** are the same as for the limited form.
3. **Interstitial pulmonary fibrosis** occurs in as many as 70% of patients. There is usually an inflammatory phase that progresses to fibrosis and scarring.
4. **Renal manifestations** include hypertension with rapidly progressive renal insufficiency, which may be associated with a microangiopathic hemolytic anemia.

C. **Laboratory testing**

1. **Positive antinuclear antibodies** are present in 90% of patients with both the limited and diffuse forms of systemic sclerosis.
2. **Positive anticentromere antibodies** occur in 50%–90% of patients with limited systemic sclerosis.
3. **Positive anti–Scl-70** (also known as antitopoisomerase) **antibodies** occur in 25%–75% of patients with diffuse systemic sclerosis, but these antibodies are highly specific when present.

SUGGESTED READING

Kremer JM (ed): Rheumatoid arthritis. *Rheum Dis Clin North Am* 21:589–852, 1995.
Petri M (ed): Systemic lupus erythematosus. *Rheum Dis Clin North Am* 26:215–406, 2000.
Steen VD (ed): Scleroderma. *Rheum Dis Clin North Am* 22:647–907, 1996.

Inflammatory Muscle Diseases

I. **Definition. Polymyositis** and **dermatomyositis** are inflammatory myopathies, which result in symmetric proximal muscle weakness of the upper and lower extremities.

II. **Diagnosis**

A. **History.** Most patients have an insidious onset of symptoms (over 3–6 months), but an abrupt onset can also occur.

1. Patients often complain of constitutional symptoms such as fever, anorexia, and weight loss.
2. Weakness begins in the muscles of the neck, shoulder girdle, and hip girdle. Involvement of the distal muscles may develop late in the disease course.

3. Patients may complain of an inability to elevate their heads against gravity (due to neck flexor weakness).

4. Patients may note difficulties in everyday tasks, such as brushing their teeth, combing their hair, rising from a chair, carrying grocery bags, or climbing stairs.

5. Myalgias and arthralgias are common.

B. Physical examination. There is weakness of the proximal muscles, including flexors and extensors of the neck, shoulder, and hip.

III. How to Confirm the Diagnosis

A. Radiographic findings. A chest radiograph may show signs of interstitial fibrosis or interstitial pneumonitis in some patients.

B. Laboratory studies. The creatine phosphokinase (CPK) is elevated at some time during the course of the disease, and it is a useful marker to follow response to treatment; however, normal CPK levels may be found very early in the course of the disease or in advanced cases with significant atrophy. Similarly, other muscle enzymes (e.g., SGOT, SGPT, LDH, aldolase) are elevated during the course of the illness.

C. Electromyogram classically shows:

1. Increased insertional activity, fibrillations, and sharp positive waves

2. Spontaneous, bizarre high-frequency discharges

3. Polyphasic motor unit potentials of low amplitude and short duration

D. Skeletal muscle biopsy shows evidence of necrosis of type 1 and 2 muscle fibers, phagocytosis, regeneration with basophilia, large sacrolemnal nuclei, and prominent nucleoli.

SUGGESTED READING

Callen JP: Dermatomyositis. *Lancet* 355:53–7, 2000.

Jaundice

History:
- Stool characteristics
- Urine characteristics
- Pain, fever, weight loss, pruritis, travel, IVDU
- Sexual promiscuity, blood transfusions, medications
- Prior biliary surgery

CBC, Reticulocytes
Platelets
Total and direct bilirubin
Alkaline phosphatase
ALT, AST
Amylase
PT
Urinalysis

Physical exam:
- Assess for stigmata of chronic liver disease (see text)
- Scleral inspection
- Hepatic exam (size, texture, auscultatory findings, tenderness), splenomegaly, palpable mass
- Stool guaiac

Direct: total bilirubin > 50%

Refer to conjugated hyperbilirubinemia

Indirect: total bilirubin ratio > 80%

Unconjugated hyperbilirubinemia

Hemolysis
CBC with:
- Reticulocytosis
- Peripheral smear with schistocytes
Serum with:
- LDH elevated
- AST elevated
Haptoglobin decreased

NO

Abnormal transaminases

YES

Review smear
Haptoglobin
PT, aPTT
FDP
Creatinine

NO

YES

*Gilbert's Syndrome
Ineffective erythropoiesis
Hematoma resorption

*Common cause for unconjugated hyperbilirubinemia, but an uncommon cause for jaundice

Diffuse hepatocellular disease

Refer to hemolytic anemia in Chapter 41

Refer to hepatocellular jaundice

501
▲

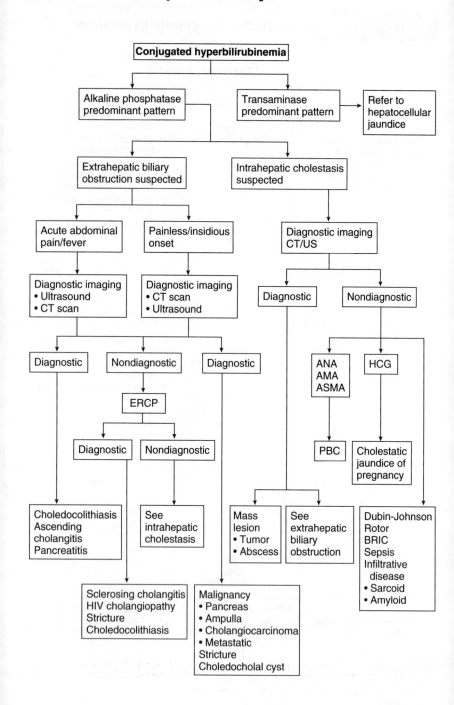

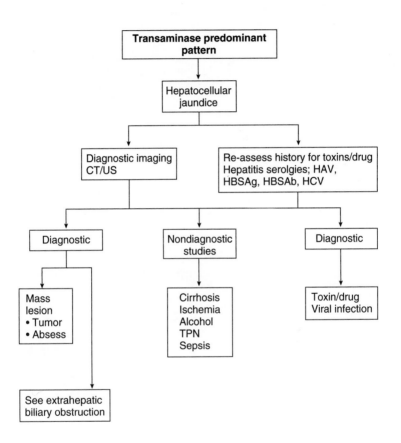

Appendix B Chronic Cough Algorithm

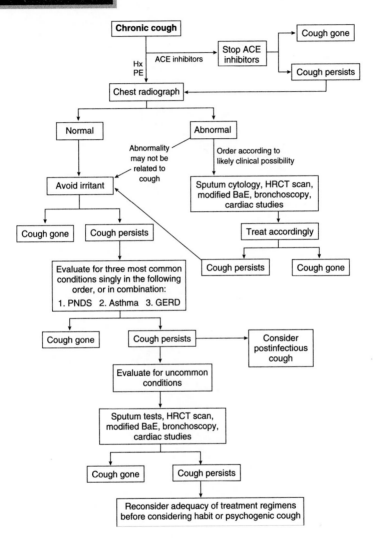

Guidelines for evaluating chronic cough in immunocompetent adults. *ACE* = angiotensin-converting enzyme; *BaE* = barium esophagography; *GERD* = gastroesophageal reflux disease; *HRCT* = high-resolution computed tomography; *Hx* = history; *PE* = physical examination; *PNDS* = postnasal drip syndrome. (Reprinted with permission. Irwin RS, Boulet LP, Cloutier MM, et al: Managing cough as a defense mechanism and as a symptom. A consensus panel report of the American College of Chest Physicians. *Chest* 114 (2 Suppl Managing): 1665, 1998.)

Index

Page numbers in *italics* denote figures; those followed by a t denote tables.

▲